Diagnostic Tests in Endocrinology and Diabetes

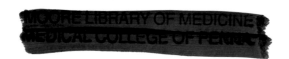
Diagnostic Tests in Endocrinology and Diabetes

Edited by

P.-M.G. Bouloux

Academic Department of Medicine
Royal Free Hospital
London

and

L.H. Rees

St Bartholomew's Hospital
London

CHAPMAN & HALL MEDICAL
London · Glasgow · New York · Tokyo · Melbourne · Madras

Published by Chapman & Hall, 2–6 Boundary Row, London SE1 8HN

Chapman & Hall, 2–6 Boundary Row, London SE1 8HN, UK

Blackie Academic & Professional, Wester Cleddens Road, Bishopbriggs, Glasgow G64 2NZ, UK

Chapman & Hall Inc., One Penn Plaza, 41st Floor, New York NY10119, USA

Chapman & Hall Japan, Thomson Publishing Japan, Hirakawacho Nemoto Building, 6F, 1-7-11 Hirakawa-cho, Chiyoda-ku, Tokyo 102, Japan

Chapman & Hall Australia, Thomas Nelson Australia, 102 Dodds Street, South Melbourne, Victoria 3205, Australia

Chapman & Hall India, R. Seshadri, 32 Second Main Road, CIT East, Madras 600 035, India

First edition 1994

© 1994   Chapman & Hall

Typeset in Hong Kong by Excel Typesetters Company

Printed in Great Britain by The Alden Press, Oxford

ISBN   0 412 35200 1

A catalogue record for this book is available from the British Library

Library of Congress Cataloging-in-Publication data available

∞ Printed on acid-free text paper, manufactured in accordance with ANSI/ NISO Z39.48-1992 (Permanence of Paper).

Contents

Contents

List of contributors

Stephanie A. Amiel, MD, FRCP
Senior Lecturer in Diabetes and
  Endocrinology
Unit for Metabolic Medicine
Guy's Hospital
London SE1 9RT
UK

D.C. Anderson MSc, MD, FRCP
Department of Medicine
The Chinese University of Hong Kong
Prince of Wales Hospital
Shatin
New Territories
Hong Kong

Pierre M. Bouloux, BSc, MD, FRCP
Senior Lecturer in Endocrinology
Academic Department of Medicine
Royal Free Hospital
Pond Street
London NW3 2QG
UK

A.M. Cotterill MD, MRCP
Wellcome Research Fellow
St Bartholomew's Hospital
51–53 Bartholomew Close
West Smithfield
London EC1A 7BE
UK

Christopher R.W. Edwards MA, MD, FRCP
University of Edinburgh
Department of Medicine
Western General Hospital
Edinburgh EH4 2XU
UK

Ray Edwards PhD
North East Thames Region Immunoassay
  Unit (NETRIA)
St Bartholomew's Hospital
51–53 Bartholomew Close
West Smithfield
London EC1A 7BE
UK

Stephen Franks, MD, FRCP
Department of Obstetrics and Gynaecology
Imperial College of Science, Technology and
  Medicine
St Mary's Hospital Medical School
London W2 1PG
UK

Edwin A.M. Gale, MB, FRCP
Professor of Diabetes
St Bartholomew's Hospital Centre for Clinical
  Research
59 Bartholomew Close
West Smithfield
London EC1A 7BE
UK

Reginald Hall, CBE, MD, FRCP
Professor Emeritus
University of Wales College of Medicine
Cardiff
UK

J.W. Honour, BSc, PhD, FRCPath
Senior Lecturer in Steroid Endocrinology
University College and Middlesex School of
  Medicine
Middlesex Hospital
Mortimer Street
London W1N 8AA
UK

I. Jialal, MD
The University of Texas at Dallas
Southwestern Medical Center
5323 Harry Hines Blvd.
Dallas
Texas 75235-9052
USA

Rhys John, BSc, PhD, MRCPath
Principal Biochemist
Department of Medical Biochemistry
University Hospital of Wales
Cardiff
UK

D.P.E. Kingsley FRCS, FRCR
Consultant Neuroradiologist
The National Hospital for Neurology and
   Neurosurgery
Lysholm Radiological Department
Queen Square
London WC1N 3BG
UK

**John H. Lazarus, MA, MD, FRCP (Lond &
   Glas)**
Senior Lecturer and Consultant Physician
University of Wales College of Medicine
Department of Medicine
Llandough Hospital
Penarth
Cardiff CF6 1XX
UK

Paul L. Padfield MD, FRCP
University of Edinburgh
Department of Medicine
Western General Hospital
Edinburgh EH4 2XU
UK

L.H. Rees MSc, MD, DSc, FRCP, FRCPath
St Bartholomew's Hospital
51–53 Bartholomew Close
West Smithfield
London EC1A 7BE
UK

P.C. Richardson MRCP
Ciba Geigy Ltd
Basel
Switzerland

Martin O. Savage, MA, MD, FRCP
Consultant Paediatric Endocrinologist
St Bartholomew's Hospital
51–53 Bartholomew Close
West Smithfield
London EC1A 7BE
UK

R.V. Thakker, MA, FRCP
MRC Clinical Scientist
Division of Molecular Medicine
Clinical Research Centre
Watford Road
Harrow
Middlesex HA1 3UJ
UK

Peter J. Trainer, MB, MRCP
Lecturer in Endocrinology
St Bartholomew's Hospital
51–53 Bartholomew Close
West Smithfield
London EC1A 7BE
UK

Ehud Ur, MB, MRCP
Lecturer in Endocrinology
St Bartholomew's Hospital
51–53 Bartholomew Close
West Smithfield
London EC1A 7BE
UK

Davinia M. White MB, MRCOG
Department of Obstetrics and Gynaecology
Imperial College of Science, Technology and
   Medicine
St Mary's Hospital Medical School
London W2 1PG
UK

Introduction

Although good clinical assessment remains, as in all branches of medicine, the cornerstone of the approach to diagnosis in patients with endocrine disorders, the highly sensitive and specific hormone assays and imaging techniques that are currently available also play an important and complementary role in modern endocrine practice.

Indeed, the accurate measurement of large arrays of hormones present in minute concentrations in body fluids, made possible by radioimmunoassay and allied techniques, have had a profound effect on the evolution of this branch of medicine, having provided powerful tools for exploring the physiology and pathophysiology of hormone secretion. With the proliferation in the number of hormones now readily measured, and the introduction of a wide range of stimulation and suppression tests, clinicians are now faced with a bewildering range of possible tests for the diagnosis of endocrine disorders. We believe this is an opportune moment to write a text focusing principally on the application of current biochemical and imaging techniques in the diagnosis of endocrinopathies. The emphasis is of necessity on the biochemical characterization of disease and its implication for the selection of appropriate diagnostic tests for the accurate diagnosis and treatment of endocrinopathies.

Each section starts with a brief review of the background physiology, pathophysiology and clinical features of the endocrine disorder under consideration, thus forming a conceptual framework in which to understand the behaviour of pathological processes. The aim is to present an accurate, critical and updated account of present day endocrine investigative techniques which will be of value to generalists as well as to practising endocrinologists. The emphasis is practical, with information on the applications, interpretations and predictive value as well as limitiations of the diagnostic tests and procedures used in evaluating specific endocrinopathies. We make use of diagnostic algorithms where they facilitate understanding.

We have started with an account of the principles and practice of biochemical measurement, particularly radioimmunoassay and allied analytical techniques. The chapters that follow are a mixture of organ-based and symptombased approaches to endocrine disorders. We have found this mix simplest in terms of ease of presentation and avoidance of duplication. We have given a selective bibliography at the end of each chapter.

Pierre Bouloux
Royal Free Hospital

Lesley Rees
St Bartholomew's Hospital

1

Radioimmunoassay and immunoradiometric assays

R. EDWARDS and L. H. REES

1.1 INTRODUCTION

The accurate measurement of the minute concentrations of hormone present in body fluids, together with imaging techniques, greatly assists clinical assessment of endocrine disorders.

In the 1950s work at two centres, one in London and the other in New York, gave rise to a technique which revolutionized clinical diagnostics in endocrinology.

At the Veterans Administrations Hospital in New York, Solomon Berson and Rosalyn Yalow were investigating the metabolic fate of intravenously administered ^{131}I-labelled insulin [1]. Insulin disappeared rapidly from the blood of normal subjects and diabetic patients not treated with insulin. In contrast, the ^{131}I-insulin persisted for much longer in the bloodstream of diabetic or schizophrenic patients who had received insulin therapy for more than a few weeks. Their studies demonstrated the presence of antibodies to insulin in the group receiving (insulin) therapy. These initial studies also demonstrated that the binding of the ^{131}I-insulin to antibody was competitively inhibited in a quantitative fashion by the presence of unlabelled insulin.

Roger Ekins, working in the radioisotope unit of the Middlesex Hospital Medical School, formulated a theory for the measurement of endogenous hormones at levels consistent with those found in blood [2]. Unfortunately, because of financial constraints, he was unable to buy the expensive radiolabelled thyroxine (T4) to apply the method to the measurement of T4 in patients' serum. He had to wait for several years until 1957, when up to 138 mCi of ^{131}I was being administered to a 46-year-old woman undergoing therapy for thyroid carcinoma metastases. It was found that the fully differentiated metastases were producing ^{131}I-radiolabelled T4. From blood samples taken to monitor treatment, Ekins was able to extract sufficient ^{131}I-T4 to validate his theory. Measurement of T4 depended upon relative binding of endogenous hormone and radiolabelled hormone to a specific binding protein, in this case the patient's own T4 binding globulin (TBG). Ekins called the method 'saturation analysis', while Berson and Yalow referred to 'radioimmunoassay' (RIA). Although the term 'saturation analysis' was intended to cover a general procedure utilizing any specific binding protein, including receptor proteins and antibodies, the term 'immuno-

1

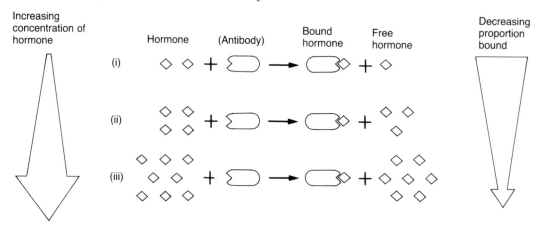

Fig. 1.1 The principle of radioimmunoassay (RIA). Different concentrations of hormone in the presence of a limited and constant concentration of antibody give rise to an inversely related proportion of bound hormone. The radioactive tracer is used to measure the proportion of bound and free.

assay' has persisted and is often used in a generic sense, antibodies being the most ubiquitous and stable of specific binding proteins.

In ensuing years, successful immunoassays were developed for many hormones and their application in practice demonstrated characteristics which were far superior to any other method available at that time.

1.2 PRINCIPLES AND APPLICATION OF RADIOIMMUNOASSAY

The specific reagent, the antibody, is used at a low or limited concentration. The hormone to be measured is reacted with the antibody. As the concentration of hormone increases, the antibody binding sites become increasingly saturated and excess 'spills over' into the 'free' fraction, as illustrated in Fig. 1.1.

The amount of 'bound' and 'free' hormone is proportional to its concentration. This proportion is measured by a trace amount of radiolabelled hormone following separation of 'bound' from 'free' by an appropriate method, such as second antibody reagent

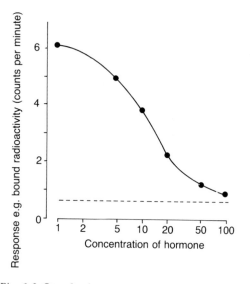

Fig. 1.2 Standard curve. A standard curve is generated by plotting the measured response, e.g. bound counts, derived from selected concentrations of hormone. The standards are usually calibrated against reference preparations. The estimated concentration of hormone in the unknown is read from the standard curve.

2

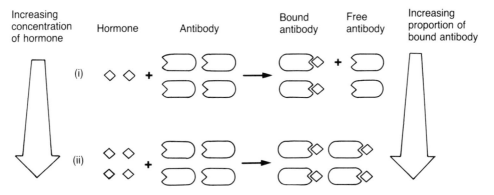

Fig. 1.3 The principle of immunoradiometric assay (IRMA). Different concentrations of hormone in the presence of 'excess' concentration of antibody give rise to a directly related proportion of bound antibody. The radiolabelled antibody is used to measure the amount of bound antibody.

or solid phase. Using known amounts of hormone or 'standards', a standard curve is constructed (Fig. 1.2) from which the concentration of unknown samples can be interpolated.

1.2.1 IMMUNORADIOMETRIC ASSAYS

In 1968, Miles and Hales published the details of an immunoassay using the antibody or reagent at a high or 'excess' concentration [3]. Increasing concentrations of hormone progressively saturate antibody binding sites (Fig. 1.3).

In this method, the immunoradiometric assay (IRMA), radiolabelled antibody measures the distribution of antibody between the 'free' antibody (unreacted) and the 'bound' antibody (reacted) fractions. Separation of 'bound' from 'free' antibody is usually carried out by solid phase reagents. Solid phase antigen is used where the IRMA measures small molecules (Fig. 1.4).

Where the analyte is sufficiently large to accommodate binding sites of two antibodies, an additional antibody attached to a solid phase may be used (Fig. 1.5).

This latter variant is commonly referred to as a 'sandwich' or 'two-site' IRMA. A curve

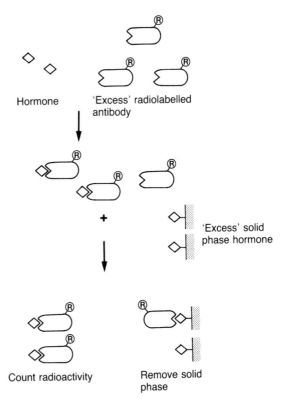

Fig. 1.4 The IRMA technique applied to small molecules, i.e. too small to bind more than one antibody. The amount of solid phase hormone needs careful optimization to avoid interfering with the equilibrium of the reaction.

3

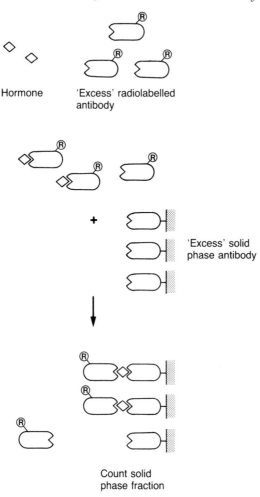

Fig. 1.5 The IRMA technique applied to large molecules, i.e. large enough to accommodate two distinct and separate epitopes; capable of binding two different antibodies. This type of IRMA is often referred to as 'two-site' or 'sandwich'.

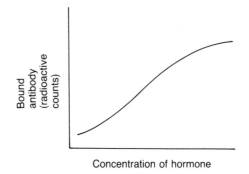

Fig. 1.6 The IRMA standard curve follows the conventional relationship of an increase in response for an increase in concentration.

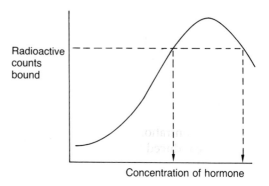

Fig. 1.7 The 'hook' effect. A potential problem with the IRMA technique is a biphasic response relationship at high concentrations. A single measurement can be read as two different concentrations. This particular problem is usually only significant at very high concentrations. Appropriate measures can be taken to eliminate the difficulty.

(Fig. 1.6) is constructed from standard concentrations of hormone, from which values of unknown samples are computed.

The IRMA is often more sensitive than its counterpart, the immunoassay, and has been shown to have an improved working range. Until recently, purification of antibodies of reproducible quality and in sufficient quan-

tities has been a major limitation. The increasing availability of monoclonal antibodies is undoubtedly encouraging wider use, especially in the use of 'two-site' IRMAs for large molecules. The method does have one major disadvantage. At very high concentrations of hormone, the standard curve becomes biphasic, or 'hooks' (Fig. 1.7).

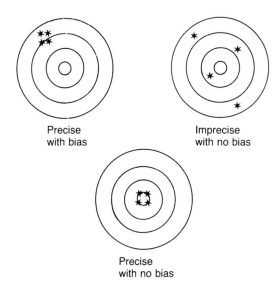

Precise
with bias

Imprecise
with no bias

Precise
with no bias

Fig. 1.8 The concepts of precision and bias illustrated by analogy with a target. An accurate result is precise without bias.

This presents a problem, because a single measurement can be interpolated as two different concentrations. This potential difficulty can be reduced by careful assay design

or by measuring high concentrations of hormone at appropriate dilutions.

1.2.2 ACCURACY

Immunoassays display a degree of accuracy not commonly found in other analytical procedures, even though they do not include several complex and technically demanding steps such as extraction and purification. Essentially, accuracy relates to correctness. However, the term embodies a number of concepts such as specificity, precision, sensitivity and bias (Fig. 1.8).

1.2.3 SPECIFICITY

The specificity of a method relates to the potency of substances, other than the specific analyte, when reacting with the antibody under assay conditions. The potency of selected substances, often referred to as 'cross-reactants' can be expressed as a single figure. For example, in a triiodothyronine (T3) RIA, T4 may cross-react with a potency of 0.25%. This means that 400 molecules of T4 have a

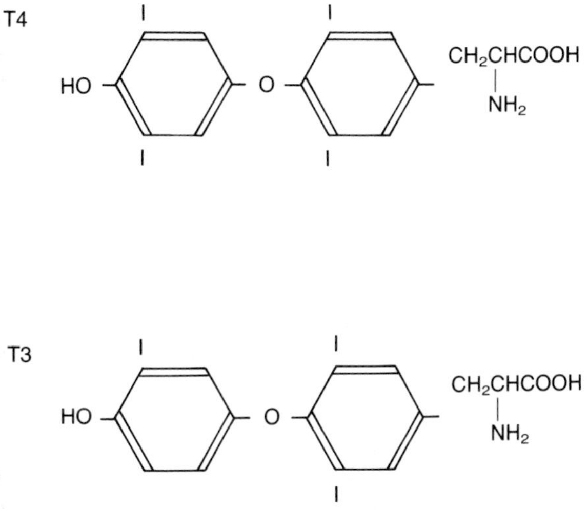

T4

$$HO - \bigcirc - O - \bigcirc - CH_2CHCOOH$$
$$\qquad\qquad\qquad\qquad\qquad\qquad NH_2$$

T3

$$HO - \bigcirc - O - \bigcirc - CH_2CHCOOH$$
$$\qquad\qquad\qquad\qquad\qquad\qquad NH_2$$

Fig. 1.9 The chemical formulae for thyroxine (T4) and triiodothyronine (T3) showing the structural similarity. A cross-reaction of 0.25% for T4 in a T3 RIA represents a discrimination of 400-fold.

5

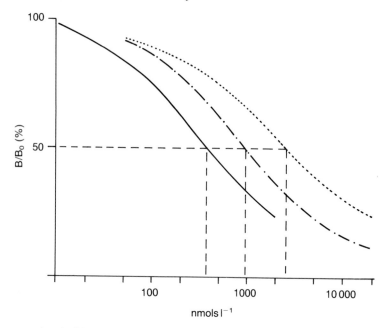

Fig. 1.10 Cross-reaction in RIA. Response curves for cortisol (——) and two cross-reactants in an assay for cortisol. Conventionally, relative potency is expressed by reference to 50% of binding at zero hormone concentration (B_0). This figure illustrates a cross-reaction of 14.5% for 11-deoxycortisol (·······) and 38% prednisolone (·—·).

similar potency to 1 molecule of T3. The close relationship between the molecular structures of T3 and T4 (Fig. 1.9) illustrates the remarkable specificity that can be achieved in RIA.

This degree of specificity, inherent in antibodies, negates the need for complex purification procedures to remove interfering substances, and predisposes RIA methods to simplicity. Cross-reactivity in RIA is not a constant factor (Fig. 1.10).

However, it is the convention to determine the degree of specificity from the relative concentrations of analyte and cross-reactant that reduce antibody binding to 50% of that at zero hormone concentration. Although it is an oversimplification, this convention has proved useful in determining the practical specificity of antibodies and assays.

Cross-reaction in the IRMA is more com-

plex. This makes a single figure irrelevant and probably misleading. Cross-reactions are subject to the biphasic response. They vary in the presence of different concentrations of analyte and may be negative rather than positive (Fig. 1.11).

All this clearly requires that a more exact definition be given for specificity in IRMAs. Cross-reactions should relate to various relevant concentrations of analyte and indicate the effect of the 'hook'.

1.2.4 SENSITIVITY AND PRECISION

Sensitivity and precision are two aspects of a single concept. Sensitivity can be defined as the minimum detectable concentration or that concentration of the hormone analyte that can be distinguished from zero concentration with a stated degree of probability. This

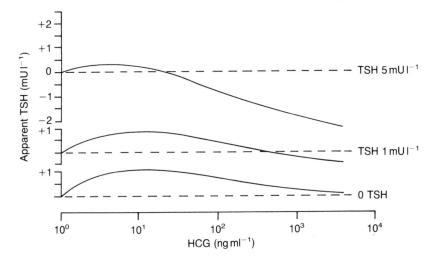

Fig. 1.11 Cross-reaction in IRMA. Specificity in an IRMA is complex. This figure illustrates cross-reaction of human chorionic gonadotropin (HCG) in an IRMA for thyrotropic hormone (TSH). A biphasic response curve is generated which includes negative interference, i.e. it reduces results rather than increasing them, to a greater or lesser extent at different basal concentrations of TSH.

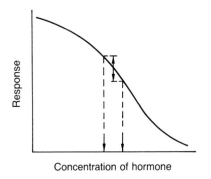

Fig. 1.12 Steps in deriving a precision profile. Statistically derived variations in the measurement, e.g. 'true' standard deviation (s.d.) in bound counts are translated into valid variations in the derived concentration (result). Thus the 'error', e.g. %cv, in the result can be calculated for any given concentration.

can be calculated from the precision at zero hormone concentration. Precision, or the inherent variation in the measurement, is best described by a precision profile. Precision profiles are calculated from a statistical analysis of the variation in the measurement, i.e.

in the counts detected, throughout the assay range. The derived standard deviation in terms of counts is then translated into the appropriate variability in terms of concentration units (Fig. 1.12).

This variability can be expressed as a coefficient of variation and plotted against concentration to give a conventional precision profile (Fig. 1.13).

Precision profiles are usually calculated by computer and often incorporate a function which relates to the closeness of fit in the standard curve. Precision profiles from different assays or methods are easily compared. They also give the significance for any given result in a form which is readily understood.

1.2.5 REPRODUCIBILITY

Reproducibility refers to the cumulative precision over a number of assays. This is frequently deduced from the repeated measurement of quality control pools in successive assays (Fig. 1.14).

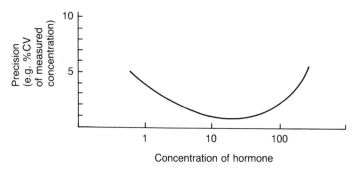

Fig. 1.13 A precision profile is derived from plotting the calculated error, e.g. %cv, in the result (in terms of concentration) for selected concentration. Then the error in any result can be interpolated from the precision profile. The precision profile is a sensitive indicator of assay quality and is extremely useful when comparing two different assays for the same analyte.

1.2.6 BINDING PROTEINS AND FREE HORMONES

A considerable portion of some hormones circulate in blood bound to specific binding proteins. In some cases, the affinity constant and concentration of these proteins is such that very little of the hormone remains unbound. For example, only 0.5% of T4 and 0.5% of T3 are unbound or free. It is generally held that only the free hormone is biologically active and that the protein-bound proportion is not active, serving only as a 'buffer' store or reserve. In general, most assays measure the total hormone, i.e. the protein-bound and the free hormone. Special sensitive assays have been developed to measure specifically the free hormone, particularly for thyroid hormones. The reference method for free T4 and free T3 is equilibrium dialysis but this is not widely available because it is cumbersome and subject to methodological errors. Two basic methods have been introduced: the 'analogue' free hormone measurement and the 'two-step' or 'back titration' free hormone measurement. Both these methods are simpler to perform and more robust than equilibrium dialysis. However, the results are sometimes equivocal, especially when using the analogue method. In situations where

the binding proteins remain constant, the total hormone measurement undoubtedly discriminates diagnostically.

In circumstances where the concentration of binding protein changes, e.g. in pregnancy, or where binding sites are blocked, e.g. patient on drug therapy, the total hormone concentration may be misleading. In these cases, a free hormone measurement would be useful. An alternative approach is either direct measurement of the binding protein, e.g. TBG, or a 'hormone uptake test'. The uptake test is a much simpler test than a direct free hormone assay. It measures the distribution of exogenous radiolabelled hormone between the sample and some non-specific absorbent, e.g. Sephadex or ion-exchange resin. It is an estimate of binding capacity in the sample and, in conjunction with the total hormone measurement, a 'free hormone index' can be derived, e.g. free T4 index (FTI). In practice, the FTI discriminates better than many of the free T4 assays.

It has also been the practice to use the term 'free steroids', e.g. free oestriol, for unconjugated steroids. This is a completely different use of the word and is confusing. Assays for unconjugated oestriol are better referred to as such, and not as 'free' oestriol.

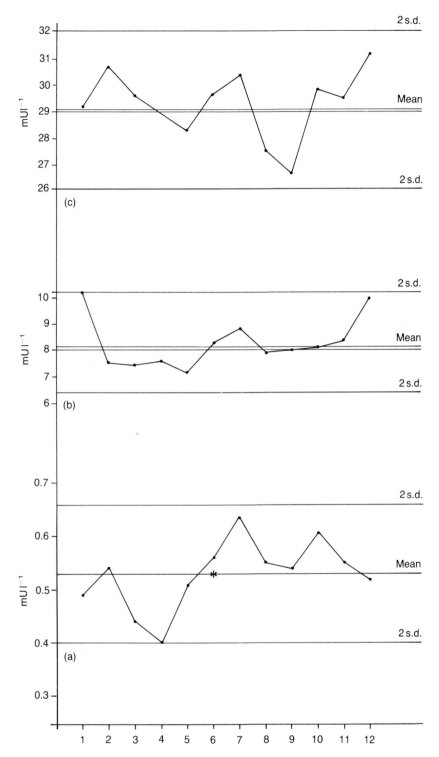

Fig. 1.14 Quality control chart for thyrotropic hormone (TSH) assay. Reproducibility is monitored by the measurement of 'quality control' pools in successive assays. The results of assaying three pools, representing (a) low, (b) medium and (c) high concentrations of analyte, are plotted against assay number.

1.2.7 ALTERNATIVE NON-RADIOISOTOPIC ASSAYS

In recent years many alternatives to radio-isotope labels have been introduced, e.g. enzymes with coloured, luminescent or fluo-rescent products, fluorophores and lumino-phores. Although these assays are sometimes more convenient, they are more susceptible to interference and their use in clinically vali-dated diagnoses is limited. In principle they should give similar results and it cannot be assumed that the vast experience gained from the use of radioisotope labelled assays can be transferred. It will require extensive evalua-tion to identify all the possible causes of interference in 'alternative' systems.

1.3 FACTORS AFFECTING THE INTERPRETATION OF HORMONE MEASUREMENT

Concentrations of hormones in biological fluids rarely, if ever, remain static. Many hormones show pronounced circadian or oscillatory rhythms. They show seasonal vari-ations and vary throughout the menstrual cycle. Variations are, of course, a reflection of the natural hormonal function, as secretion is stimulated or suppressed by many factors, both external and internal. For accurate diag-nosis in many cases, it is imperative that certain precautions are taken in preparing the patient and collecting samples. Some analy-ses require special precautions in the handling of the sample and in its storage.

1.3.1 PATIENT PREPARATION

For some analytes no special preparations or precautions are necessary prior to taking the sample. In these instances, it is only necessary to take a blood sample by simple venepunc-ture and to collect either a plasma or serum sample. It is usually convenient to have the patient seated and relaxed.

For many hormone measurements, e.g. pancreatic, gut and growth hormone (GH), patients should be fasted overnight and sampled before being allowed to eat. In a few cases, patients must be recumbent or up-right after a period of recumbency. Where stress is a potent stimulator, an indwelling catheter may be inserted and left for 30 minutes before samples are taken. As a pre-caution, it is always useful to note when patients are highly stressed during sampling. A list of requirements for specific analytes is given in Table 1.1.

1.3.2 MEDICATION

Medication affects hormone results in two ways. Firstly, medication may affect the hor-mone concentration *in vivo* by suppressing or stimulating biosynthetic pathways leading to release and, in the second instance, medi-cation may give rise to substances that cross-react or interfere with the analysis *in vitro*.

Thus, for analysis of aldosterone, all drugs are discontinued for two weeks prior to sampling and, if necessary, the patient must receive additional sodium and potassium to ensure an adequate intake. Failure to do this makes it difficult to give accurate interpre-tations. Medication with prednisolone causes problems in interpreting cortisol results be-cause it cross-reacts in most immunoassays for cortisol. In these circumstances the drug is stopped before a sample is taken. Details of medication and any relevance to accurate interpretation of results will be found in the appropriate chapters.

1.3.3 STRESS, ACTIVITY AND POSTURE

The stress mechanism is a powerful stimu-lator of some hormones, e.g. cortisol and GH. Very high levels of cortisol may be achieved following physical or psychological stress, much higher than those seen when the subject is at rest.

Table 1.1 Patient preparation

Analyte	Preparation
Adrenal steroids	
Aldosterone	All drugs discontinued for 2 weeks, ensure adequate intake of sodium (100–150 mmol/day) and potassium (50–100 mmol/day)
	Overnight recumbency
Cortisol	Fasting
Dehydroepiandrosterone (DHEA)	No special preparation
DHEA-sulphate	No special preparation
11-Deoxycortisol	No special preparation
17-Hydroxyprogesterone	Before emergency corticosteroid treatment, preferably in the morning
Pancreatic and gut hormones	
Gastrin	Fasting
Insulin	Fasting
Insulin C-peptide	Fasting
Carcinoembryonic antigen (CEA)	Note whether smoker or non-smoker
Vasoactive intestinal peptide (VIP)	Overnight fast, patient at rest
Pancreatic polypeptide (PP)	Fasting
Glucagon	Fasting
Gonadal steroids	
Androstenedione	Avoid stress
Oestradiol	No special preparation
Progesterone	No special preparation
Testosterone	No special preparation (note time of day)
Dihydrotestosterone (DHT)	No special preparation
Anterior pituitary hormones	
Adrenocorticotropic hormone* (ACTH)	Before morning dose of corticosteroids
Follicle stimulating hormone (FSH)	No special preparation
Growth hormone (GH)	Fasting, indwelling venous needle for repetitive sampling
Luteinizing hormone (LH)	No special preparation
Prolactin (PRL)	Avoid stress
Thyroid stimulating hormone (TSH)	No special preparation
Thyroid hormones	
Thyroxine (T4)	No special preparation
Triiodothyronine (T3)	No special preparation
Catecholamines	
Adrenaline (epinephrine)	Patient lying down with cannula in place
Noradrenaline (norepinephrine)	Patient lying down with cannula in place
Miscellaneous	
Parathyroid hormone (PTH)	Fasting
Alphafoetoprotein (AFP)	No special preparation
Human chorionic gonadotropin (HCG)	No special preparation
Calcitonin	Fasting
Renin/angiotensin	See Aldosterone; replacement therapy, any time during the day

* Failure to take blood may invalidate results from subsequent venepuncture.

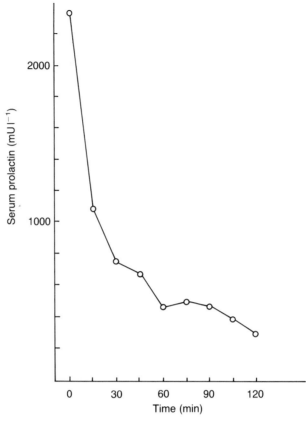

Fig. 1.15 Stress. Sequential blood sampling using an indwelling catheter shows elevated prolactin values falling to within the normal range over a two-hour period. The elevation was assumed to be stress-related.

Where interpretation may be compromised because of the stress phenomenon, time should be allowed for the stress response to die down. An indwelling catheter inserted and left for 30 minutes is recommended to avoid stress-related problems, particularly when sampling for adrenocorticotropic hormone (ACTH), cortisol, catecholamines and renin, or when repeated sampling may induce a stress response.

Stimulation of a hormone following exercise is classically demonstrated by GH. Strenuous exercise leading to a sufficient degree of fatigue, with elevation of the pulse and sweating, usually increases GH to values $>20\,mU\,l^{-1}$ from a basal value of $<2\,mU\,l^{-1}$. Indeed, this phenomenon has been used as the basis of a diagnostic test for GH deficiency.

A singular example of a very high prolactin value presumed to be stress-provoked (patient felt very faint!) which slowly fell to normal values over 2 hours is given in Fig. 1.15.

Posture is important in a few instances. For accurate results in catecholamine measurements, it is necessary to ensure that the patient is lying down with a cannula in place before sampling. Plasma renin activity changes diagnostically in response to the change in posture from a supine to an upright position. Table 1.2

Table 1.2 Timing

Analyte	Preparation
Adrenal steroids	
Aldosterone	8 a.m. before sitting up (before breakfast); 8.30 a.m. after 30 min out of bed (before breakfast); 12 noon out of bed since 8 a.m. (before lunch)
Cortisol	9 a.m.
11-Deoxycortisol	9 a.m.
17-Hydroxyprogesterone	For diagnosis, in the early morning; for monitoring treatment, 8–9 a.m. and 2 h after first dose of corticosteroid
Gonadal steroids	
Androstenedione	HCG stimulation, 9 a.m.
Dihydrotestosterone (DHT)	HCG stimulation, 9 a.m.
Anterior pituitary hormones	
Adrenocorticotropic hormone (ACTH)	Between 9 and 10 a.m. or at 9 a.m.
Growth hormone (GH)	Basal 8.30 a.m.; four point day curve 8.30 a.m., 1 p.m., 5 p.m., 7 p.m.
Miscellaneous	
Renin/angiotensin	See Aldosterone

gives details of analytes where precautions are necessary to avoid inaccuracies.

1.3.4 EFFECT OF TIME

Many hormones are secreted episodically throughout a 24-hour period, frequently with an increase in secretion at night or during the sleep period. A typical pattern in the circadian variation of thyroid stimulating hormone (TSH) is given in Fig. 1.16.

Often samples taken during the day will miss the peak values and for such hormones the variations during normal hours is minimal. It is important to note that a shift in the circadian rhythm can take place following an alteration in sleep–wake patterns, such as may occur with jet travel. It may take at least one week before the 'normal' pattern is re-established. Circadian rhythms in prolactin levels from four normal subjects, three males and one female, illustrate considerable individual variation (Fig. 1.17).

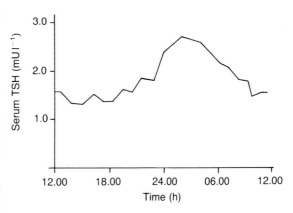

Fig. 1.16 Circadian rhythm. Blood samples taken every 30 minutes and assayed for thyrotropic hormone (TSH) show a marked circadian variation. This is typical of a number of hormones.

Another point to note is the occasional very high value found in the males during the evening and night rise. Figure 1.18 shows a shift in the acrophase of prolactin rhythm

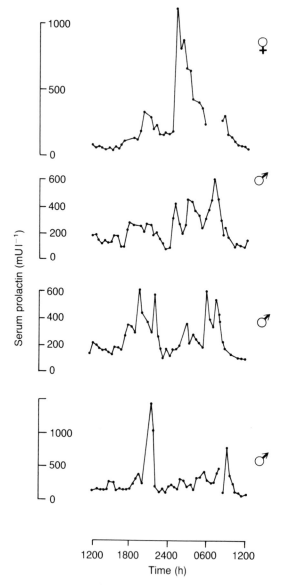

Fig. 1.17 Circadian rhythm in prolactin. The patterns seen in prolactin values measured in blood samples taken every 30 minutes from four normal subjects (three male, one female) show considerable variation between individuals, although all subjects show an evening and night rise.

in a normal female subject, possibly related to a difference in sleep–wake behaviour.

The significance here is that a sample taken in the morning may give an elevated value.

Frequently, hormone concentrations vary seasonally. These variations are often insignificant within the variations used for reference ranges, particularly where reference ranges are deduced from data taken throughout at least one year.

Details of situations where timing is critical are given in Table 1.2.

1.3.5 AGE, SEX AND WEIGHT

Hormones are involved in growth, development and ageing processes, so it is reasonable to expect changes in concentrations of certain hormones with different age groups. Some hormones, e.g. thyroid hormones, remain relatively consistent throughout life, although they do fall slightly with old age, when a slight increase in TSH is also observed. Basal plasma renin activity and the increase on changing from a supine to upright position gradually decline with increasing age. It is reported that both these values for 60-year-olds are half those for young adults.

Weight may also be relevant in interpreting results. Specific details are found in the relevant chapters.

1.3.6 PREGNANCY

Pregnancy is a condition with profound changes in many hormone concentrations. A notable change is the large increase in TBG and the accompanying increase in thyroid hormones. Both cortisol binding protein and cortisol increase as pregnancy advances. Aldosterone shows a marked increase from the sixteenth week of gestation. It is likely that special reference ranges are necessary for pregnant patients and particular details will be noted in the relevant chapters.

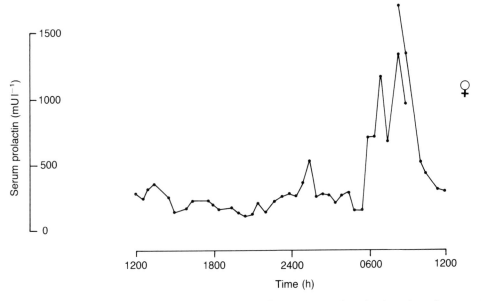

Fig. 1.18 Acrophase shift in circadian rhythm. The circadian pattern of prolactin values from a subject with a delayed sleep–wake routine shows a shift in the position of the peak. This shift could compromise prolactin measurements in blood samples taken in the morning.

1.3.7 SAMPLES

Many types of samples are specified and, generally speaking, each analytic method requires a specific type of sample. Measurement of certain hormones in blood can be performed on either plasma or serum, and where they are relatively stable, no strict precautions are necessary for storage or transport to the laboratory. Where a choice is possible, serum samples are usually handled more simply in the laboratory, especially as less particulate material is formed during freezing. After separation of the blood as either serum or plasma, the sample is usually refrigerated for short-term storage and transported to the laboratory at ambient temperature. The samples are frozen at −20°C if they are to be stored for longer than a day.

A number of hormones are less stable. Samples are separated quickly in a refrigerated centrifuge (cold spin) and immediately frozen. These must remain frozen during transport to the analytical laboratory. Special containers for transporting samples in the frozen state are usually available from the specialist laboratory or the Supraregional Assay Service (SAS).

Plastic tubes are specified for some hormones because they are absorbed onto glass surfaces, e.g. ACTH. Specific details of samples are given in Table 1.3.

Transport of samples through the post must comply with Post Office (PO) regulations. All specimens must be sent by first class post only. Details of suppliers of PO approved boxes and special containers for the transport of frozen specimens are given in the booklet 'Specialized Assay Services for Hospital Laboratories' provided by the SAS.

It is advisable to alert the laboratory when a specialized investigation is taking place and confirm the details of the current protocol. Many laboratories do not have special facil-

15

Table 1.3 Sample details

Sample	Details
Adrenal steroids	
Aldosterone	Plasma; freeze at $-20°C$ after separation
Cortisol	Serum/plasma
Dehydroepiandrosterone (DHEA)	Serum/plasma
DHEA-sulphate	Serum/plasma
11-Deoxycortisol	Serum/plasma
17-Hydroxyprogesterone	Serum/plasma
Pancreatic and gut hormones	
Gastrin	Heparin plasma containing Trasylol; cold spin, freeze within 15 min of venepuncture
Insulin	Plasma/serum; prompt cold spin, store and transport frozen
Insulin C-peptide	Plasma; prompt separation, store and transport frozen
Carcinoembryonic antigen (CEA)	Serum
Vasoactive intestinal peptide (VIP)	Heparin plasma containing Trasylol; cold spin, freeze within 15 min of venepuncture
Pancreatic polypeptide (PP)	Heparin plasma containing Trasylol; cold spin, freeze within 15 min of venepuncture
Glucagon	Heparin plasma containing Trasylol; cold spin, freeze within 15 min of venepuncture
Gonadal steroids	
Androstenedione	Serum/plasma
Oestradiol	Serum/plasma
Progesterone	Serum/plasma
Testosterone	Serum/plasma
Dihydrotestosterone (DHT)	Serum/plasma
Anterior pituitary hormones	
Adrenocorticotropic hormone (ACTH)	Heparin plasma, plastic tubes only, cold spin, freeze at $-20°C$
Follicle stimulating hormone (FSH)	Serum; portion into fluoride oxalate tube for glucose
Growth hormone (GH)	Serum
Luteinizing hormone (LH)	Serum
Prolactin (PRL)	Serum
Thyroid stimulating hormone (TSH)	Serum
Thyroid hormones	
Thyroxine (T4)	Serum preferred, keep free T4 and free T3 samples frozen during transport
Triiodothyronine (T3)	Serum preferred, keep free T4 and free T3 samples frozen during transport
Catecholamines	
Adrenaline (epinephrine)	Heparin plasma tube containing sodium metabisulphite (contact laboratory), transfer to laboratory on ice immediately; laboratory: immediate cold spin and freeze plasma

Table 1.3 Continued

Sample	Details
Noradrenaline (norepinephrine)	
Miscellaneous	
Parathyroid hormone (PTH)	Serum; store and transport frozen
Alphafoetoprotein (AFP)	Serum
Human chorionic gonadotropin (HCG)	Serum
Calcitonin	Heparin plasma; avoid glass tube
Renin/angiotensin	Plasma

Note: Avoid haemolysis and lipaemia in all samples.

Table 1.4 Analyte information and reference ranges

Analyte	Volume (ml)	Reference ranges	Notes
Tests: blood			
ACTH	10	$<10-80 \, ng \, ml^{-1}$ (circadian rhythm)	Collect on ice, deliver immediately
Aldosterone	10	Recumbent: $100-500 \, pmol \, l^{-1}$ Ambulant: $900-1500 \, pmol \, l^{-1}$	Collect on ice, deliver immediately
Alkaline phosphatase	5	$35-130 \, U \, l^{-1}$ (adults)	Increased in children
Androstenedione	5	Age and sex related	
Anti-diuretic hormone	10	$2-6 \, pmol \, l^{-1}$	Collect on ice, deliver immediately
Apo-lipoprotein A1	10	$0.7-1.7 \, mg \, l^{-1}$	
Apo-lipoprotein A2	10	$0.2-0.6 \, mg \, l^{-1}$	
Apo-lipoprotein B	10	$0.6-1.4 \, mg \, l^{-1}$	
Calcitonin	10	Up to $0.08 \, \mu g \, l^{-1}$	Collect on ice, deliver immediately
Calcium	5	$2.1-2.6 \, mmol \, l^{-1}$	
Cholesterol	5	Age and sex related; adults in range $3.0-5.6 \, mmol \, l^{-1}$	
Cortisol	5	At 9 a.m.: $200-650 \, nmol \, l^{-1}$ At midnight: $30-120 \, nmol \, l^{-1}$	
DHEA-sulphate	5	Age and sex related	
Dihydrotestosterone	5	In adult males: $1.0-2.9 \, nmol \, l^{-1}$	
FSH	5	Males: $0.5-6.0 \, IU \, l^{-1}$ Females, cyclical: Early: $2-8 \, IU \, l^{-1}$ Mid: $6-25 \, IU \, l^{-1}$ Luteal: $2-6 \, IU \, l^{-1}$ Menopausal: $10-50 \, IU \, l^{-1}$	
Gastrin	10	Up to $40 \, pmol \, l^{-1}$	Collect on ice, deliver immediately
Glucagon	10	Up to $50 \, pmol \, l^{-1}$	Collect on ice, deliver immediately

Continued

Table 1.4 Continued

Analyte	Volume (ml)	Reference ranges	Notes
Glucose	5	2.9–5.3 mmol l^{-1} (if fasting)	
Glycated haemoglobin	5	2.8%–4.9%	
Growth hormone	5	Up to 10 mU l^{-1} (if fasting)	
HDL cholesterol	5	Males: 0.9–1.7 mmol l^{-1}	
		Females: 1.0–2.2 mmol l^{-1}	
Lipoprotein lipase	10	5–25 mmol l^{-1} h^{-1}	
Magnesium	5	0.7–1.0 mmol l^{-1}	
Neurotensin	10	Up to 100 pmol l^{-1}	Collect on ice, deliver immediately
Oestradiol	5	Prepubertal: 37–92 pmol l^{-1}	
		Males: 55–92 pmol l^{-1}	
		Females, cyclical:	
		Early: 110–183 pmol l^{-1}	
		Mid: 550–1650 pmol l^{-1}	
		Luteal: 550–845 pmol l^{-1}	
		Menopausal: up to 200 pmol l^{-1}	
Osmolality	5	275–295 mmol kg^{-1}	
Pancreatic polypeptide	10	Up to 300 pmol l^{-1}	Collect on ice, deliver immediately
Phosphate	5	0.70–1.25 mmol l^{-1}	
Potassium	5	3.5–5.0 mmol l^{-1}	
Progesterone	5	Males: average 2.0 nmol l^{-1}	
		Females, cyclical:	
		Early: up to 5 nmol l^{-1}	
		Luteal: 20–80 nmol l^{-1}	
17OH-progesterone	5	Prepubertal: <1.1 nmol l^{-1}	
		Males: 0.6–6.0 nmol l^{-1}	
		Females, cyclical:	
		Early: 0.6–3.0 nmol l^{-1}	
		Luteal: 3–12 nmol l^{-1}	
Prolactin	5	30–400 mU l^{-1}	
PTH	10	10–55 pg ml^{-1}	Collect on ice, deliver immediately
Renin	10	Recumbent: 1.14–2.65 pmol l^{-1} h^{-1}	Collect on ice, deliver immediately
		Ambulant: 2.82–4.49 pmol l^{-1} h^{-1}	
Reverse T3	5	250–650 pmol l^{-1}	
SHBG	5	Males: 10–50 nmol l^{-1}	
		Females: 30–90 nmol l^{-1}	
Sodium	5	135–145 mmol l^{-1}	
IgF-I	10	Males: 9–46 nmol l^{-1}	
		Females: 12–48 nmol l^{-1}	
Somatostatin	10	Up to 120 pmol l^{-1}	Collect on ice, deliver immediately
TBG	5	7–17 g l^{-1}	
Testosterone	10	Males: 9–30 nmol l^{-1}	
		Females: 0.5–2.5 nmol l^{-1}	

Table 1.4 Continued

Analyte	Volume (ml)	Reference ranges	Notes
Triglycerides	5	Males: 0.7–2.2 mmol l^{-1} Females: 0.6–1.7 mmol l^{-1}	
TSH	5	0.5–4.7 mU l^{-1}	
Urea	5	3.0–6.5 mmol l^{-1}	
VIP	10	Up to 30 pmol l^{-1}	Collect on ice, deliver immediately
25OH vitamin D	10	19–107 nmol l^{-1}	Restricted availability
Tests: urine			
Adrenaline		0.05–0.20 µmol per 24 h	
ADH		10–20 pmol l^{-1}	
Aldosterone		10–50 nmol per 24 h	
Calcium		2.5–7.5 mmol per 24 h	
Cortisol (urinary free)		Males: up to 350 nmol l^{-1} Females: up to 290 nmol l^{-1}	
HMMA (VMA)		10–35 µmol per 24 h	
Magnesium		3–5 mmol per 24 h	
Noradrenaline		0.53–1.80 µmol per 24 h	
Osmolality		40–1400 mmol kg^{-1}	
Oxalate		30–240 µmol per 24 h	
Phosphate		15–50 mmol per 24 h	
Potassium		40–120 mmol per 24 h	
Sodium		100–250 mmol per 24 h	

Source: Royal Free Hampstead NHS Trust, Department of Chemical Pathology and Human Metabolism, laboratory handbook.

ities to handle category 3 pathogens, such as hepatitis B virus or AIDS virus. In such cases, always consult the laboratory prior to sending the sample. Where patients are considered to be at risk, it may be necessary to show the absence of either pathogen or specific antibody. Always consult the laboratory where there is any doubt.

For specialized investigations take two samples: one to be sent to the laboratory, the other to be retained in reserve. Store the second sample frozen for use if necessary, for example in case the first is lost or spilt.

Analyte information and reference ranges are given in Table 1.4.

REFERENCES

1. Yalow, R.S. and Berson, S.A. (1960) Immunoassay of endogenous plasma insulin in man. *J. Clin. Invest.*, **39**, 1157.
2. Ekins, R.P. (1960) The estimation of thyroxine in human plasma by an electrophoretic technique. *Clin. Chim. Acta*, **5**, 453.
3. Miles, L.E.M. and Hales, C.N. (1968) Labelled antibodies and immunological assays systems. *Nature*, **219**, 186.

Investigation of hypothalamo-pituitary disorders

P.M. BOULOUX

2.1 INTRODUCTION

The hypothalamus regulates anterior pituitary hormone secretion through production and hypothalamo-pituitary portal venous delivery of stimulatory and inhibitory hormones. Because of the anatomical and functional interrelationship of the hypothalamus and pituitary, it may be difficult on clinical grounds alone to determine whether defective pituitary function is caused primarily by pituitary disease or whether it is of hypothalamic origin. However, the presence of diabetes insipidus (DI), resulting from insufficiency of vasopressin production, strongly suggests the presence of a hypothalamic or stalk lesion.

In addition to alterations in anterior and posterior pituitary function, lesions of the hypothalamus may present with abnormal cerebral function and behavioural disturbance. In general, hypothalamic disease leads to deficiency of anterior pituitary hormone production. However, withdrawal of inhibitory dopaminergic tone to the lactotrophs will cause hyperprolactinaemia, with its diverse manifestations. Some cells of the hypothalamus are under similar restraint; thus, loss of restraint on the gonadotropin releasing

hormone (GnRH) secreting cells of the hypothalamic arcuate and supraoptic nuclei in the prepubertal child may trigger off precocious puberty, as occurs in lesions of the posterior hypothalamus (for example, pinealoma, hamartoma).

Pituitary disease usually presents with symptoms and signs of hormone excess or insufficiency, or as a result of the space-occupying effect of a tumour.

The usual clinical features of hypothalamic disease are:

Evidence of hypogonadism
Menstrual disturbance
Precocious puberty
Poor or arrested growth
Cranial DI
Feeding disorders (obesity and hyperphagia).

Disorders of thirst perception, somnolence, emaciation, anorexia and disturbance of thermoregulation may also occur, reflecting the large number of physiological functions regulated by the hypothalamic nuclei. The close proximity of the optic chiasm to the anterior wall of the hypothalamus makes this structure particularly susceptible to damage from an expanding lesion in this area.

DI is almost invariable in hypothalamic

Table 2.1 Classification of hypothalamic disorders

1. *Tumours*
   Craniopharyngioma
   Glioma
   Hamartomas
   Dysgerminoma
   Histiocytosis X
   Leukaemia
   Neuroblastoma
   Meningioma
   Colloid cyst of third ventricle
   Ependymoma
   Angioma
   Lymphoma
   Teratoma
   Secondary deposits
   Pineal tumours: germ cell tumours, pineal
      parenchymal tumours
2. *Trauma*
   Subarachnoid haemorrhage
   Arteriovenous malformations
   Aneurysms
   Surgical or traumatic stalk section
3. *Inflammatory*
   Meningitis
   Encephalitis
   Sarcoidosis
   Hydatid disease
   AIDS
4. *Miscellaneous*
   Chronic hydrocephalus
   Raised intracranial pressure
   Radiotherapy damage
   Anorexia nervosa
   Exercise induced amenorrhoea
   Poor growth due to psychosocial deprivation
   Depression

disease, and is often the presenting feature. Full expression of DI requires the presence of adequate amounts of circulating cortisol, and may thus be masked in the presence of coincidental adrenocorticotropic hormone (ACTH) deficiency. Trauma, granulomas (TB and sarcoid) and tumours (primary and secondary) are the usual causes of acquired DI, but in a significant number of cases no structural lesion is revealed. In such cases, autoimmune processes may be operative, or, possibly, vascular events within the hypothalamus. Rarely, demyelinating processes have affected hypothalamic function.

A classification of hypothalamic disorders is given in Table 2.1.

2.1.1 HORMONE DEFICIENCY RESULTING FROM HYPOTHALAMIC DISEASE

Deficiency of one or more hypothalamic-pituitary releasing hormones can lead to selective pituitary insufficiency. Selective deficiency of thyrotropin releasing hormone (TRH) is rare and leads to 'tertiary hypothyroidism'. In such cases, an intravenous TRH test ($200–500\,\mu g$) will give a characteristic pattern of response, with the 60 minute thyroid stimulating hormone (TSH) response being higher than the 20 minute value. GnRH deficiency may occur either singly or in combination with other releasing hormone deficiencies. In Kallmann's syndrome, hypogonadotropic hypogonadism due to GnRH deficiency is associated with anosmia.

Isolated growth hormone releasing hormone (GHRH) deficiency underlies many cases of idiopathic GH deficiency in childhood. These children frequently demonstrate a GH response to the exogenous administration of GHRH but not to physiological stimuli (sleep, exercise), or to dynamic tests of the pituitary (for example, insulin-induced hypoglycaemia).

Corticotropin releasing hormone (CRH) deficiency, though rare, causes tertiary hypoadrenalism. There is no cortisol response to insulin-induced hypoglycaemia, although ACTH release can be stimulated by exogenous CRH administration. Defective dopamine synthesis and delivery to the lactotroph is associated with hyperprolactinaemia.

2.2 DIAGNOSTIC EVALUATION OF HYPOTHALAMO-PITUITARY DISORDERS

Diagnostic evaluation has two principal objectives: (i) to identify and characterize the nature of the lesion in the area, and (ii) to document associated hypothalamo-pituitary dysfunction.

The patient's history and physical examination will reveal much useful information. Thereafter, a combination of biochemical, hormonal, neuro-ophthalmological and neuro-radiological assessments is indicated.

2.2.1 HORMONAL EVALUATION

Basal

Ideally, measurement of basal pituitary and target hormones is required. In practice this means a 9 a.m. sample for cortisol, TSH, thyroxine (T4) and triiodothyronine (T3), luteinizing hormone (LH), follicle stimulating hormone (FSH), oestradiol and testosterone (where appropriate), prolactin, GH, and paired plasma and urine osmolalities. A low circulating target hormone level associated with a low pituitary tropic hormone pinpoints the lesion to either the hypothalamus or pituitary, or both.

Dynamic

(a) Tests of GH and ACTH release

Physiological tests

GH secretion

GH levels are undetectable throughout most of the day in normal subjects, episodic day-time bursts occurring with a periodicity of about 4 hours, and at night during sleep stages III and IV (slow wave sleep). Sleep associated GH release correlates well with that seen following insulin-induced hypoglycaemia. In practice, physiological GH secretion is only performed as a research investigation, and requires 20-minute blood sampling from a peripheral vein during daytime and night-time. In view of the difficulties in performing this, it is more usual to carry out provocative testing.

Insulin tolerance test (ITT)

Procedure

Soluble insulin in a dose of $0.15\,U\,kg^{-1}$ is administered intravenously to a fasting individual, although patients with insulin resistance (for example, those with Cushing's syndrome or acromegaly) may require a dose of $0.2-0.3\,U\,kg^{-1}$. Hypopituitary patients are usually very sensitive to hypoglycaemia. Children below eight years are given a dose of $0.1\,U\,kg^{-1}$. The test is seldom performed in children younger than five years of age. The nadir of blood sugar response occurs 20-30 minutes after injection, and should be equal or inferior to $2.2\,mmol\,l^{-1}$. The patient should be seen to be clinically hypoglycaemic, with sweating, tachycardia and pallor.

Blood is sampled at 0, 30, 45, 60, 90 and 120 minutes following insulin injection, and analysed for glucose, GH and cortisol. A glucose meter should be available for immediate measurement of glucose. In the event of a severe reaction, such as loss of consciousness or seizure, the test is terminated by intravenous administration of 20 ml 50% dextrose, followed by a 5% dextrose drip. However, sampling should continue as an adequate stress stimulus will have been achieved.

Interpretation

The ensuing neuroglycopaenia stimulates ACTH and GH release (via CRH, vasopressin and GHRH release, and reciprocal inhibition of somatostatin release, respectively). The peak GH response should exceed $20\,mU\,l^{-1}$ ($10\,ng\,ml^{-1}$). However, prepubertal children (especially those with bone age of 10 years or over) should receive priming with stilboestrol 1 mg twice daily for 48 hours prior to the test, as even normal children may otherwise have a borderline response. In some centres testosterone is used, although the priming effect may take a few days.

Cortisol response to ITT

Clinically, the ITT is of especial value in the assessment of pituitary GH reserve and ACTH, although it does test the integrity of the hypothalamo-pituitary axis. The peak cortisol response should exceed $550\,nmol\,l^{-1}$. However, an abnormal response to ITT can result from either pituitary or hypothalamic dysfunction.

Contraindications

1. History of epilepsy, known ischaemic heart disease or abnormal ECG.
2. Hypothyroidism. This is associated with an impaired GH and ACTH response, and should be corrected before an ITT.
3. Hypocortisolaemia. This is associated with severe and prolonged hypoglycaemia following insulin administration, due to inadequate hepatic glycogen stores and failure of increased glucose efflux in response to the acute glucose counter-regulatory hormones, adrenalin and glucagon.

Other tests of GH reserve

Glucagon test

This stimulates the release of insulin, and subsequently of GH and ACTH. The GH response occurs 120–180 minutes after the start of the test. Poor GH and cortisol responses may occur in some normal individuals, but prior administration of propranolol reduces this to 10%–15%. Peripubertal children should receive oestrogen priming, usually stilboestrol 1 mg bd for 48 hours prior to the test. This test may be used in patients with a history of epilepsy and ischaemic heart disease.

Procedure

Following an overnight fast, 1 mg glucagon is given subcutaneously (0.5 mg for children and 1.5 mg for patients whose weight exceeds 90 kg). Blood is sampled before glucagon is given and at 30-minute intervals for 240 minutes, for glucose, GH and cortisol. Nausea and vomiting may occur during the second half of the test.

Interpretation

The peak GH response should exceed $20\,mU\,l^{-1}$, and the peak cortisol response should exceed $550\,nmol\,l^{-1}$.

Arginine test

Several amino acids, including arginine, histidine, lysine, phenylalanine, leucine, valine, methionine and threonine, can stimulate GH secretion, when given either as an infusion or as part of a protein meal or beef extract. The most commonly used test is the arginine test.

Procedure

Following an overnight fast, a 10% arginine solution in saline in a dose of $0.5\,g\,kg^{-1}$ (to a maximum of 30 g) is infused over 30 minutes. Blood is sampled over a 2-hour period at 30 minute intervals.

Interpretation

Women and children respond more consistently than men, with peak values usually occurring at around 60 minutes. Peripubertal children should receive oestrogen priming prior to the test. GH response should rise to at least $15\,\mathrm{mU\,l^{-1}}$.

L-Dopa

Dopamine agonists increase GH levels in normal subjects. If L-Dopa is given orally in a dose of 500 mg (or $10\,\mathrm{mg\,kg^{-1}}$), peak GH levels are achieved 60–120 minutes later. Prior administration of propranolol $0.75\,\mathrm{mg\,kg^{-1}}$ (maximum 40 mg) increases the response rate to 80%–90%. Unfortunately, the drug causes nausea and vomiting.

Clonidine

This α_2 adrenoceptor agonist, administered orally in a dose of $0.15\,\mathrm{mg\,m^{-2}}$ or intravenously in a dose of $0.2\,\mathrm{\mu g\,kg^{-1}}$ over 10 minutes, leads to GH release after 30 minutes. Side effects include drowsiness and hypotension, lasting for several hours.

(b) Tests of the hypothalamo-pituitary gonadal axis

Clomiphene test

Clomiphene citrate is an oestrogen antagonist with partial agonist properties. It tests the integrity of the negative feedback regulation of hypothalamic GnRH secretion by circulating gonadal steroids. The increased GnRH activity cannot be measured, but the pituitary response (LH/FSH) to it can. The response takes up to four days to occur. Its direct hepatic agonist effect causes stimulation of sex hormone binding globulin (SHBG) production.

Procedure

Oral clomiphene citrate $3\,\mathrm{mg\,kg^{-1}}$ per day is given in divided doses for 7–10 days and the LH/FSH response is measured at 0, 4, 7 and 10 days. Measurement of the oestradiol response gives additional information on the ovarian sensitivity to endogenous gonadotropins. In women, a day 21 progesterone test is carried out to ascertain ovulation.

Interpretation

Both LH and FSH rise in response to clomiphene, and a doubling of basal levels is considered normal by day 10. However, the qualitative and quantitative responses are dependent upon the ambient circulating gonadal steroid levels (and thus upon stage of puberty).

Clomiphene may act as an agonist in patients with low or absent oestrogen levels, and in such cases the LH and FSH responses may actually be depressed following its administration (for example, in prepubertal children and in patients with weight-related amenorrhoea, Kallmann's syndrome or hypothalamic disease). Failure of LH and FSH response to clomiphene can result from both hypothalamic and pituitary disorders.

Contraindications

The drug should be avoided in patients with liver disease and a recent history of depression. Flickering at the periphery of the visual fields is a common complication.

(c) Pituitary releasing hormone tests

Synthetic TRH, GnRH, GHRH and CRH are available for clinical testing of TSH, LH/FSH, GH and ACTH reserves, respectively. These releasing hormones will stimulate only the readily releasable pools of pituitary hormones.

TRH test

Administration of synthetic TRH is associated with release of the readily releasable pool of TSH in the thyrotroph.

Procedure

A TRH dose of 200–500 µg is administered intravenously and the TSH response measured at 0, 20 and 60 minutes.

Interpretation

Patients with destructive pituitary lesions show no rise in TSH, whereas those with hypothalamic disease show a delayed peak response, with the 60-minute TSH value exceeding the 20-minute value. A flat TSH response to TRH occurs in thyrotoxicosis due to Graves' disease or any other cause. The test is of particular value in ruling out thyroid autonomy.

Patients with Cushing's syndrome of any cause have an attenuated TSH response to TRH. In primary hypothyroidism, the basal TSH is elevated and the TSH response to TRH exaggerated.

Side effects

Mild and transient nausea, a metallic taste in the mouth, the urge to micturate, and transient pressor and tachycardic effects occur after intravenous TRH administration.

GnRH test

Procedure

The synthetic decapeptide GnRH is given intravenously in a dose of 100 mcg, and blood is sampled for LH and FSH at 0, 30 and 60 minutes.

Interpretation

The response of LH and FSH to 100 µg of intravenous GnRH depends on age, sex, degree of sexual maturation and, in women, the phase of the menstrual cycle. In the normal subject, the maximum LH rise occurs at 20–30 minutes, falling significantly by 60 minutes, whereas the peak FSH rise may take longer. In the prepubertal child, the FSH response exceeds the LH response, whereas the opposite is observed in sexual maturity.

In situations of prolonged GnRH deficiency (for example, Kallmann's syndrome) there may be no LH or FSH response to intravenous GnRH initially, but after a suitable period of priming with GnRH the pituitary responsiveness is restored. An absent LH/FSH response to clomiphene, accompanied by an LH/FSH response to GnRH, is suggestive of a hypothalamic disturbance.

GHRH test

Administration of exogenous GHRH tests the readily releasable pool of GH in the pituitary. Although native GHRH is a 40-amino acid peptide, the 1–29 form is just as potent.

Procedure

After an overnight fast, two basal GH samples are taken at 15-minute intervals. After 100 µg GHRH (or 1.5 µg kg^{-1} in a child) administration, samples for GH are collected at 15-minute intervals for 120 minutes. Transient facial flushing may occur.

Interpretation

The GH response to GHRH depends on the stage of puberty of the individual being tested. Failure of GH release with the insulin hypoglycaemia test, yet a GH response to GHRH, suggests the presence of hypothalamic GHRH deficiency. This appears to underlie many cases of idiopathic GH deficiency in childhood. A flat GH response to GHRH occurs in destructive pituitary lesions and in patients with Cushing's syndrome of any cause. Some patients with acromegaly have an exaggerated GH response to GHRH despite an elevated basal GH level.

CRH test

This also tests the readily releasable pool of ACTH from the pituitary.

Procedure

A dose of 100 µg CRH is given intravenously and blood is sampled for cortisol at 15-minute intervals for 120 minutes.

Interpretation

Failure of ACTH/cortisol response to hypoglycaemia in the presence of responsiveness to exogenous CRH suggests a hypothalamic disturbance with CRH deficiency. An exaggerated ACTH/cortisol response to CRH is seen in most cases of Cushing's disease. In normal individuals, the ACTH/cortisol response depends on the initial basal cortisol level, the largest incremental rises occurring in subjects with the lowest basal cortisols. Failure of a cortisol response will occur in patients with atrophic adrenals.

2.2.2 INVESTIGATION OF POSTERIOR PITUITARY FUNCTION

Plasma osmolality is maintained within a narrow physiological range (285 plus 3 mmol kg^{-1}). This constancy is achieved through osmoregulation of thirst and vasopressin secretion. Vasopressin reduces urinary excretion of water by stimulating its reabsorption in the renal collecting tubules.

Physiologically, plasma osmolality regulates both thirst and vasopressin secretion by acting on specialized osmotically sensitive neurons (osmoreceptors) present in the anterior hypothalamus, close to the organum vasculosum lamina terminalis. Under physiological conditions, if osmolality falls below 280 mmol kg^{-1}, vasopressin secretion levels fall to low or undetectable levels, resulting in the passage of urine of low osmolality (less than 100 mmol kg^{-1}).

Conversely, when plasma osmolality exceeds a critical threshold value, vasopressin is secreted and the urine becomes more concentrated. In normal subjects, the level of osmoconcentration at which maximal antidiuresis occurs (295 mmol kg^{-1}) is also the thirst threshold. Provided that the subject is conscious, this mechanism is exquisitely sensitive and will maintain normal hydration even in the face of high urinary water loss. Not all solutes exert the same effect on vasopressin secretion. Salt is the most effective, but urea has little or no effect; glucose stimulates vasopressin secretion in the absence – but not in the presence – of insulin.

Clinically, hypotonic polyuria, polydipsia, hypodipsia and hypernatraemia, and hyponatraemia are the three ways in which disturbances of thirst and vasopressin secretion occur.

Polyuria and polydipsia

This can result from three main mechanisms:

1. Deficient vasopressin secretion (central, cranial, neurogenic or vasopressin sensitive DI).
2. Decreased renal sensitivity to vasopressin (nephrogenic DI).
3. Primary polydipsia (hysterical polydipsia) or excessive water intake.

Clinical presentation

Thirst, polyuria and polydipsia are the usual clinical manifestations of DI. Nocturia is present and enuresis occurs in children. Dehydration is only present if water intake becomes inadequate for any reason (see Table 2.2).

Diagnosis

Glycosuria and other causes of solute diuresis are excluded. The diagnosis is made by

Table 2.2 Causes of diabetes insipidus

Central/cranial DI
Idiopathic: Familial (autosomal dominant)
              Sporadic
Secondary: Trauma (RTA, surgical)
              Tumours (primary and metastatic)
              Granuloma (neurosarcoid, histiocytosis X)
              Infections (encephalitis, syphilis, meningitis)
              Vascular (aneurysms, hypoxic brain damage, vasculitis)
              Autoimmune

Nephrogenic DI
Idiopathic: Familial (X linked recessive)
              Sporadic
Secondary: Drug/toxic (demethylchlorotetracycline, lithium,
                colchicine)
              Hypercalcaemia and hypokalaemia
              Vascular (sickle cell disease)
              Pyelonephritis
              Post-obstructive uropathy

Primary polydipsia
Compulsive water drinking

Pregnancy associated
Vasopressin resistant (secondary to placental vasopressinase)

demonstrating the presence of hypotonic polyuria in the presence of concentrated plasma. Plasma sodium is at the upper limit of the normal range in cranial and nephrogenic DI but is low in primary polydipsia. Hypercalcaemia and hypokalaemia need to be excluded.

Water deprivation test

The 8-hour water deprivation test (Dashe test) or, in equivocal cases, the Miller and Moses test, is used. In both instances, the aim is to ascertain whether the patient is capable of secreting vasopressin and thus concentrating the urine in response to a rising plasma osmolality.

Precautions

1. Care is essential in patients with severe DI, who may become dangerously dehydrated during the test.
2. Thyroid and adrenal function must be normal, and patients on replacement therapy if necessary.

Procedure

In the Dashe test, patients are allowed fluid *ad libitum* up to the start of the test. Tea, coffee, alcohol and cigarettes, all of which can interfere with vasopressin secretion, are specifically excluded after midnight on the day before the test. If a patient is on a vaso-

Table 2.3 Water deprivation test

URINE					
Time	Hours	Sample	Weight	Time	Hours
07.30	0	Discard	+		
				08.00	0.5	P1
08.30	1	U1			
10.30	3	Discard			
				11.00	3.5	P2
11.30	4	U2	+		
13.30	6	Discard	+		
				14.00	6.5	P3
14.30	7	U3	+		
15.30	8	U4	+	15.30	8.0	P4
16.30	9	U5	+	16.30	9.0	P5

After DDAVP 2 mcg im: 1 h (allow to drink freely)
　　　　　　　　　　 2 h
　　　　　　　　　　 3 h
　　　　　　　　　　 4 h

pressin preparation, this is discontinued the night before the test.

The patient empties the bladder at a set time, and is weighed, then 97% of the body weight is calculated. An intravenous cannula is inserted and water intake is restricted for 8 hours. The patient is weighed before the beginning of the test and after 4, 6, 7 and 8 hours. Five urine samples are collected in the hour prior to and at intervals during the 8-hour period of water restriction (see Table 2.3).

Normal response

Urine osmolality rises, and urine volume and free water clearance fall progressively with water deprivation. The U:P ratio should exceed 2.0 at the completion of the test. Plasma osmolality rises but remains below 295 mosm kg^{-1}.

Interpretation

1. Cranial DI: urine osmolality fails to rise appropriately and urine volume remains inappropriately high despite rising plasma osmolality. Plasma osmolality exceeds 295 by the end of the test, but the U:P ratio is less than 2.0. Urine concentrates after the DDAVP. If the plasma osmolality has not risen to over 295, the U:P ratio of less than 2.0 is not diagnostic since the patient has not been adequately water deprived. U5 and P5 should be collected before DDAVP administration.

2. Nephrogenic DI: plasma osmolality rises and urine osmolality fails to rise appropriately (as for central DI), but urine fails to concentrate after DDAVP.

3. Primary polydipsia: U:P ratio exceeds 2.0 at the end of the test, provided that adequate dehydration has been achieved. Patients are frequently overloaded with fluid at the start of the test; however, 8 hours may not be an adequate period of water deprivation to stimulate vasopressin release and hence urine concentration. If P4 and P5 are below 295 mosm kg^{-1} and the U:P ratio is under 2.0, a Miller and Moses test should be performed.

Prolonged water deprivation test (after Miller and Moses)

This is carried out when equivocal results have been obtained with the standard water deprivation test.

Precautions

Adrenal and thyroid function should be normal.

Procedure

The patient should have fasted completely from 6 p.m. on the day before the test, be weighed on the day of the test, then 97% of weight calculated. An intravenous cannula is inserted. The general arrangement is as for a water deprivation test. Blood and urine are sampled from 8 a.m., and the patient is weighed every 2 hours. If the patient loses more than 3% of body weight, a plasma osmolality should be carried out urgently where more than 305 mosm kg^{-1} DDAVP had been given, and the patient should be allowed to drink.

If the osmolality is lower, then the patient was probably overloaded with fluid prior to the test. Urine and plasma osmolality are measured immediately and the period of water deprivation continued until the urine osmolality reaches a plateau (<30 mosm kg^{-1} increase for three consecutive samples). DDAVP 2 mcg is given when a plateau is reached, and the patient is allowed to drink (see Table 2.4).

Table 2.4 Collection procedure

Time	Hours	Urine	Plasma	Weight
08.00	0	U1	P1	Yes
09.00	1	U2	–	–
10.00	2	U3	P3	Yes
11.00	3	U4	–	–
etc.				

Normal response

Urine osmolality rises to reach a plateau; there is no further increase in urine osmolality following DDAVP.

Interpretation

A rise in urine osmolality of 9% or more following DDAVP suggests partial cranial DI. A normal urine osmolality response in the presence of a high plasma osmolality is compatible with a subtle defect of vasopressin secretion or 'reset osmostat'. No rise in urine osmolality after DDAVP in the presence of polydipsia and polyuria suggests primary polydipsia.

Hypertonic saline infusion

Indications

Assessment of subtle defects of vasopressin secretion.

Procedure

The test is started at 9 a.m. The bladder is emptied, the volume recorded and osmolality measured. Volume and osmolality of any further urine passed are recorded. Blood pressure is recorded at 15-minute intervals during the test. Saline 5% is infused at 0.06 ml kg^{-1} min^{-1} for 2 hours from 0 to 120 minutes. The time of onset of thirst is recorded.

After 135 minutes, the patient is asked to void urine and any volume is recorded together with osmolality. Blood for plasma osmolality and vasopressin are taken at −15, 0, 30, 60, 90, 120 and 135 minutes.

Interpretation

Plasma osmolality rises during infusion and plasma vasopressin begins to rise at about

285 mosm kg^{-1}. Onset of severe thirst is at about 295 mosm kg^{-1}. The study may reveal a reset osmotic threshold for vasopressin secretion and/or onset of thirst, compatible with the clinical finding.

2.2.3 NEURO-OPHTHALMOLOGICAL EVALUATION

Visual field testing by confrontation

Bedside visual field testing using a small red target and a confrontation technique is extremely valuable in determining the presence and extent of a visual field defect. A typical pituitary lesion that extends upwards compresses the body of the optic chiasm and decussating fibres from below, causing a characteristic bitemporal (initially superior quadrantinopia) hemianopia. Lesions expanding downwards (for example, anterior communicating artery aneurysm) may also produce a similar visual field defect. Early lesions cause an inferior bitemporal quadrantinopia, progressing eventually to a bitemporal hemianopia. Optic atrophy may ensue. Papilloedema is rare unless there has been compression of the third ventricle with interruption of CSF pathways and hydrocephalus.

Pituitary tumours and visual field defects

Visual loss associated with pituitary tumours is usually gradual, although it may be sudden in cases of haemorrhage into a pre-existing tumour (apoplexy). The visual field defect associated with a pituitary tumour depends on four factors:

1. Tumour size
2. Direction of tumour growth
3. Anatomical relationship of the visual pathways to the pituitary
4. Rate of tumour growth.

By definition, only macroadenomas cause visual field defects if the direction of expan-

sion is upwards. In cases of a prefixed chiasm, the posterior angles of chiasm and optic tract are primarily involved, whereas in a post-fixed chiasm the tumour expansion may be between the optic nerves.

Perimetry

Formal perimetry should be carried out using a Goldmann perimeter. Targets of different sizes and intensity are used for mapping out individual visual fields, with the patient's gaze fixed on a central target. An electronic buzzer is used to indicate when the patient has seen the target. The operator has to ensure that the patient's gaze remains fixed to the central target throughout the visual field charting procedure.

Visual evoked response

The use of visual evoked response is advocated in cases where there is equivocal evidence of optic pathway compression. Compressive involvement of pathways causes distortion of the waveform. The major advantage of using this test is its capacity to evaluate individual portions of the visual field.

2.3 DIAGNOSIS OF PITUITARY TUMOURS

These are primarily benign lesions which constitute between 10% and 15% of intracranial tumours in surgical material, and up to 23% of unselected adult autopsies. Most lesions originate from within the sella turcica and are slow growing, although occasionally lesions can expand very rapidly. Extension of such tumours to the suprasellar region may cause visual field defects, headache and cranial nerve palsies. Rarely, inferior extension into the sphenoid sinus may cause CSF rhinorrhoea.

Pituitary adenomas may be function-less or lead to oversecretion of hormones. GH hypersecretion is associated with gigant-ism in childhood and acromegaly in adult-hood; ACTH hypersecretion is associated with Cushing's disease; and hyperprolactin-aemia is associated with the amenorrhoea–galactorrhoea syndrome and infertility. TSH hypersecretion is a rare cause of thyro-toxicosis. LH-FSHomas are usually large tumours which may be associated with normal gonadal function.

2.3.1 PROLACTIN SECRETING TUMOURS

Hyperprolactinaemia is a common endocrine problem and has several causes. It is defined as persistent elevation of prolactin above $360\,\mathrm{mU}\,\mathrm{l}^{-1}$ in the absence of pregnancy or postpartum lactation.

Prolactin secretion from the pituitary is under predominantly inhibitory control from hypothalamic dopamine, which is trans-ported to the lactotrophs via the hypotha-lamohypophyseal portal circulation. Thus, lesions that destroy the dopamine synthesiz-ing neurons, lesions that impair the normal delivery of dopamine to the lactotroph, or those that inhibit the action of dopamine on

Table 2.5 Causes of hyperprolactinaemia

Hypothalamic disorders
Tumours:
    Craniopharyngioma
    Germinoma
    Glioma
    Colloid cyst of the third ventricle
    Hamartoma
    Metastatic tumour
Infiltrative disorders:
    Sarcoidosis
    Tuberculosis

Table 2.5 Continued

    Histiocytosis X infection
    Hydatid disease
    Encephalitis
Radiotherapy
Pituitary disorders:
    Prolactinoma
    Acromegaly
    Pituitary stalk section
    Empty sella syndrome
    Functional stalk section (pseudoprolactinoma)
    Lymphocytic hypophysitis
Drugs:
    Neuroleptics:
        Perphenazine
        Fluphenazine
        Chlorpromazine
        Haloperidol
        Metoclopramide
        Sulpiride
        Domperidone
    Antidepressants:
        Imipramine
        Amitriptyline
    Other drugs:
        Methyl dopa
        Reserpine
        Oestrogens
        Opiates
        Intravenous cimetidine
Miscellaneous:
    Hypothyroidism
    Chronic renal failure
    Cirrhosis
    Chest wall lesions
    Spinal cord lesions
    Breast stimulation (acting by stimulation of afferent sensory mechanism of suckling)
Idiopathic:
    Physiological
    Pregnancy (slow increase in first two trimesters; sharp rise in third trimester to 6000–$10\,000\,\mathrm{mu}\,\mathrm{l}^{-1}$)
    Lactation (initially hyperprolactinaemia with large pulses during suckling; gradual normalization, despite continuation of suckling)
    Stress (exercise, pain, surgery, anaesthesia, hypoglycaemia)

its lactotroph receptor (for example, dopamine antagonists) will cause pathological hyperprolactinaemia.

The causes of hyperprolactinaemia are diverse, and are listed in Table 2.5.

Clinical features

Gonadal dysfunction is the most common manifestation of hyperprolactinaemia in the female, with disruption of menstrual cyclicity (amenorrhoea, oligomenorrhoea, luteal insufficiency), loss of libido and galactorrhoea. Infertility is a common presentation. For the most part, the tumours are small at the time of presentation (prolactin secreting microadenoma), and the remainder of anterior pituitary function tends to be preserved.

In a proportion of patients, a suprasellar extension is evident at the time of presentation, and a visual field defect may be present. In addition to the hormonal changes, patients with this disorder appear to have a higher incidence of psychological disturbance (hostility, anxiety, depression).

Men with hyperprolactinaemia tend to present later in the course of their disease. Gonadal dysfunction is gradual and patients may not readily admit to problems with impotence and loss of libido. Seminal emissions tend to be of low volume, but sperm count is maintained until significant gonadotropin deficiency occurs. Impotence is frequent. Among unselected impotent males, hyperprolactinaemia is found in 2–5%.

Because of delayed presentation, tumours are frequently large (macroadenomas) at the time of presentation, and visual field defects due to chiasmatic compression may occur. Macroadenomas tend to cause headaches because of dural stretch.

In both sexes, prolactinomas may be a cause of delayed sexual maturation. The larger tumours may also inhibit growth by impaired growth hormone secretion.

Biochemical features

Several prolactin levels should be determined to confirm the diagnosis of hyperprolactinaemia, particularly when levels are only marginally raised. This is to avoid spurious elevations consequent upon the occurrence of a spontaneous peak or the effect of a stressful venipuncture.

The finding of hyperprolactinaemia should prompt a search for underlying causes such as hypothyroidism, pregnancy, renal failure and drug ingestion. When these causes have been ruled out, the diagnosis is most commonly found to be due to a prolactin secreting tumour. However, a larger number of intracranial lesions may cause hyperprolactinaemia (see Table 2.5), and computerized tomography (CT) scanning is mandatory.

High resolution CT with contrast enhancement, reformatted pictures in the coronal and sagittal plane and the use of 1.5 mm collimations will usually reveal the presence of a pituitary tumour.

In general, space-occupying lesions that cause effective stalk section do not induce hyperprolactinaemia exceeding $2500 \, \text{mU} \, \text{l}^{-1}$. Patients with macroadenomas usually have prolactin levels exceeding $4000 \, \text{mU} \, \text{l}^{-1}$.

Differential diagnosis

A number of dynamic tests have been advocated to differentiate between hyperprolactinaemia caused by a prolactin secreting adenoma and that due to hypothalamic causes or effective stalk section. Physiological causes need to be ruled out.

TRH test

The most popular test involves the evaluation of prolactin response to intravenous TRH (200 µg i.v. and blood for prolactin at 0, 20 and 60 minutes).

Interpretation

Normal subjects demonstrate a small rise in prolactin following TRH, whereas the response is blunted in patients with pro-lactinomas. However, this test lacks both sensitivity and specificity, and should not be used to rule out tumours.

Domperidone and metoclopramide tests

Administration of dopamine antagonists, such as domperidone (10 mg i.v.) and meto-clopramide (10 mg i.v.), has also been ad-vocated to distinguish between tumorous and non-tumorous causes of hyperprolactin-aemia.

Interpretation

Failure of prolactin rise following adminis-tration of these agents has been taken to indicate the presence of a pituitary tumour.

2.3.2 ACROMEGALY

Acromegaly is the clinical syndrome pro-duced by prolonged, inappropriate and ex-cessive secretion of GH. It is most usually associated with a pituitary tumour and more rarely with GHRH secretion from an ectopic source, with consequent somatotroph hyper-plasia. In the population, prevalence is esti-mated to be 4–5 : 100 000.

Acromegaly is a disease of middle age with a predilection for women. Gigantism is the term given to describe the sequelae of GH excess before skeletal maturation is complete.

Clinical features

The systemic manifestations of acromegaly result from the bony and soft tissue enlarge-ment caused by GH or insulin-like growth factors I (IGF-I) excess. A typical patient presents with thickening of the skin, coarse facial features, large nose, thick lips and deep facial folds (particularly frontal furrows). There is progressive enlargement of the hands and feet, and patients have to keep changing shoe and glove size. Hyperhidrosis is in-variably present and the skin is oily. Cuta-neous fibromas, fleshy tags, sebaceous cysts and acanthosis nigricans (also hirsutism in females) may occur.

The voice is deep and resonant. An en-larged tongue (rarely to the point of causing obstruction) and overgrowth of buccal soft tissue can impair mastication. The jaw pro-trudes and there is widening of interdental separation so that food tends to become trapped between the teeth. Patients usually have a barrel chest due to the failure of osteo-chondral junctions to close. Kyphosis is fre-quent. Sinuses are enlarged, particularly the frontal sinuses. The supraorbital ridges are prominent and may limit the upper visual fields. There is a tendency to premature osteoarthritis, affecting not only the weight-bearing joints, but also the glenohumeral joint. The width of cartilage is increased. Soft tissue overgrowth is thought to be respon-sible for the tendency to peripheral nerve compression syndromes, particularly the median nerve at the wrist. Hypertension occurs in up to 30% of patients, and does not necessarily resolve with treatment. Left ventricular hypertrophy is common, but dilated 'acromegalic cardiomyopathy' asso-ciated with congestive cardiac failure and arrhythmias is more rare. Glucose intolerance is common (up to 70%).

Rarely, acromegaly may represent one component of the MEN1 syndrome, with hyperparathyroidism and pancreatic islet cell tumours. Left untreated, cardiovascular morbidity and mortality (tenfold risk) are the dominant consequences. Earlier series showed that up to 89% of acromegalic patients die before the age of 60. Treatment has been shown to improve the prognosis significantly.

Biochemical findings

In acromegaly, the pulsatile nature of normal GH secretion is maintained, but the GH spikes are higher and GH levels fail to return to normal (i.e. are undetectable) between bursts. Although the total amount of GH secreted over 24 hours is increased in acromegaly, there appears to be no direct relationship between the clinical severity of the disease and circulating growth hormone levels.

Dynamics of GH secretion in acromegaly

GH dynamics are also abnormal in acromegaly, and in 50% of cases there is a paradoxical rise in GH secretion following oral glucose administration (the hormone is normally suppressed after glucose is given).

Oral glucose tolerance test

Procedure

Following an overnight fast, 75 g glucose is given orally, and blood samples are taken at 15-minute intervals for 120 minutes for glucose and GH.

Interpretation

Oral administration of glucose normally suppresses GH to less than $2\,mUl^{-1}$ in practically all normal subjects within 30–120 minutes. Typically in acromegaly, GH levels remain elevated, increase (50% of cases) or fall slightly, but never to less than $2\,mUl^{-1}$.

TRH test

In normal individuals, intravenous TRH (200 µg) does not cause an elevation of GH, whereas in acromegaly it may do so.

Procedure

Following an overnight fast, TRH (200 µg) is given intravenously and blood is taken at 20 and 60 minutes for GH.

Interpretation

In acromegaly, the GH level is acutely elevated by more than 50% of the basal value in 60%–80% of patients within 20–30 minites. The test is sometimes helpful in patients with low circulating levels of GH. Unfortunately, false positives can occur in patients with malnutrition, uncontrolled diabetes mellitus, in cases of renal failure and in some tall adolescents.

Dopamine infusion

Administration of dopamine or a dopamine agonist to a normal patient will lead to an elevation of GH, whereas in 50%–80% of acromegalics, there is suppression of GH. The test may sometimes be used for confirmation of abnormal GH dynamics in patients with suspected mild acromegaly, but low mean GH.

Contraindications

Dopamine infusion is contraindicated in patients with severe ischaemic heart disease.

Procedure

The patient is fasted from midnight, and intravenous cannulae are placed in both arms at −30 minutes. Dopamine is infused at $4\,\mu g\,kg^{-1}\,min^{-1}$ for 3 hours from +60 minutes to +240 minutes. Pulse and blood pressure are recorded every half hour during the test. GH and prolactin are sampled at 0, 30, 60, 90, 120, 150, 180, 210, 240, 270 and 300 minutes.

Interpretation

In a normal person serum prolactin falls promptly to $<60\,mUl^{-1}$ during dopamine infusion. GH shows a transient rise. A fall in GH during the dopamine infusion is characteristic of acromegaly.

IGF-I measurement

GH exerts its biological actions partly by induction of IGF-I (somatomedin C), produced predominantly, but not exclusively, by the liver, and partly by a direct action (see Table 2.6). Direct actions of GH are the diabetic actions, lipolysis, amino acid transport and phosphate retention. IGF-I reflects an index of integrated GH over time. IGF-I levels are better correlated with the severity of acromegaly than GH levels.

Measurement of IGF-I in acromegaly

Since IGF-I is not subject to pulsatile secretion, it was previously thought to be a convenient tool for assessing normality of GH secretion. Earlier studies reported a near 100% accuracy of IGF-I measurement in differentiating between acromegaly and non-acromegaly. Studies have indeed shown excellent cor-

Table 2.6 Actions of growth hormone and IGF-I

Protein synthesis, nitrogen retention
Amino acid transport
Phosphorus retention
Increased muscle mass
Growth of cartilage
Stimulation of soft tissue and bone growth
Anti-insulin:
    Antagonism of peripheral insulin action
    Lipolysis, ketogenesis
    Hyperinsulinaemia
Electrolyte metabolism:
    Sodium retention
    Calciuria
    Increased bone turnover
Others:
    IGF production in peripheral tissues
    Bone elongation
    Promotes lactation

---

relations between integrated 24-hour GH measurements and IGF-I. However, the measurement of IFG-I can only be interpreted provided the concentrations of the IGF-I binding proteins are known, and some of these are also regulated by GH.

2.3.3 GONADOTROPINOMAS

These secrete gonadotropins and/or their subunits. The normal gonadotroph secretes both LH and FSH. Glycoproteins are composed of two subunits, alpha and beta. The alpha subunit is common to all glycoprotein hormones (TSH, human chorionic gonadotropin (HCG)), whereas the beta subunit is unique to each hormone. It has been shown that under normal circumstances the alpha subunit is synthesized in excess of the beta subunit, so that the latter is the rate limiting step in the synthesis of intact glycoprotein hormone.

In one series, up to 17% of 139 consecutive men with previously untreated pituitary macroadenomas were found to have a gonadotropin secreting tumour. Although this represents an overestimate of the proportion of gonadotropin secreting tumours in all pituitary tumours (i.e. microadenomas and macroadenomas), gonadotropinomas are certainly not rare. Tumours secrete intact LH, FSH and alpha subunit, alone or in combination. Hypersecretion of intact FSH is most commonly seen.

Clinical features

The typical patient is a middle-aged man referred for visual field impairment. There is no history of impaired gonadal function, and puberty has been normal. There is no history of infertility. By the time of presentation the tumours are frequently enormous, with suprasellar extension and invariably a visual field defect. This late presentation presumably reflects the absence of gonadal dysfunction in males. Hypopituitarism with ACTH and TSH hyposecretion may be present. Clinical hypopituitarism in the presence of normal or, often, enlarged testes should suggest the underlying diagnosis.

Biochemical features

Intact FSH and hypersecretion of alpha and beta FSH subunits is found in the serum. The latter is never found in the serum of normal men. Hypersecretion of intact LH is more rare but causes supranormal levels of circulating testosterone. These tumours frequently secrete LH (beta subunit) and FSH (intact molecule) in response to exogenous TRH. In some patients, testosterone levels are subnormal despite the presence of elevated LH levels in the serum. In such instances, this represents spurious LH elevation due to cross-reactivity of uncombined alpha and beta subunits.

Such patients respond to exogenous HCG administration by a normal incremental testosterone rise, showing that there is no primary gonadal failure.

2.3.4 THYROTROPIN SECRETING PITUITARY TUMOURS

These may occur as feedback tumours in cases of primary hypothyroidism (most frequently), or *de novo*, causing thyrotoxicosis. Both types are extremely rare.

Feedback tumours

In primary hypothyroidism the pituitary gland enlarges, this being due to thyrotroph hyperplasia. Most often this is caused by diffuse hyperplasia, and less frequently by nodular hyperplasia. Radiological enlargement of the gland is evident in cases where a feedback tumour has occurred.

Clinical features

Hypothyroidism is typically long-standing in these cases, and is caused predominantly by autoimmune thyroiditis (83%), lingual thyroids and athyrotic cretinism. Headaches (68%) and visual field defects (37%) are frequent. The condition is more common in females, reflecting the higher incidence of autoimmune disorders in this sex.

Precocious puberty secondary to hypothyroidism has been observed, with menstrual bleeding in girls, breast development, labial and uterine maturation, but scant pubic hair. The mechanism of sexual precocity in these instances is unknown. Suggested mechanisms include premature activation of the hypothalamo-pituitary ovarian axis and enhanced sensitivity to gonadotropins. In adults, gonadal dysfunction is also present, with loss of libido and amenorrhoea–galactorrhoea. Hyperprolactinaemia may be present.

Virtually all patients with feedback tumours are clinically and biochemically hypothyroid at the time of presentation. There may be GH, ACTH and gonadotropin deficiency.

2.3.5 TSH SECRETING TUMOURS AND THYROTOXICOSIS

This condition occurs as a result of a pituitary TSH secreting adenoma. Unlike Grave's disease, the usual female to male preponderance is lacking. The disorder is described with an age range of 17–76 years. In all cases there is thyroid enlargement, but in addition to the usual features of thyrotoxicosis, pretibial myxoedema and ophthalmopathy are absent.

Biochemical features

Circulating TSH is elevated in the presence of raised total and free T4 and T3. The condition must be distinguished from TSH elevation resulting from central resistance to thyroid hormone. Patients with thyrotropinomas usually have an excess of circulating alpha subunit. Furthermore, the elevation of TSH levels may be inversely related to the biological potency.

These paradoxical characteristics are thought to be related to abnormal glycosylation of TSH. Co-secretion of GH and prolactin is common in these tumours, and more rarely gonadotropins. The TSH response to TRH is usually flattened in patients with thyrotropinomas, and only approximately 15% show an incremental rise. T3 suppression tests are generally ineffective in reducing TSH levels. Paradoxically, initiation of antithyroid medication in such patients has been noted to cause a rise in TSH in 70% of cases. Furthermore, dopamine agonists, which generally suppress TSH in normal subjects, have no effect in patients with thyrotropinomas.

However, the sensitivity of tumorous thyrotrophs to the suppressive effects of exogenous glucocorticoids is maintained, or even enhanced, in patients with thyrotropinomas. In some patients, TSH as well as the circulating alpha subunit are completely suppressed. Somatostatin or its analogue (octreotide) has been beneficial only in suppressing TSH secretion in some cases. There have been anecdotal reports of TSH suppression in patients with cholinergic agonists and acetylcholinesterase inhibitors.

Differential diagnosis

The major differential diagnosis is from the syndrome of inappropriate TSH secretion. In such patients there may be a generalized resistance to the actions of T4. In cases where the pituitary is most affected there may be clinical hyperthyroidism, whereas patients with generalized tissue resistance are euthyroid or frankly hypothyroid.

2.3.6 NON-SECRETING PITUITARY TUMOURS

These account for up to 30% of pituitary tumours. As they do not produce the characteristic clinical syndrome associated with hormone excess, these tumours tend to present because of mass effects such as headache, visual loss and symptoms of hypopituitarism.

Pathology

Although these tumours were previously thought to be functionless, it is now recognized that they do, in fact, synthesize and occasionally secrete glycoprotein subunits.

Clinical features

These tumours tend to be macroadenomas and thus present with symptoms of suprasellar or extrasellar extension. Therefore, visual field defects and cranial nerve palsies are not uncommon. Occasionally, patients present with pituitary apoplexy with a sudden severe headache and visual embarrassment.

Biochemical features

Patients may present with partial or total hypopituitarism. GH and gonadotropin deficiency are most frequently seen. Modest hyperprolactinaemia (up to $2000-3000\,\mathrm{mU\,l}^{-1}$) is caused by effective stalk compression and impairment of delivery of dopamine to the lactotrophs. Impaired pituitary adrenal function is usually demonstrable on dynamic testing.

FURTHER READING

1. Afrasiabi, A., Valents, L. and Gwinup, G. (1979) A TSH-producing pituitary tumour causing hyperthyroidism: presentation of a case and review of the literature. *Acta Endocrinol.*, **92**, 448.
2. Besser, G.M. and Ross, R.J.M. (1989) Are

hypothalamic releasing hormones useful in the diagnosis of endocrine disorders? *Recent Adv. Endocrinol. Metab.*, **3**, 135.

3. Bouloux, P.M. and Grossman, A. (1987) Hyperprolactinaemia and sexual function in the male. *Br. J. Hosp. Med.*, June, 503.

4. Bruno, O.D., Ross, M.A., Contreras, L.N., Gomes, R.M., Galparsola, G., Cazado, E., Krai, M., Leber, B. and Arias, D. (1985) Nocturnal high dose dexamethasone suppression test in the etiological diagnosis of Cushing's syndrome. *Br. Acta Endocrinol.*, **109**, 158.

5. Chrousos, G.P., Schulte, H.M., Oldfield, E.H., Gold, P.W., Cutler, A.G., Jr. and Loriaux, D.L. (1984) The corticotrophin-releasing factor stimulation test: an aid in the evaluation of patients with Cushing's syndrome. *New Engl. J. Med.*, **310**, 622.

6. Clemmons, D.R., Van Wyk, J.J., Ridgeway, E.C., Kliman, B. and Kjellberg, R.W. (1979) Evaluation of acromegaly by radioimmunoassay of somatomedin C. *New Engl. J. Med.*, **301**, 1138.

7. Ferrari, C., Rampin, P., Benco, R., Caldara, R., Scardvelli, C. and Crosigniani, P.G. (1982) Functional characterisation of hypothalamic hyperprolactinaemia. *J. Clin. Endocrinol. Metab.*, **55**, 897.

8. Findling, J.W., Aron, D.C., Tyrrel, J.B., Shinsako, J.H., Fitzgerald, P.A., Norman, D., Wilson, C.B. and Forsham, P.H. (1981) Selective venous sampling for ACTH in Cushing's syndrome: differentiation between Cushing's disease and the ectopic ACTH syndrome. *Ann. Intern. Med.*, **94**, 647.

9. Grossman, A., Howlett, T.A., Perry, L., Coy, D.H., Savage, M.O., Lavender, P., Rees, L.H. and Besser, G.M. (1988) CRF in the differential diagnosis of Cushing's syndrome: a comparison with the dexamethasone suppression test. *Clin. Endocrinol.*, **29**, 167.

10. Liuzzi, A., Chiodini, P.G., Botalla, A., Cremascoli, G. and Silvestrini, F. (1972) Inhibitory effect of L-dopa on GH release in acromegalic patients. *J. Clin. Endocrinol. Metab.*, **39**, 941.

11. Snyder, P.J. (1985) Gonadotropin cell adenomas of the pituitary. *Endocrine Rev.*, **6**, 552.

3

Thyroid disorders

J.H. LAZARUS, R. JOHN and R. HALL

3.1 THE PRODUCTION AND REGULATION OF THYROID HORMONE SECRETION

3.1.1 PHYSIOLOGY OF THE HYPOTHALAMIC-PITUITARY-THYROID AXIS

Thyroid stimulating hormone (TSH), a glycoprotein produced and secreted from the thyrotroph cells of the anterior pituitary, stimulates the thyroid follicular cell to produce thyroid hormones. The secretion of TSH is under tonic control of the hypothalamic tripeptide thyrotropin releasing hormone (TRH). However, the major factor regulating the secretion of TSH is the negative feedback of the thyroid hormones thyroxine (T4) and triiodothyronine (T3) on the anterior pituitary gland. The effects of other regulators of TSH (somatostatin and dopamine) are shown in Fig. 3.1.

There may be a negative effect of T4 and T3 at the hypothalamic level.

Thyroid hormone biosynthesis

Iodine is an essential substrate for thyroid hormone biosynthesis. Humans require 150 µg of iodine daily, currently obtained from milk, fish and other foodstuffs. Following ingestion, iodine is absorbed mainly in the stomach and jejunum and concentrated by the thyroid follicular cell at the basal cell membrane approximately 10–20 times the plasma level.

Iodine not trapped is excreted by the kidneys, with a small amount being found in the faeces. There are extrathyroidal sites of iodine concentration (e.g. salivary glands, stomach, choroid plexus), but there is no known functional association. Other ions in Table VII of the periodic table (e.g. perchlorate and thiocyanate) can compete with iodide for the trapping mechanism, resulting in goitre. Thiocyanate derived from cassava, for example, is an important co-factor in goitre development in parts of Africa.

Regulation of TSH biosynthesis

The primary factors involved in the regulation of TSH biosynthesis are thyroid hormones and TRH, acting along with the secondary modulators, dopamine, catecholamines and somatostatin.

There is a circadian rhythm of TSH secretion, levels rising during the evening, even before the onset of sleep. The nadir of TSH levels is seen at about 11 a.m., when basal levels should be taken for critical studies. The

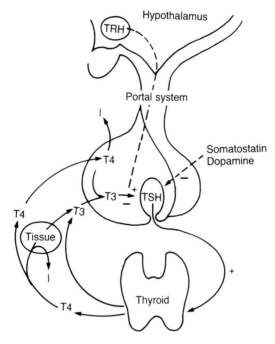

Fig. 3.1 Control of thyroid hormone secretion by hypothalamic TRH, pituitary TSH and thyroidal T4 and T3 iodine (I) is by monodeiodination of T4 in the tissues and the pituitary (after L. Van Middlesworth (ed.) *The Thyroid Gland*, Year Book Medical Publishers, with permission).

mechanism controlling the circadian rhythm is unknown.

Disorders of TSH biosynthesis

Disorders are rarely seen, but excess production of alpha subunit is a characteristic of a thyrotroph adenoma.

TSH action

TSH binds to a specific membrane receptor recently cloned [1], leading to activation of adenylate cyclase and a rise in cyclic adenosine 3',5'-monophosphate (cAMP), which activates a series of protein kinases responsible for mediating the various effects of TSH.

Thyroid hormone action

This occurs after the binding of thyroid hormones to high affinity nuclear receptors. The nuclear T3 receptor has recently been shown to be a protein encoded by the proto-oncogene c-erb-A [2]. The hormone receptor complex binds to specific areas of DNA whose activation leads to transcription of specific messenger RNAs coding for proteins known to be stimulated by T3, e.g. growth hormone (GH), malic enzyme and others.

Diseases of the thyroid present as goitre either in the euthyroid state or in the hyperthyroid or hypothyroid situation. Some patients do not have goitre. In the western world, goitre has an average prevalence of around 5%–10%, but this may vary markedly in iodine deficient areas. Hyperthyroidism (treated and untreated) occurs in 1%–1.5% of the population, and hypothyroidism at about half that rate.

3.2 TESTS DETERMINING THE LEVEL OF THYROID FUNCTION

Improvements in assay technology to detect even subclinical disease has led to a dramatic increase in the workload of a laboratory, as clinicians have become increasingly aware of the ability to screen for thyroid disease.

3.2.1 ROUTINE TESTS OF THYROID FUNCTION

Total T4/T3

Procedure

Before the advent of free T4 (FT4) and free T3 (FT3) assays, the standard approach to the assessment of thyroid function was the measurement of total T4 (TT4) and total T3 (TT3) by radioimmunoassay (RIA).

Interpretation

Although these methods were fairly reliable, their major limitation has been the many conditions other than thyroid disease which alter total concentrations of T4 and T3. These include altered concentrations of thyroxine binding globulin (TBG) as well as increased and decreased binding to albumin and pre-albumin, decreased binding to TBG and increased binding to antibodies to T4 or T3.

An attempt to overcome this was the derivation of the FT4 index, which was the product of TT4 and the T3 uptake – an estimate of unoccupied binding sites on TBG. Although this reflected the patients's euthyroid state when TT4 and TBG were elevated due to the contraceptive pill or pregnancy, the FT4 index had limitations at extremes of TBG concentration and failed to correct for abnormal binding to the other serum proteins.

Plasma FT3 (normal range 3–9 pmol l^{-1}) and plasma FT4 (normal range 8–26 pmol l^{-1})

Procedure

It was for these reasons that a large number of centres have now abandoned TT4 and TT3 assays in favour of one of the free hormone assays for FT4 and FT3. These are largely of two types:

1. Analogue RIA: these utilize a chemically modified analogue of T4 which competes in the assay with T4. This method produces results that are valid in patients with normal albumin and pre-albumin, but is affected to variable extents when these binding proteins are abnormal.
2. Two-step RIA: these methods produce results that agree with equilibrium dialysis techniques and appear to be the most valid, although because of their greater complexity and cost they are not in widespread use.

Interpretation

The main advantage that FT4 and FT3 assays have over the TT4 and TT3 methods is that they are independent of TBG concentrations so that patients on oestrogen therapy or taking the oral contraceptive pill, or individuals with inherited excess or deficiency of TBG, will have normal FT4 and FT3 concentrations if they are euthyroid.

Plasma TSH (normal range 0.36–5.4 mU l^{-1})

Procedure

The application of monoclonal antibodies to measure TSH in serum has produced immunometric assays that can distinguish the suppressed levels found in hyperthyroidism from normal levels. These sensitive TSH assays provide the most reliable first-line test of thyroid dysfunction, as they produce fewer abnormal results in euthyroid patients with various nonthyroidal illnesses and those on drug therapy.

Undetectable TSH concentrations may also be found in apparently euthyroid subjects who are severely ill or suffer from subclinical diseases, such as non-toxic multinodular goitre or a solitary autonomous nodule.

Interpretation

The ability of TSH assays to separate normal and low levels depends on the TSH methodology in use. Some sensitive TSH assays will be reliable only down to $0.2\,\text{mU}\,\text{l}^{-1}$, whereas with other assays thyrotoxicosis will have TSH concentrations of less than $0.02\,\text{mU}\,\text{l}^{-1}$ [3]. Because some normal patients may also show a suppressed or undetectable TSH concentration, it is essential to perform a confirmatory test in all patients with abnormally low TSH concentrations.

Biochemical tests can only categorize patients as euthyroid, hypothyroid or hyperthyroid, and can give no indication of the nature of the disease.

Thyroidal radioisotope uptake measurements: (i) technetium $^{99m}TcO_4$ pertechnetate

Procedure

Measurement of technetium ^{99m}Tc uptake by the thyroid 20 minutes after an intravenous dose provides rapid information about the patient's level of thyroid function, with low thyroidal, gonadal and whole body radiation. Technetium is trapped by the thyroid but is not converted to an organic form. Like isotopes of iodine, its uptake is affected by drugs which alter the trapping of iodine and by alterations of the body's iodide pool.

Interpretation

^{99m}Tc uptake is of no value in the diagnosis of hypothyroidism but it does provide good discrimination in separating hyperthyroid patients from normal. Uptake measurements can be combined with scanning of the thyroid at 20–30 minutes.

Thyroidal radioisotope uptake measurements: (ii) radioiodine ^{131}I and ^{123}I

Procedure

^{123}I and ^{131}I are used for uptake measurements of the thyroid. ^{123}I (half-life 13 hours) has a much lower effective dose equivalent than ^{131}I and therefore is preferred, particularly for repeat measurements and in children. Uptakes are carried out at early intervals (2–6 hours) in the diagnosis of hyperthyroidism and at later intervals (24–48 hours) for hypothyroidism. Plasma can be obtained for measurement of protein bound ^{131}I (^{123}I) 24–48 hours following ^{131}I or ^{123}I

administration. Scans can be performed at 2–4 hours or later.

Indication

^{123}I is the radionuclide of choice in neonatal hypothyroidism, retrosternal extensions and suspected ectopic or lingual thyroids. ^{131}I for scanning is now usually confined to looking for secondary deposits following thyroidal ablation in carcinoma of the thyroid. Uptakes are also useful as a diagnostic test in suspected dyshormonogenetic goitres where serial measurements of uptake are valuable.

Many centres find uptake values useful in determining the dosage of ^{131}I therapy for hyperthyroidism, although others do not. Other indications for radioisotope uptakes include the confirmation of the low uptake seen in subacute viral thyroiditis, thyrotoxicosis factitia and postpartum thyroiditis.

Interpretation

Low iodide uptake is seen in the thyroid trapping defect. Rapid early uptake with spontaneous or perchlorate-induced discharge of radioactivity is seen in organification defects. Rapid uptake and spontaneous discharge are seen in dehalogenase defects. Rapid and sustained uptake values are seen in some patients whose thyroids secrete iodoalbumin.

High uptakes are seen in hyperthyroidism and iodine deficiency. Values of protein bound $^{123}I > 0.3\%$ dose l^{-1} plasma are seen in hyperthyroidism and in conditions where there is a low intrathyroidal iodine pool, in Hashimoto's disease or following destructive therapy to the thyroid. Thyroid and renal iodide clearances, thyroid absolute iodide uptake and plasma inorganic iodide can be measured after ^{131}I or ^{123}I (see below).

In North America, silent thyroiditis is a cause of hyperthyroidism which is associated with suppressed thyroid uptake measurements – an important observation if radio-iodine therapy is being considered.

3.3 THYROID DISEASE

3.3.1 OVERT PRIMARY THYROID DISEASE

Hypothyroidism

In primary hypothyroidism, plasma FT4 concentration will be low with an elevated plasma TSH concentration. Plasma FT3 concentration need not be measured, as in less severe disease FT3 concentration usually remains within the normal range.

Hyperthyroidism

In hyperthyroidism, plasma FT4 will be increased with a suppression of TSH to undetectable concentrations. It is a wise precaution to confirm hyperthyroidism by a plasma FT3 measurement, as an increased FT4 with a suppressed TSH concentration may be seen in conditions other than hyperthyroidism.

In developing hyperthyroidism, both FT4 and FT3 are elevated before TT4 and TT3. There may be the occasional patient in whom plasma FT4 remains within the reference range and plasma FT3 becomes elevated. Again, this increased thyroidal secretion of T3 will be accompanied by a suppression of plasma TSH to low levels.

3.3.2 COMPENSATED HYPOTHYROIDISM AND HYPERTHYROIDISM

Detection of mild cases of thyroid disease is difficult because the clinical examination may reveal non-specific or conflicting symptoms, particularly in the elderly. In a patient developing hypothyroidism, the decreasing production of T4 by the thyroid gland causes the serum FT4 concentration to decrease, which produces an increased TSH output from the pituitary. This increased TSH drive can be sufficient to maintain plasma FT4 concentration within the bottom end of the reference range. The only biochemical abnormality, therefore, will be an increased plasma TSH concentration. In a patient developing hyperthyroidism, a slight increase in T4 and T3 production can be enough to decrease plasma TSH concentration below the normal range, with only minimally increased FT4 and FT3 concentrations.

3.4 EFFECT OF NON-THYROIDAL DISEASE ON THYROID FUNCTION TESTS

Not all abnormalities in thyroid function tests are due to thyroid disease, and before any therapy is commenced confirmation should be sought by a back-up assay. When results are at variance with the clinical state of the patient, the laboratory should be contacted to discuss the possibility of a non-thyroidal cause of an abnormal thyroid function test result [4]. Some of the conditions that can give rise to difficulty in interpretation of thyroid function tests are considered below.

3.4.1 NON-THYROIDAL ILLNESS

Interpretation

The most common finding is a low serum FT3 concentration due to a decreased peripheral conversion of T4 to T3 as well as a decreased cellular uptake of T4. Serum FT4 concentration can be low, normal or high, and can be method-related.

In those ill patients with a high FT4 concentration, a normal TSH concentration will rule out hyperthyroidism. Those with a normal FT4 usually have a mild illness, whereas those with a low FT4 concentration can be quite sick. Those with the lowest FT4 concentration have the worst prognosis for survival.

The best indicator of euthyroidism in the majority of sick patients is the sensitive TSH concentration, which will be normal apart from drug effects (dopamine and glucocorticoids) and suppression from very severe illness, as seen with some malignancies. In conditions such as chronic renal failure, both FT4 and FT3 can be substantially decreased, but TSH is usually normal.

With the sometimes conflicting results seen when more than one thyroid function test is done in severe non-thyroidal illness, the best advice is to refrain from requesting thyroid function tests in ill patients unless there are clear clinical signs of a thyroid disorder.

A particular problem may occur in the elderly, in whom there will be a high incidence of illness and drug therapy, which may cause decreased FT4 and FT3 concentrations and may also have decreased TSH concentrations. Some centres have found a high incidence of suppressed TSH concentrations in elderly patients admitted to a geriatric ward, but others have not found this high incidence.

Again, the utility of the TRH test is not as great in the sick elderly patient, as failure to respond to TRH does not necessarily indicate hyperthyroidism [5]. When these elderly sick patients were re-investigated six weeks after their illness, a recovery of TSH responsiveness to TRH was seen in some patients.

3.4.2 EFFECT OF DRUGS IN THE INTERPRETATION OF THYROID FUNCTION TESTS

A variety of drugs have *in vivo* effects on thyroid hormone metabolism, cause abnormal binding to thyroid hormone binding proteins, or reduce thyroid hormone availability as well as having an *in vitro* effect on thyroid function tests.

Amiodarone

This anti-arrhythmic drug has more than one effect [6]. It causes a decreased peripheral conversion of T4 to T3, therefore serum FT4 concentrations are commonly increased, with normal or decreased FT3 concentrations and an increased TSH concentration in the first few weeks of treatment, followed by a normal or suppressed TSH concentration on longer term treatment.

Because amiodarone contains two atoms of iodine per molecule and is only very slowly eliminated from the body, there is an excess iodine load which can cause hypothyroidism in subjects who may have pre-existing thyroid abnormalities. Hyperthyroidism can occur in areas with iodine deficiency and is best diagnosed by increased FT3 concentration combined with a suppressed TSH and absent response to TRH.

Thyroid investigations are difficult to interpret in patients taking amiodarone, and before commencing treatment, basal thyroid hormones, TSH concentration and thyroid autoantibodies should be assessed to identify any with occult thyroid disease.

Propranolol

Patients on a high dose of propranolol of greater that 160 mg per day may also have decreased FT3 with increased FT4 concentrations due to inhibition of T4 to T3 conversion.

Cholecystographic media

These may also lower FT3 concentrations, but FT4 concentrations remain within their reference range.

Lithium

This inhibits the release of T4 and T3 from the thyroid gland and can cause primary hypothyroidism in some patients.

Phenytoin

This both inhibits T4 binding to plasma proteins and increases cellular uptake of T4, thus reducing FT4 concentrations.

Salicylate, carbamazepine and corticosteroids

These have complex effects and may lower FT4 concentrations by some methods.

Heparin

Heparin administered *in vivo* causes the release of free fatty acids, which can interfere in analogue FT4 methods, causing spuriously decreased FT4 concentrations.

In patients taking drugs, serum TSH concentrations appear to be far less affected than free hormone measurements, apart from a suppression of TSH seen with L-dopa, dopamine or glucocorticoids. Patients taking these drugs may have the typical findings of secondary hypothyroidism with decreased FT4 and TSH concentrations.

3.4.3 EFFECT OF PREGNANCY ON THYROID FUNCTION TESTS

During pregnancy, serum FT4 concentrations are approximately 25% lower than the euthyroid reference range. FT3 concentrations mimic this fall in FT4 concentrations but to a lesser extent. There is a concomitant small increase in TSH concentrations in the second and third trimesters, but not sufficient to cause any diagnostic confusion.

In hyperemesis gravidarum, there may be a temporary and spontaneous reversible increase in FT4 and FT3 concentrations with a suppressed TSH concentration. To distinguish this temporary hyperthyroid state from pre-existing thyrotoxicosis, red blood cell zinc concentration is decreased in pre-existing thyrotoxics and has been found to be useful

in deciding whether to treat with antithyroid drugs.

3.4.4 PAEDIATRICS AND THE NEONATE

Thyroid function tests are difficult to interpret within the first 24 hours of birth, as TSH concentrations rise rapidly to peak within 1 hour of birth and fall gradually to normal within 3 days of birth. FT4 and FT3 concentrations in response to TSH stimulation also increase, but the decrease to normal values takes longer.

In well and sick preterm infants, FT4 and FT3 concentrations will be lower than in normal infants. The detection of congenital hypothyroidism, if blood spot screening has not been performed by 6 days after birth, is best done by measuring serum TSH concentration.

3.4.5 ASSAY INTERFERENCE

Many instances are now described of substances present in plasma which can interfere with the hormone assays to cause spuriously low or high results. This can occur in subjects who are euthyroid, hypothyroid or hyperthyroid (a 'normal' result in a hypothyroid or hyperthyroid patient is clearly abnormal and warrants further investigation). To arrive at the correct classification requires an ordered approach to the investigation of any assay artefact.

Endogenous antibodies to T4 and T3

These are usually detected when thyroid function tests are at variance with the clinical state of the patient. Although antibodies that interfere in TT4 and TT3 assays appear to be rare, interference in FT4 and FT3 analogue assays occurs more commonly [7]. In patient samples sent for thyroid function testing the incidence of interfering samples in an FT4

45

analogue assay was 1 in 2460. Interference can occur in either FT4 or FT3 assays with grossly increased free hormone estimations. It can be seen in hypothyroid patients who have evidence of autoimmune disease, in hyperthyroid patients, particularly after treatment with ^{131}I, or in euthyroid individuals with no illness, or very rarely in patients with Waldenstrom's macroglobulinaemia, Sjogren's syndrome or hepatocellular carcinoma. TSH assays are unaffected by this interference and FT4 and FT3 two-step assays are valid.

3.5 EFFECT OF OTHER THYROIDAL DISEASE ON THYROID FUNCTION TESTS

3.5.1 FAMILIAL DYSALBUMINAEMIC HYPERTHYROXINAEMIA (FDH)

Some normal individuals have a genetically determined variant, possessing albumin or pre-albumin with a greater affinity for T4 than normal individuals. Others have a variant albumin which has a greater affinity for T3. In either case, FT4 and FT3 determined with an analogue method may be spuriously increased, but TSH is normal in a euthyroid individual. Free hormones measured by a two-step procedure will not be affected and will give normal results.

3.5.2 ENDOGENOUS ANTIBODIES TO TSH

Rarely, some normal individuals have endogenous antibodies which bind to TSH. These can be detected in subjects who have an inappropriately high TSH for their FT4 and FT3 concentrations. The subjects are usually euthyroid and the artefact can be confirmed by precipitating the antibody from serum after labelling with ^{125}I-TSH.

An interference in some two-site immunometric assays has been observed if non-immune serum is left out, or in assays that use mouse monoclonal antibodies if mouse serum is not incorporated. Endogenous antibodies in serum which bind to reagent antibodies can mimic TSH, thus producing a spuriously high TSH result. Using TSH as a front-line screen may cause a thyrotoxic patient to be missed if this interference produces a 'normal' result.

3.5.3 THYROID HORMONE RESISTANCE

There is a group of individuals who display varied end organ resistance to thyroid hormones. The clinical presentation varies depending upon where the defect occurs. Resistance can be generalized with findings of an increased FT4 and FT3 concentration, with a normal or increased TSH concentration.

3.5.4 PITUITARY TSH-SECRETING TUMOURS

Another rare cause of increased FT4 and FT3 concentration with normal or increased TSH concentrations is a pituitary TSH-secreting tumour. Patients are usually thyrotoxic. Confirmation of the source of the TSH can be made radiologically and by measuring an excess of alpha subunit, which usually occurs in thyrotropic adenomas.

3.6 TESTS DETERMINING THE CAUSE OF THYROID DYSFUNCTION

Having established the thyroid status of the patient, the following tests may be used to determine the aetiology of the condition (Table 3.1).

3.6.1 THYROID ANTIBODIES

Antibodies directed against thyroid follicular test components

Circulating antibodies to components of the thyroid follicular cell were described nearly

Table 3.1 Appropriate diagnostic thyroid tests

Condition	First choice	Others
Graves' hyperthyroidism	TsAb TBII	Thyroid ^{123}I scan
Toxic multinodular goitre	FNA	[123]I scan
Plummer's disease (toxic adenoma)	[123]I scan	T3 suppression with scan
Hashimoto's disease	Tg and TPO antibody	Ultrasound FNA Iodide perchlorate discharge
Cancer of thyroid	FNA	Calcitonin (medullary cancer only)
Diagnosis of 'single' nodule	FNA	Ultrasound
Presence of metastases	Tg (differentiated thyroid cancer) Calcitonin (medullary cancer)	Isotope scan CT/MRI scan

Note: Not all thyroid states or conditions are considered. It is assumed that the thyroid status has been evaluated by standardized biochemical testing. The first choice is considered to be the most reliable in terms of specificity and sensitivity but may require to be supplemented by one or more of the other tests

35 years ago and led to the concept of auto-immunity in relation to Hashimoto's disease. The first antibodies to be described were antithyroglobulin antibodies (TgAb) and the so-called antimicrosomal antibodies, now referred to as anti-thyroid peroxidase (TPO) antibodies.

The original tests for anti-Tg and anti-TPO were by haemagglutination inhibition and complement fixation, respectively. The sensitivity of the tests has been improved considerably by the use of enzyme-linked immunosorbent assay (ELISA) and RIA.

High titres of antibodies are seen in Hashi-moto's disease and lower titres in Graves' disease. It is useful to measure anti-Tg and anti-TPO antibodies in all patients present-ing with hypothyroidism and goitre. In the management of Graves' disease with ^{131}I or surgery there is some evidence that high titres of antibodies may predict the develop-ment of post-therapy hypothyroidism.

The role of anti-TPO antibody in the de-structive process associated with autoimmune thyroiditis is probably more important than that of anti-TgAb, as the TPO antigen can be expressed on the surface of the follicular cell. Another intracellular antibody, the second colloid antibody, has also been described, but its pathogenic significance is less clear.

Antibodies directed against the TSH receptor

The TSH receptor is located within the thyroid follicular cell membrane and has a domain protruding from it. Long acting thyroid stimu-lator (LATS) was first described as a serum factor from patients with Graves' disease that caused a delayed increase in the radioiodine release from the mouse thyroid, compared to TSH.

Subsequently, the recognition [8] that this factor was an immunoglobulin (IgG) anti-body and that there was species specificity has allowed the development of various types of assay [9]. The most common is the binding assay in which the ability of the IgG to compete with radiolabelled TSH to binding sites on solubilized thyroid membranes is measured.

The stimulatory (or inhibitory) nature of

the antibody can be assessed by the measurement of cAMP following addition of the IgG to a suitable thyroid slice preparation and comparing the effect to that of TSH. The results are expressed as thyrotropin binding inhibitory immunoglobulin (TBII), thyroid stimulating antibody (TSAb) or thyrotropin blocking antibody (TBAb), depending on the test used.

Other tests using different physiological effects of TSH action have been described. TBII is positive in most patients with Graves' hyperthyroidism. Thus, TSH receptor antibody measurements can confirm a diagnosis of Graves' disease when obvious clinical features are absent. TSAb is of value in euthyroid Graves' ophthalmopathy, as well as in predicting the likelihood of neonatal thyrotoxicosis in a pregnant patient with Graves' disease.

Antibodies related to thyroid cell growth

Drexhage and colleagues have described the occurrence of antibodies mediating thyroid follicular cell growth [10]. These antibodies are thought to interact at or near the TSH receptor but not to cause stimulation via the cAMP pathway. Measurement is complex and is performed by cytochemical bioassay and other methods.

It has been shown that these antibodies are present in sporadic non-toxic goitre and in endemic goitre, as well as in autoimmune thyroid disease. These workers also describe antibodies which block the growth of thyroid cells and postulate their presence in some cases of cretinism. It should be stated that, while there is increasing evidence for the presence of these antibodies, there is controversy about their role in the pathophysiology of thyroid disease. The measurements are not available on a routine basis.

Other antibodies

Antibodies against circulating T4 and T3 have been described in patients with Hashimoto's disease. This may result in false results in routine assays for these hormones (see below).

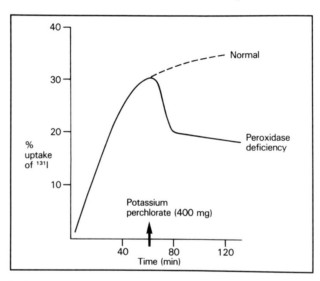

Fig. 3.2 Perchlorate discharge test. Potassium perchlorate is given orally 1 hour after radioiodine administration. The decrease in thyroidal iodine uptake is expressed as a percentage discharge from the gland relative to the uptake at 1 hour. (This figure is reproduced from *Hospital Update*, December 1988, p. 2246, by kind permission of Update-Siebert Publications Ltd).

48

3.6.2 RADIOIODINE STUDIES

In addition to the routine radioiodine studies, several procedures are available for diagnosing specific conditions.

Perchlorate discharge test

The principle is that the anion perchlorate will discharge any unbound iodide from the thyroid gland. In practice, the most common cause of unbound iodide is the presence of an organification defect due to deficiency or malfunction of the peroxidase enzyme system.

Procedure

The test is performed by giving 1 g potassium perchlorate orally, 2 hours after a tracer dose of radioiodine, and observing the subsequent thyroid counts (Fig. 3.2) measured at 30 minutes and 60 minutes following the perchlorate dose.

Interpretation

A positive test occurs when the radioiodine uptake declines by more than 10% of the 2-hour value. A modification of this test, which will uncover latent organification defects, is the iodide-perchlorate test in which 500 μg of iodide is given at the time of the radioiodine. This test is positive in many cases of Hashimoto's thyroiditis.

Stable iodine studies

The plasma inorganic iodine (PII) exists in too small a concentration to be readily measured, but may be derived from the concentrations of radioiodine in urine and plasma and the urinary concentration of stable ^{127}I iodine. If the thyroid iodide clearance rate (thyroid clearance) is also calculated, the absolute iodine uptake (AIU) may be calculated thus:

$$AIU = PII \times thyroid\ clearance$$

These measurements may be useful in cases where the standard radioiodine uptakes do not correlate with the clinical state, but they are now mostly reserved for research purposes.

Other tests

Goitre due to an iodide transport defect is rare, and the failure of the iodide concentrating mechanism may be diagnosed by measuring salivary radioiodine levels following ^{131}I administration.

The T3 suppression test has been used to aid the diagnosis of thyrotoxicosis and to assess the function of a single hot nodule (see 'Radioisotope thyroid scanning', p. 51).

3.6.3 THYROGLOBULIN AND CALCITONIN

Thyroglobulin is released from the thyroid gland in small quantities and may be measured in serum by RIA. The presence of anti-TgAb may distort the assay but more specific assays are available to circumvent this problem. Serum thyroglobulin concentrations are elevated in Graves' disease and thyroid cancer (see Section 3.10).

Absence of serum Tg is seen in agenesis of the thyroid and following total removal of the gland. Calcitonin, which arises from the C cells within the thyroid, is measured by RIA and is raised in medullary carcinoma of the thyroid. It may also be raised non-specifically in other conditions and, like Tg, is more useful for following the progress of the patient than in diagnosis.

3.6.4 FINE NEEDLE ASPIRATION BIOPSY OF THE THYROID

Fine needle aspiration (FNA) biopsy has been employed in Scandinavia for over 25 years.

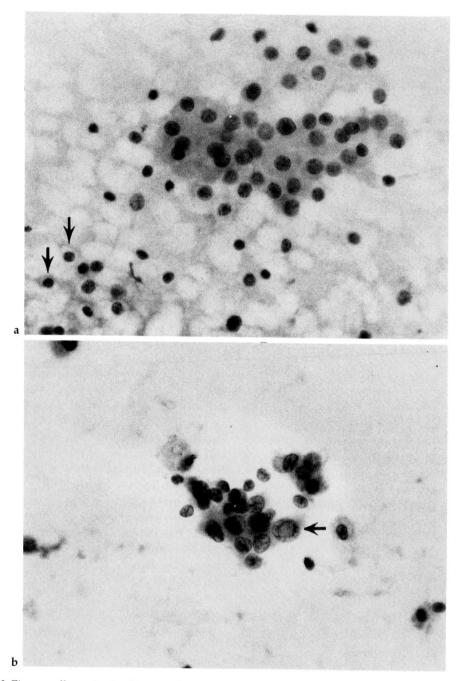

Fig. 3.3 Fine needle aspiration biopsy of thyroid. (a) Hashimoto's thyroiditis: a cluster of oxyphiltype epithelial cells with associated lymphoid cell infiltrate including plasma cells (arrows). (b) Papillary carcinoma: tumour cells exhibit delicate nuclear grooves and pseudo-inclusions (arrow).

Thyroid follicular cells, together with lymphocytes and other cells if present, are sucked into the hub of a fine needle and subsequently smeared on a slide and stained. Its use has now become widespread in thyroid clinics in the USA, the UK, Japan and elsewhere. It is the investigation of choice in patients presenting with non-toxic goitre, particularly single nodules. A cyst may be aspirated to dryness. A confident diagnosis of colloid goitre or autoimmune thyroiditis may be made, and a positive diagnosis of papillary, medullary and anaplastic cancers is possible (Fig. 3.3).

It is important to note that it is not possible to diagnose follicular cancer because of the absence of a capsule in the FNA sample. The appearance of adenomatous cells is therefore an indication for surgery. FNA is easy to perform, repeatable and remarkably free from side effects. An experienced cytologist is essential, but the material may be placed in formalin and examined as a histological specimen.

3.6.5 THYROID IMAGING

There are many techniques for imaging the thyroid [11]. The results give information on the position of the gland, its size and to some extent its consistency. Information about the function of the gland and diagnosis in a particular patient is not usually obtained.

Radiology of the thyroid

Standard radiography of the chest and soft tissue views of the neck in antero-posterior and oblique views may show the size and extent of a retrosternal goitre, as well as indicating the degree of both tracheal deviation and compression (Fig. 3.4).

In the case of superior caval compression by a large goitre, infrared photography with subtraction techniques may clearly show the venous engorgement (Fig. 3.5).

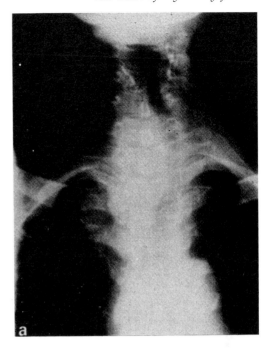

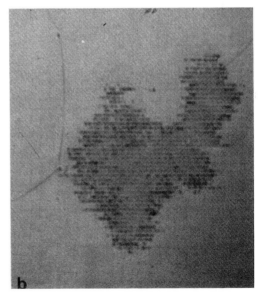

Fig. 3.4 Plain radiograph (a) showing marked lateral tracheal deviation in a patient with a large goitre. In this case the isotope (b) confirms the thyroidal nature of the mass.

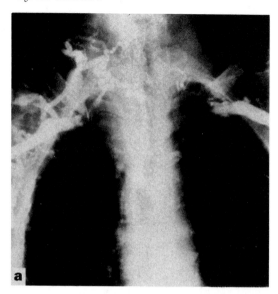

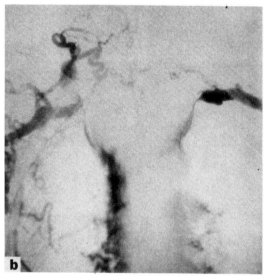

Fig. 3.5 Infrared photography of the venous drainage of the neck viewed directly (a) and by a subtraction technique (b) to show venous obstruction by large non-toxic goitre in a male.

Radioisotope thyroid scanning

Procedure

The isotopes normally used are technetium (^{99m}Tc; half-life 6 hours) and ^{123}I iodide.

Thyroid scintigraphy may visualize functioning thyroid tissue in normal or abnormal positions.

Interpretation

The qualitative function of one or more thyroid nodules may be determined. Thus, nodules may be 'cold' (no isotope uptake), 'warm' (some uptake) or 'hot' (Fig. 3.6).

The latter term usually describes the high uptake in a single nodule which is autonomous. In this situation, the rest of the thyroid is suppressed and no uptake is observed.

No tissue diagnosis is possible with this technique; note that thyroid cancer may occur in a 'warm' or 'hot' nodule as well as in a nodule with no uptake. Furthermore, a nodule which takes up ^{99m}Tc may not take up ^{123}I. An autonomous 'warm' or 'hot' nodule will not suppress isotope uptake when the patient is given T3 20 µg four times per day for 8 days, unlike the normal surrounding thyroid.

Whole body 'profile' scanning is useful in delineating metastases from differentiated thyroid carcinoma and the rare struma ovarii causing hyperthyroidism. The other use of thyroid scanning is to confirm the suggestion of Graves' disease as the cause of hyperthyroidism when a diffuse thyroid is observed.

Ultrasound examination

The thyroid may be readily visualized by modern ultrasound equipment, using a 7.5 Hz probe. Differentiation of a non-functioning nodule from a cyst is possible, and if necessary the cyst may be aspirated under ultrasonic guidance. Distinctive ultrasonic patterns in the thyroid are seen in patients with Hashimoto's thyroiditis, and this technique may even be used to diagnose the condition (Fig. 3.7).

In general, however, the diagnostic value of ultrasound in patients with non-toxic

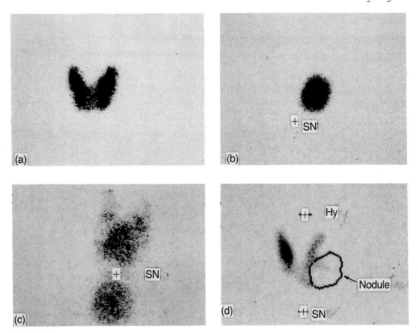

Fig. 3.6 Thyroid isotope scans showing (a) normal thyroid, (b) uninodular goitre, (c) multinodular goitre, and (d) 'cold' nodule. SN, sternal notch; Hy, hyoid bone.

goitre is very limited. Recently, quantitative volumetric ultrasonography has enabled subtle changes in thyroid volume to be ascribed to factors such as cigarette smoking. Ultrasound measurements of the extraocular muscles have been used in assessing Graves' ophthalmopathy.

Computerized tomography

Computerized tomography (CT) scanning of the neck and upper thorax may be useful in defining the extent of an intrathoracic goitre prior to surgery, and in delineating the extent of malignant spread in cases of thyroid carcinoma.

Magnetic resonance imaging

Magnetic resonance imaging (MRI) is a very good technique for imaging the mediastinum, producing high resolution, three-dimensional or tomographic images. No ionizing radiation is involved, and contrast agents are not required. It is probably the technique of choice for visualizing thyroid cancer and its spread in the neck and mediastinum.

Both MRI and CT have been used to evaluate quantitatively the eye muscles in Graves' ophthalmopathy. Serial studies are best done with MRI, which avoids the radiation exposure associated with CT scanning.

Other isotopic scan techniques

Thallium chloride 201 can successfully image thyroid carcinoma and has been used in cases

53

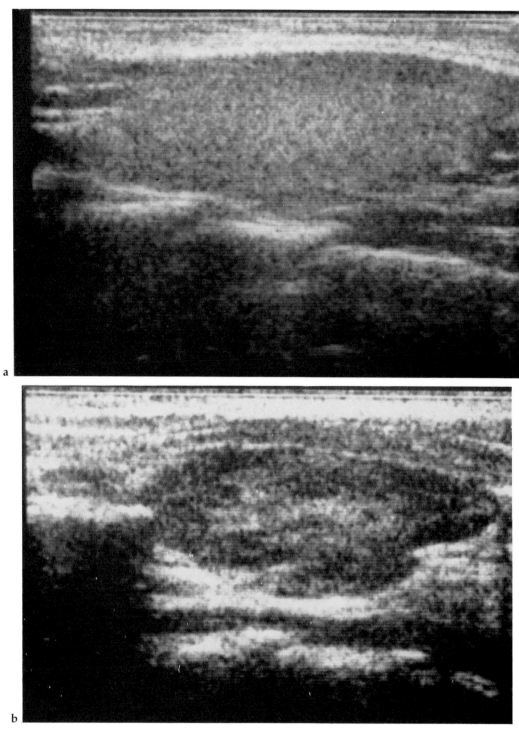

Fig. 3.7 (a) Normal thyroid, sagittal scan through the right lobe. The echotexture is homogeneous. (b) Autoimmune thyroid disease, sagittal scan through the right lobe. There are multifocal hypoechoic areas.

which did not concentrate [131]I. However, it is not of diagnostic help in patients with thyroid nodules.

[131]I metaiodobenzylguanidine (^{131}I MIBG) and [99m]Tc (V dimercaptosuccinic acid; DMSA) are compounds used for localization of medullary carcinoma of the thyroid. However, their efficacy is disputed, especially in diagnosis. The best that can be said is that if there is uptake with these isotopes then tumour will be present.

X-ray fluorescence

The quantitative X-ray fluorescence (XRF) scanning technique can compare the stable iodine ([127]I) in one area of the thyroid with another. No radioactivity is involved, but the technology is relatively expensive. In studies of patients with solitary cold nodules, an iodine content ratio of less than 0.6 (that is, the iodine content of the area of interest compared to that of nearby normal thyroid tissue) was shown to be a good discriminant for thyroid cancer.

If available, this technique is useful in paediatric practice and in pregnant patients where radioactivity is to be avoided.

3.7 GOITRE

3.7.1 CLINICAL FEATURES

A goitre is an enlargement of the thyroid gland. Clinically, the thyroid is enlarged if one or both lobes are larger than the terminal phalanx of the examiner's thumb. In practice, there may be considerable observer error in the description of goitre. A classification of the causes is shown in Table 3.2.

In the UK, the normal thyroid gland weighs between 10 g and 15 g, the right lobe usually being larger than the left.

In addition to noting the presence of goitre, the following features should also be described: consistency (soft, firm or hard),

Table 3.2 Classification of non-toxic goitre

Diffuse
Iodine deficiency
Iodine excess
Goitrogens: chemicals, e.g. shale oils
            drugs, e.g. lithium
            foodstuffs, e.g. cassava (thiocyanate)
Congenital defect in thyroid hormone
  biosynthesis

Nodular
Non-toxic multinodular colloid goitre
Autonomous follicular adenoma
Thyroid cyst
Hashimoto's thyroiditis
Carcinoma of thyroid
Metastatic carcinoma (rare)
Long-standing causes of 'diffuse' goitre

nodularity (nodular or diffuse), pain, stridor, or any other clinical evidence of compression of the structures at the root of the neck, in particular tracheal deviation and vascularity.

3.7.2 INVESTIGATION

Thyroid status should be evaluated both clinically and biochemically. A careful history should be taken to exclude any exogenous goitrogen administration or iodine contamination. In some parts of the world endemic goitre due to iodine deficiency is a well known public health problem. Areas of endemic goitre due to iodine excess have also been described.

Goitrogens may occur in the diet, as in medication for other illnesses, or as a by-product of industrial processes. In some cases, proof of the goitrogenic action of a compound may be difficult and extensive animal work may be required [12].

Measurement of urinary iodine is useful in defining areas of iodine deficiency. Great care must be taken to collect the sample in iodine-free containers. The results are normally expressed as urinary iodine per gram of creatinine, and group data are generally more informative than single-patient samples. There is a relationship between the degree of iodine deficiency and the degree of developmental retardation.

If a congenital defect in thyroid hormone biosynthesis is suspected, the perchlorate discharge test will be helpful in delineating a peroxidase deficiency. Deafness should be looked for and a family history of recessive disorder should be sought. In Pendred's syndrome there is a high tone deafness with a positive perchlorate discharge test, but the patient is euthyroid.

Further tests involve more sophisticated studies of stable iodine metabolism and the ability of the patient to handle labelled mono-iodotyrosine. Further analysis of congenital hormone defects can be performed by obtaining thyroid tissue at operation. Biochemical studies can then indicate the ratio of all the iodinated amino acids and may help to pinpoint the biochemical lesion.

Appropriate enzyme activities can also be measured. In some instances, all enzyme studies are normal and the defect may reside in an abnormality of thyroglobulin. The gene for thyroglobulin has been cloned, and any goitre due to a defective primary structure of thyroglobulin can now be traced to a specific gene defect.

In the investigation of nodular goitres, it is important to note that for practical purposes cancer is very unusual in multinodular goitre. It should also be remembered that when clinical examination suggests a single nodule, further evaluation by scanning or other techniques shows that this assessment is wrong in up to 50% of patients, and the gland is really multinodular.

However, if there is a strong clinical suspicion of a single nodule, the investigation of choice is FNA biopsy. If fluid is obtained,

Table 3.3 Causes of hyperthyroidism

Graves' disease and its variants
Toxic nodular goitre
Thyroid adenoma
Jod–Basedow
Postpartum thyroiditis
Silent thyroiditis
Thyrotoxicosis factitia, including hamburger hyperthyroidism
De Quervain's thyroiditis
Molar hyperthyroidism
Functioning thyroid carcinoma
Pituitary hyperthyroidism
Struma ovarii

Table 3.4 Symptoms and signs of hyperthyroidism

Symptoms[a]	Signs
Nervousness	Warm moist palms
Irritability	Tremor
Sweating	Tachycardia (may be atrial fibrillation)
Palpitations	
Tremor	Goitre (with bruit)
Heat intolerance	Hyperkinesis
Increased appetite	Eye signs:[b] lid retraction, lid lag, exophthalmos, diplopia
Weight loss	Thyroid acropachy[b]
	Pretibial myxoedema[b]

[a] Rather non-specific; rarer ones (e.g. proximal myopathy and thirst) occur
[b] Signs of Graves' disease. These do not necessarily indicate hyperthyroidism

a carcinoma in the wall of the cyst is not excluded and careful follow-up is advised. When FNA cytology is performed, the results will fall into three categories: benign, malignant or uncertain. It is implicit in the 'uncertain' group that operation should be advised, as carcinoma, especially of the follicular type, cannot be excluded.

3.8 HYPERTHYROIDISM

A classification of the causes of hyperthyroidism is shown in Table 3.3. and the signs and symptoms of hyperthyroidism are presented in Table 3.4.

By far the most common cause in western countries and iodine replete areas is Graves' disease, but in areas of moderate or severe iodine deficiency toxic nodular goitre and toxic adenoma are more common. Probably the most usual cause of biochemical hyperthyroidism is postpartum thyroiditis which affects 5%–10% of women a few months after giving birth, but this tends to be asymptomatic.

3.8.1 GRAVES' DISEASE AND ITS VARIANTS

The term 'classical Graves' disease' is used to describe patients with a goitre, hyperthyroidism and eye signs, who in addition may exhibit thyroid acropachy and localized myxoedema. Neonatal Graves' disease occurs in children born to mothers with the disease. The mother has stimulating thyrotropin receptor antibodies which cross the placenta and stimulate the foetal thyroid [13]. Juvenile Graves' disease is a persistent form of the disease in which one or both parents are often affected by autoimmune thyroid disease. Ophthalmic Graves' disease is the condition in which the eye signs of the disease develop in a patient who is not and has never been clinically or biochemically thyrotoxic. Thyroid tests may show minimal elevation of

T3 and impaired, absent or exaggerated TSH response to TRH, depending on the level of thyroid function.

The term 'latent Graves' disease' applies to patients in remission from the disease either as a result of spontaneous remission or previous therapy. 'Potential Graves' disease' refers to the first degree relatives of patients with Graves' disease, particularly those with circulating thyroid antibodies.

Investigations

Procedure

The tests shown in Table 3.5 may be carried out. A minimum requirement would be an FT4 or FT3 and a TSH assay.

Interpretation

Typical results of thyroid function tests in classical Graves' disease and ophthalmic Graves' disease are shown in Table 3.5. The syndrome of T3 toxicosis can occur in any variety of hyperthyroidism and is characterized by a raised total and free T3 in the presence of a normal total and free T4, and normal thyroid hormone binding proteins. It is seen particularly in iodine deficient areas, in the early stages of hyperthyroidism and in relapsed hyperthyroidism.

A low TSH level when measured by a sensitive assay is helpful in the diagnosis of hyperthyroidism, but some euthyroid normal and sick patients have undetectable TSH levels, so this test should not be relied upon on its own.

All patients with hyperthyroidism have an impaired or absent response following 100 µg of TRH intravenously. A normal TSH response to TRH virtually excludes hyperthyroidism, although an impaired or absent response is not necessarily diagnostic of hyperthyroidism, which also occurs in ophthalmic Graves' disease, thyroid autonomy in

Table 3.5 Thyroid function test results in the different varieties of hyperthyroidism

	FT4	FT3	TSH	TRH	4-hour ^{123}I uptake	Other
Classical Graves' disease	↑	↑	↓	Absent	N or ↑	
Ophthalmic Graves' disease	N	N or ↑	↑ N ↓	Normal Impaired Absent	N	
T3 toxicosis	↑ N	↑	↓	Absent	N or ↑	
Toxic nodular goitre	↑ or N	N or ↑	↓	Absent	N or ↑	
Toxic adenoma	N or ↑	↑	↓	Absent	N or ↑	
Postpartum thyroiditis	↑	N or ↑	↓	Absent	↓	
Silent thyroiditis	↑	↑	↓	Absent	↓	
Jod–Basedow	↑	N or ↑	↓	Absent	N ↑ or ↓	
Thyrotoxicosis factitia	N or ↑	N or ↑	↓	Absent	↓	
De Quervain's thyroiditis	↑	↑	↓	Absent	↓	
Molar hyperthyroidism	↑	↑	↓	Absent	↑	
Functioning thyroid carcinoma	↑	↑	↓	Absent	↑	Very rare
Pituitary hyperthyroidism	↑	↑	↓	Absent	↓	Due to thyrotroph adenoma or congenital pituitary resistance to T4
Struma ovarii	↑	↑	↓	Absent	↓	Increased radioiodine uptake in pelvis

N, normal.

a nodular goitre and thyroid adenoma, and for some months following remission of hyperthyroidism due to pituitary suppression.

A measurement of the 4-hour thyroidal radioiodine uptake is helpful if the FT4 and FT3 are normal in the elderly or sick patient with suspected hyperthyroidism.

3.8.2 TOXIC NODULAR GOITRE

This condition is most common in areas of iodine deficiency and in elderly patients in whom cardiovascular features, e.g. atrial fibrillation or heart failure, predominate. The possibility of iodine exposure as a precipitat-

ing cause of hyperthyroidism should always be considered in a patient with a pre-existing nodular goitre, but this is often difficult to confirm.

Thyroid ultrasound reveals a nodular goitre and radiation studies show a patchy uptake. Since these patients are often elderly or sick, FT4 and FT3 levels may be suppressed into the normal or subnormal range, and radio-iodine studies can sometimes be helpful.

3.8.3 TOXIC ADENOMA

Autonomous thyroid nodules make up approximately 5% of cases with hyperthyroidism in the UK, but are more common in areas of iodine deficiency. Whether a nodule causes hyperthyroidism depends on its size and its iodine supply. Such nodules may go through a phase of subclinical hyperthyroidism with mildly elevated thyroid hormone levels and an impaired response to TRH before causing frank hyperthyroidism. The syndrome of T3 toxicosis is commonly associated with thyroid nodules. Hyperfunctioning nodules are rarely malignant.

3.8.4 JOD–BASEDOW PHENOMENON

This term is applied to iodine-induced hyperthyroidism, usually occurring in patients with pre-existing goitres, especially if they are nodular and exhibit thyroid autonomy. The sources of iodine are many and varied, e.g. from radiological studies using iodine contrast media, iodine-containing cough medicine, or vitamin tablets (although it is rare to define the source with accuracy). The FT4 level is usually raised but the FT3 may be normal. Radioiodine uptake values are variable, depending on their timing relative to the iodine ingestion.

3.8.5 POSTPARTUM THYROIDITIS

Transient biochemical hyperthyroidism occurs in some 10% of women following delivery as the first feature of postpartum thyroiditis. The condition is much more common than Graves' disease at this time and remits spontaneously, to be followed by a hypothyroid phase. Women who develop postpartum thyroiditis more usually show circulating microsomal (TPO) antibodies and have a small goitre. The condition is a destructive thyroiditis characterized by a suppressed radioiodine uptake and a leak of iodine in the urine. Thyrotropin receptor antibodies are rarely detected unless the patient has pre-existing Graves' disease, which can also be complicated by postpartum

thyroiditis. The latter tends to recur in subsequent pregnancies and is occasionally followed by permanent hypothyroidism.

3.8.6 SILENT THYROIDITIS

This term probably embraces a group of different conditions apart from Graves' disease and toxic nodular goitre. It is characterized by mild hyperthyroidism, a small goitre and no typical features of Graves' disease. Circulating thyroid hormone levels are raised and the radioiodine uptake suppressed. Remission occurs with symptomatic therapy in a few months. Some patients have previously suffered from postpartum thyroiditis or De Quervain thyroiditis, and others have been exposed to thyroglobulin and thyroid hormones in the form of hamburgers.

3.8.7 THYROTOXICOSIS FACTITIA

Hyperthyroidism is occasionally seen as a result of self-medication with thyroid hormones. Such patients are usually found to have had access to this medication as prior therapy for goitre, or to be members of the medical or nursing professions. An epidemic of inadvertent thyrotoxicosis factitia has recently been described in North America as a result of the ingestion of hamburgers prepared from neck strap muscles contaminated by thyroid tissue. In such patients, the radioiodine uptake is suppressed by the ingested thyroid.

3.8.8 DE QUERVAIN'S THYROIDITIS

This typically causes pain in the thyroid, which is tender, the areas of tenderness flitting through the enlarged gland. There is often systemic upset with fever and a raised erythrocyte sedimentation rate and white cell count. In the early stages the patient may be hyperthyroid, and later on hypothyroidism, which is rarely permanent, may develop. The hyperthyroidism is distinctive in type with a low radioiodine uptake, and thyroglobulin can be detected in the circulation.

3.8.9 MOLAR HYPERTHYROIDISM

This condition is rare in the UK but is much more common in the Far East. It is caused by chorionic thyroid stimulators, e.g. high levels of human chorionic gonadotropin (HCG) in hydatiform mole or choriocarcinoma. High levels of HCG, because of the similarities in structure with TSH, interact with the TSH receptor in the thyroid.

3.8.10 FUNCTIONING THYROID CARCINOMA

Rarely, functioning follicular carcinoma of the thyroid can produce hyperthyroidism. Small incidental papillary carcinomas are present in some thyroids removed in the treatment of hyperthyroidism.

3.8.11 PITUITARY HYPERTHYROIDISM

The greater use of sensitive TSH assays has led to increased awareness of pituitary hyperthyroidism characterized by raised FT4 and FT3 levels, and a normal or raised serum TSH. The condition may be due either to a TSH-secreting pituitary thyrotroph adenoma, sometimes associated with increased levels of other pituitary hormones (e.g. GH, prolactin or alpha glycoprotein subunit), or to congenital pituitary resistance to thyroid hormone. The latter condition is lifelong and often familial, and may be largely confined to the pituitary.

3.8.12 STUMA OVARII

The presence of hyperfunctioning thyroid tissue in an ovarian teratoma is very rare. It is recognized by the occurrence of hyperthyroidism without goitre and a low thyroidal radioiodine uptake. Scanning over the pelvis reveals an increased iodine uptake in this area.

3.9 HYPOTHYROIDISM

A classification of the causes of hypothyroidism is shown in Table 3.6.

Table 3.6 Causes of hypothyroidism

Autoimmune thyroid disease
Neonatal hypothyroidism due to transplacental
 passage of blocking TSH-receptor antibodies
Juvenile hypothyroidism
Lymphocytic thyroiditis
Postpartum thyroiditis
Hashimoto's disease
Myxoedema

Iatrogenic
Postoperative
Post-radioiodine
Goitrogens

Developmental abnormalities
Agenesis and maldevelopment
Ectopic thyroid (maldescent)

Dyshormonogenesis
Trapping defect
Organification defects
Dehalogenase defect
Thyroglobulin synthesis defects

Iodine deficiency
Endemic goitre and cretinism

Peripheral hypothyroidism
Familial peripheral resistance to thyroid hormone
Thyroid hormone binding antibodies

Pituitary hypothyroidism
Hypopituitarism
Selective thyrotropin deficiency
Abnormal thyrotropin
Hypothalmic disease

Abnormalities of the TSH receptor
Pseudohypoparathyroidism

Table 3.7 Clinical and laboratory features of the different grades of hypothyroidism

Grade	Clinical features	FT4	FT3	TSH	Serum cholesterol	Thyroid antibodies
Overt	++	L	L or N	H	H or N	+ or O
Mild	+	L or N	N	H	N	+ or O
Subclinical	O	N	N or H	B	N	+ or O

+, present; ++, strongly present; O, absent; N, normal; L, low; H, high; B, borderline.

By far the most common cause in non-iodine deficient areas is autoimmune thyroid disease, which presents differently at different ages.

3.9.1 CLINICAL FEATURES

Hypothyroidism is a graded phenomenon ranging from overt hypothyroidism or myxoedema, through mild hypothyroidism, to asymptomatic subclinical hypothyroidism. The clinical and laboratory features of the different grades of hypothyroidism are shown in Table 3.7.

Overt hypothyroidism or myxoedema is always symptomatic, with lethargy, cold intolerance, depression, a puffy face, dry skin and prolonged relaxation phase of the tendon reflexes. The T4 is low, as occasionally is the FT3, and the serum TSH is clearly elevated ($>20\,mU\,l^{-1}$). Mild hypothyroidism can cause diagnostic problems since the symptoms, often lethargy and depression, are non-specific and the serum FT4 borderline, but response to T4 is usually impressive.

The syndrome of subclinical hypothyroidism has caused some controversy. Such patients are asymptomatic, have a normal FT4, though often at the lower end of the normal range, and a modestly elevated TSH (for example $<10\,mU\,l^{-1}$). The only way to differentiate them clearly from mildly hypothyroid patients is to give a therapeutic trial of T4.

A low FT4 coupled with a raised TSH is diagnostic of primary thyroid failure. A low FT4 with a normal TSH may rarely indicate pituitary hypothyroidism, but can also be seen in some euthyroid patients and those receiving a variety of drugs (e.g. aspirin).

3.9.2 AUTOIMMUNE THYROID DISEASE

Neonatal hypothyroidism

This is rarely due to the transplacental passage of blocking TSH-receptor antibodies from the mother who has myxoedema or Hashimoto's disease [13]. The condition is self-limiting, although T4 may be required for a few months.

Juvenile hypothyroidism

This is rare and often presents as shortness of stature. It is easily overlooked, and FT4 and TSH measurements are mandatory in short children in the absence of a clear family history of shortness.

Lymphocytic thyroiditis

This is usually asymptomatic and is recognized by the coincidental presence of a small firm goitre. Circulating TPO antibodies are usually present. It is from the pool of these patients that cases of silent thyroiditis and postpartum thyroiditis are probably derived.

Their thyroid function tests are usually normal, but the serum TSH may be minimally elevated.

Postpartum thyroiditis

This affects 5%–10% of all women in the first six months postpartum. Asymptomatic biochemical hyperthyroidism often precedes either symptomatic or asymptomatic hypothyroidism some four to six months after giving birth. The FT4 is low and TSH elevated, and TPO antibodies are commonly detected. Some symptomatic patients require T4, while others remit spontaneously. Therapy is withdrawn after 6 months since only about one-third develop permanent hypothyroidism.

Hashimoto's disease

This typically affects middle-aged women, who present with a firm, finely nodular goitre and sometimes symptoms of hypothyroidism. The FT4 is normal or low, and the TSH level is usually elevated. ^{123}I uptake values may be elevated in the early phase. Circulating TPO and often thyroglobulin antibody levels are usually high and are negative in only about 5% of cases.

Myxoedema

Myxoedema is the term used to refer to patients, often elderly, with overt symptomatic thyroid failure without thyroid enlargement. Serum FT4 and often FT3 levels are clearly low, and the TSH is markedly elevated.

3.9.3 IATROGENIC HYPOTHYROIDISM

Postoperative hypothyroidism

This occurs in about 20% of patients operated on for Graves' hyperthyroidism, usually within the first 2 years of operation. Minor degrees of thyroid failure may also be seen with a normal FT4, as well as a modest elevation of TSH which does not require therapy.

Post-radioiodine hypothyroidism

This is the major complication of this form of therapy, largely depending on the dose of radioiodine administered. In ablative regimes where a standard high dose of radioiodine (for example 15 mCi (555 mBq)) are given, approximately 80% of patients have clear thyroid failure within a few months. All patients given radioiodine, whatever the dose, must be followed up until they become hypothyroid and are stabilized on T4; annual measurements of FT4 and TSH are required in most cases.

Goitrogens

Many drugs have a goitrogenic action by blocking thyroid hormone biosynthesis. Carbimazole and propylthiouracil, the standard antithyroid drugs, cause hypothyroidism: hence the value of blocking replacement regimes when T4 is added to the antithyroid drug regime. Iodide in its various forms and drugs containing iodine (e.g. amiodarone) can cause thyroid failure. Amiodarone acts by its iodine content at the thyroid level, and also peripherally, to block conversion of T4 to T3.

3.9.4 DEVELOPMENTAL ABNORMALITIES

These are a common cause of neonatal hypothyroidism, and are now screened for 5–10 days after birth by TSH measurements on filter paper spots in all western countries. Spot TSH levels above $50 \, \text{mUl}^{-1}$ are confirmed by serum TSH and FT4 measurements. The prevalence of hypothyroidism is of the order of 1 in 3500 in non-iodine-deficient areas. Ectopic thyroids may fail at any age and cause mild low grade thyroid failure over many years.

3.9.5 DYSMORPHOGENESIS

Children with goitres and any degree of thyroid failure, particularly those with a family history of goitre, thyroid failure or a hearing defect, should be suspected of dysmorphogenesis. There are many congenital defects of thyroid hormone biosynthesis leading to a low FT4 and raised TSH.

The most common of these occurs in the group of organification defects often associated with nerve defects, termed Pendred's syndrome, which leads to a low FT4, often an elevated FT3 and a raised TSH. These have in common a positive perchlorate discharge test (see p. 48).

3.9.6 IODINE DEFICIENCY

Globally this is the most common cause of primary thyroid failure, often associated with endemic goitre in areas with an iodine intake $<50\,\mu g\,g^{-1}$ creatinine per day. This is well reviewed in the monograph by Hetzel [14].

3.9.7 PERIPHERAL HYPOTHYROIDISM

Peripheral resistance to thyroid hormones

This is a rare familial condition caused by a mutation in the gene coding for the thyroid hormone receptor, resulting in a single amino acid substitution in the receptor. It is characterized by elevated levels of thyroid hormones and TSH. A goitre may be present, and the patient may be euthyroid or hypothyroid, depending on the degree of tissue resistance. In the original family, speckled epiphyses were present, indicating tissue hypothyroidism.

Thyroid hormone binding antibodies

Binding of thyroid hormones to immunoglobulins or to specific T4 and T3 antibodies has been described in a variety of thyroid disease. In some patients with autoimmune thyroid disease, thyroglobulin antibodies are responsible for this binding phenomenon. The presence of T3 and T4 antibodies interferes with the measurement of FT3 and FT4, the deviation of the measurement depending on the particular method employed. Rarely, impaired thyroid function may result from the effect of these antibodies.

3.9.8 PITUITARY HYPOTHYROIDISM

This rare condition, which is due to deficient thyrotroph function or to secretion of biologically inactive TSH, usually occurs in the context of pituitary disease. It is usually mild and difficult to diagnose clinically, diagnosis usually resting on a low FT4 level. There is often evidence of pituitary disease, e.g. acromegaly or a scar from pituitary surgery, and other hormone deficiency is apparent (for instance, amenorrhoea and lack of body hair). Isolated familial TSH deficiency has rarely been described.

In the absence of TRH due to hypothalamic disease, hypothyroidism can occur with normal or slightly elevated immunoreactive TSH levels. It has been shown that the TSH is abnormally glycosylated and can be restored to a normally glycosylated form by TRH administration.

3.9.9 ABNORMALITIES

Pseudohypoparathyroidism is characterized by excessive parathyroid hormone (PTH) secretion and reduced target hormone responsiveness due to an abnormality of the PTH receptor. It may also affect other hormone receptors involving cAMP, for example TSH, causing hypothyroidism.

3.10 THYROID CANCER

Cancer of the thyroid gland accounts for 1.5% or less of all malignancies. The spectrum ranges from benign tumours with a prognosis almost the same as normal life expectancy to one of the most malignant tumours known [15].

3.10.1 CLINICAL FEATURES

The patient almost invariably presents with a goitre. The male to female ratio is 1. Normally, the patients are euthyroid. Only in cases of thyroid lymphoma where the whole thyroid has been replaced by tumour will the patient be hypothyroid. A uninodular goitre is the usual situation.

Clinical features strongly suspicious of carcinoma include rapid onset, stony hard consistency, immobility with fixation to underlying tissues, and the presence of lymph node metastases or other evidence of distant spread.

The advanced clinical picture is now rare, and the common clinical problem is that of differentiating thyroid cancer in the many patients presenting with a small lump in the thyroid gland which is mobile without any evidence of metastases or lymph node enlargement.

3.10.2 CLASSIFICATION

A working classification is given in Table 3.8 along with some pertinent clinical notes.

The aetiology of thyroid cancer remains unclear, but there are factors which may predispose to the condition.

1. Sex: overall the sex ratio is about equal, but papillary cancer is more common in females. As non-toxic goitre is much more frequent in females, it follows that in any male presenting with a single nodule there should be a strong index of suspicion for thyroid cancer.

2. Age: follicular cancer occurs in the middle-aged to elderly, as does anaplastic carcinoma and lymphoma. Other cancers

Table 3.8 Thyroid cancer

Histological type		Notes
Papillary	Good prognosis	Lymphatic spread to regional lymph nodes
Follicular	Fair prognosis	Haematogenous spread to bone and lung
Anaplastic	Fatal in one year	Widespread metastases
Medullary	From C cells	Secretes calcitonin
		Prognosis related to lymph node spread and distant metastases
		May be sporadic or inherited as in MENII
Lymphoma	Arises in Hashimoto gland	Usually radiosensitive
		May cause obstructive symptoms
Others	Secondary tumour, for example bronchus	

may occur in any age group. All single nodules in children must be regarded suspiciously.

3. Iodine status: there is evidence that papillary cancer is more common in areas of high iodine intake, as opposed to those areas which are iodine deficient.

3.10.3 RADIATION

Previous therapeutic external irradiation to the head and neck, especially in children, is associated with an increased risk of subsequent development of thyroid carcinoma. Cancer has occurred after intervals as long as 20–30 years. The risk of developing carcinoma is proportional to the radiation dose received.

3.10.4 CLINICAL FEATURES

Papillary cancer

This may present as a single nodule in the thyroid gland or as a lymph node metastasis in the neck. Diagnosis may be made by FNA cytology. Other diagnostic tests, such as thyroid scanning, are not helpful in the diagnostic process.

The disease may be multifocal, so optimal treatment is by total or near-total thyroidectomy. This may require a two-stage procedure if the initial lobectomy was not done specifically for cancer. T4 treatment sufficient to suppress TSH to undetectable levels should be instituted. Further metastases usually occur in the neck and can be removed surgically.

Following total thyroidectomy, serum thyroglobulin should be checked annually, and if found to be raised a thyroid scan may show the presence of metastases. Treatment is by surgical excision, ^{131}I administration or even external irradiation in some cases.

Follicular carcinoma

Although this usually presents as a single nodule in the neck, it may also present as a distant metastasis such as a pathological fracture. This tumour is more likely to be functional compared to other tumour types, and sometimes it even causes hyperthyroidism.

Following total thyroidectomy, any residual tumour is treated with a large dose of ^{131}I and the patient placed on suppressive T4 therapy. Subsequent metastases are easily located by the fact that they will take up ^{131}I on scanning. Treatment is with high dose ^{131}I.

Anaplastic carcinoma

This undifferentiated tumour spreads rapidly, particularly to bone and lung. Mortality is virtually 100% at one year.

Medullary carcinoma

This accounts for 10% of thyroid cancers. It occurs as a sporadic event (80%) and also as part of the familial multiple endocrine neoplasia type 2 (MEN2) syndrome (see Chapter 8). A non-MEN familial variety has also been described. Sporadic disease occurs at any age and presents as a non-toxic goitre. Metastatic spread may be local or distant.

These tumours tend to be more aggressive than those of MEN, but prognosis is 85% at 5 years if no nodes are involved. Treatment is by total thyroidectomy. The tumour is not radiosensitive. A careful family history should be obtained to exclude any suggestion of hereditary tumour, and the histology should be expertly reviewed.

The MEN2a syndrome comprises medullary carcinoma of the thyroid, hyperparathyroidism and phaeochromocytoma (often bilateral). The thyroid tumours are preceded by evidence of C cell hyperplasia (not seen in the sporadic form) and they are bilateral).

MEN2b consists of these features (except hyperparathyroidism) as well as cutaneous and tongue neuromas and other skeletal deformities.

Investigation includes the measurement of calcitonin and localization of the thyroid tumour with appropriate scanning techniques, if necessary. Calcitonin may be raised in other malignant diseases, for example breast, lung and kidney cancers. Phaeochromocytoma must be excluded by measurement of urinary metanephrines prior to surgery.

As MEN is inherited in an autosomal dominant manner, screening of relatives of an index case, especially children, is of vital importance (see Chapter 8). Follow-up of patients treated for medullary cancer must include regular measurements of calcitonin to detect metastases, together with scanning and radiographic examination, as necessary. Carcino-embryogenic antigen (CEA) levels are also raised in metastatic disease.

REFERENCES

1. Parmentier, M., Libert, F., Maenhaut, C., LeFort, A., Gerard, C., Perret, J., van Sande, J., Dumont, J.E. and Vassart, G. (1989) Molecular cloning of the thyrotrophin receptor. *Science*, **26**, 1620–2.
2. Sap, J., Munoz, A., Damm, K., Goldberg, Y., Ghysdael, J., Leutz, A., Beug, H. and Vennstrom, B. (1986) The c-erb A protein in a high affinity receptor for thyroid hormone. *Nature*, **32**, 635–40.
3. Klee, G.G. and Hay, I.D. (1987) Assessment of sensitive thyrotrophin assays for an expanded role in thyroid function testing: proposed criteria for analytic performance and clinical utility. *J. Clin. Endocrinol. Metab.*, **6**, 61–71.
4. Chopra, I.J. (1983) Thyroid function in non-thyroidal illnesses. *Ann. Intern. Med.*, **98**, 946–57.
5. Davies, A.B., Williams, I., John, R., Hall, R. and Scanlon, M.F. (1985) Diagnostic value of thyrotropin releasing hormone tests in elderly patients with atrial fibrillation. *Br. Med. J.*, **291**, 773–6.
6. Kennedy, R.L., Griffiths, H. and Gray, T.A. (1989) Amiodarone and the thyroid. *Clin. Chem.*, **35**, 1882–7.
7. John, R., Henley, R. and Shankland, D. (1990) Concentrations of free thyroxine and free triiodothyronine in patients with thyroxine- and triiodothyronine-binding autoantibodies. *Clin. Chem.*, **36**, 170–3.
8. Volpe, R. (1989) Autoimmune thyroiditis. In *Thyroid Function and Disease* (ed. G.N. Burrow, J.H. Oppenheimer and R. Volpe), W.B. Saunders, Philadelphia, pp. 191–207.
9. Marshall, N.J. and Ealey, P.A. (1986) Recent developments in the *in vitro* bioassay of TSH and thyroid stimulating antibodies. In *Immunology of Endocrine Diseases* (ed. A.M. McGregor), MTP Press, Lancaster, pp. 25–49.
10. Drexhage, H.A., Bottazo, G.F., Doniach, D. *et al.* (1980) Evidence for thyroid growth stimulating immunoglobulins in some goitrous thyroid diseases. *Lancet*, **ii**, 287–92.
11. Sandler, M.P., Patton, J.A. and McCook, B.M. (1989) Multimodality imaging of the thyroid gland. In *Imaging Endocrine Disorders. Bailliere's Clinical Endocrinology and Metabolism*, Vol. 3 (ed. F.L. Chan and C. Wang), Bailliere Tindall, London, pp. 89–119.
12. Gaitan, E. (1988) Goitrogens in hyperthyroidism and goitre. In *Bailliere's Clinical Endocrinology and Metabolism*, Vol. 2 (ed. J.H. Lazarus and R. Hall), Bailliere Tindall, London, pp. 783–802.
13. McKenzie, J.M. and Zakarija, M. (1989) The clinical use of thyrotropin receptor antibody measurements. *J. Clin. Endocrinol.*, **69**, 1093–6.
14. Hetzel, B.S. (1989) *The Story of Iodine Deficiency: An International Challenge in Nutrition.* Oxford University Press, Oxford, pp. 236ff.
15. Robbins, J. (1986) Thyroid cancer. In *The Thyroid Gland* (ed. L. van Middlesworth), Year Book Medical Publishers, Chicago, pp. 405–28.

4

Cushing's syndrome: Diagnosis and differential diagnosis

P.J. TRAINER and L.H. REES

4.1 INTRODUCTION

The diagnosis of Cushing's syndrome is dependent on the clinical and biochemical evidence of prolonged inappropriate hypercortisolaemia. The signs and symptoms are well known to clinicians (Fig. 4.1).

On initial examination, bruising, muscle weakness and hypertension have the greatest discriminatory value in the diagnosis of Cushing's syndrome [1].

4.2 PHYSIOLOGY

Plasma cortisol secretion has a free-running circadian rhythm of 25 hours, which is adapted to the normal 24-hour sleep–wake cycle. Peak plasma levels occur between 5 a.m and 9 a.m. and the nadir is around midnight, when cortisol should be undetectable. In Cushing's syndrome this pattern is lost such that, although the morning cortisol may be normal, the nocturnal levels are raised.

Superimposed on the circadian rhythm are additional pulses of cortisol secretion in response to exercise, food or stress. Cortisol secretion is regulated by pituitary adrenocorticotropic hormone (ACTH), which in

turn is controlled principally by the hypothalamic peptides corticotropin-releasing-hormone (CRH) and vasopressin. The integrity of the hypothalamo-pituitary-adrenal axis is maintained by the negative feedback of cortisol on its own secretion (Fig. 4.2), a process which operates both at hypothalamic and pituitary levels.

Psychological stress, inflammation, infection and pain, principally acting via catecholamine and opiate neurotransmitter pathways, stimulate CRH release. Evidence is now accumulating that cytokines can act directly on the hypothalamus to stimulate CRH secretion; this may be a particularly important mechanism in the well documented cortisol response to inflammation.

Ninety per cent of plasma cortisol is protein bound, the majority (70%) to the cortisol binding globulin (CBG) and the remainder to albumin (20%). States of high circulating oestrogen levels, either exogenous or during pregnancy, increase plasma CBG levels, while liver disease can result in reduced synthesis. Conventional plasma cortisol assays are for total cortisol, therefore variations in CBG will affect measured cortisol [2], hence the potential for spuriously high values, resulting in inappropriate investi-

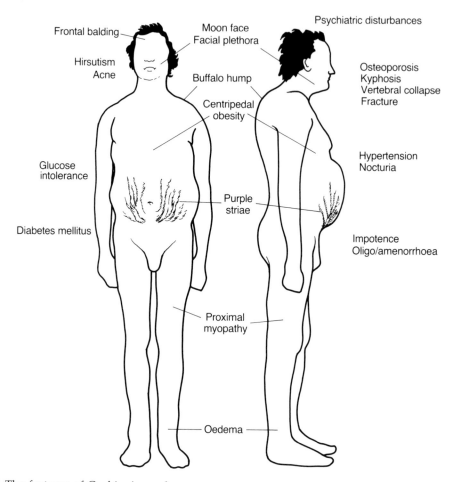

Fig. 4.1 The features of Cushing's syndrome.

gation. Only the 10% of plasma cortisol that is free is physiologically active.

4.3 DIAGNOSIS

The investigation of suspected Cushing's syndrome can be divided essentially into two stages: confirmation of the diagnosis, and establishment of the precise aetiology (Table 4.1).

The biochemical diagnosis relies upon the demonstration of abnormal regulation of the hypothalamo-pituitary-adrenal axis and excess cortisol secretion.

4.3.1 URINARY STEROIDS

The original urinary steroid assay was for 17-oxosteroids, which are principally androgen derived, and was therefore superseded by 17-hydroxycorticosteroids (17-OHCS, Porter–Silber urinary chromogens) which are a measure of the cortisol and cortisone metabolites tetrahydrocortisol (THF) and tetrahydrocor-

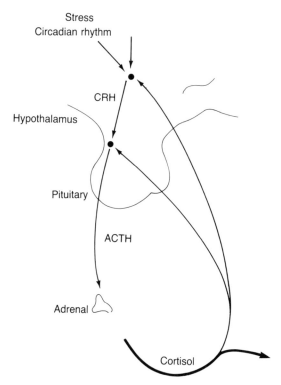

Stress
Circadian rhythm

CRH

Hypothalamus

Pituitary

ACTH

Adrenal

Cortisol

Fig. 4.2 The regulation of cortisol secretion by the hypothalamo-pituitary axis.

Table 4.1 The aetiology of Cushing's syndrome, showing the frequency of non-iatrogenic Cushing's syndrome (based on 210 patients seen at St Bartholomew's Hospital, London)

ACTH dependent	*84%*
1. Pituitary (Cushing's disease)	79%
2. Ectopic	14%
3. ACTH uncertain source	6%
4. Adrenal nodular hyperplasia (partially ACTH-dependent)	1%
5. Ectopic CRH or related peptides	Very rare
Non-ACTH dependent	*16%*
1. Adrenal adenoma	58%
2. Adrenal carcinoma	42%
Iatrogenic	
1. Glucocorticoid therapy	
2. ACTH therapy	
Pseudo-Cushing's	
1. Alcohol	
2. Depression	

tisone (THE). The measurement of urinary 17-ketogenic steroids which include cortisols and cortolones enabled greater diagnostic sensitivity, but at the expense of specificity.

Urine sampling has the disadvantage of relying on a complete and uncontaminated collection; this is a major drawback in the use of urinary cortisol assays in the diagnosis of Cushing's syndrome.

4.3.2 URINARY FREE CORTISOL

Twenty-four hour urinary free cortisol (UFC) collection produces an integrated measure of serum cortisol, 'smoothing out' the variation in plasma cortisol during the day. Radio-immunoassay (RIA) for plasma cortisol measures the total rather than the free portion; this makes interpretation difficult, particularly in conditions of abnormal CBG levels, such as pregnancy. UFC measurement circumvents this problem. Using UFC to screen for Cushing's syndrome, a false negative rate of 5.6% has been reported, with false positive results in 1% of non-obese individuals and 5% of the obese [3]. In a series of 146 patients with Cushing's syndrome, 11% have been reported to have had at least one out of four false negative 24-hour UFC collections [4].

UFC has superseded all other urinary steroid assays in the investigation of Cushing's syndrome. It can be performed on an out-patient basis [5,6], although at least three 24-hour collections are recommended. The normal range for a 24-hour UFC is 55–250 µmol.

4.3.3 CORTISOL PRODUCTION RATES

The rate of cortisol secretion can be measured by intravenous administration of a known dose of tritiated cortisol and subsequent urine collection for 24 hours. The urinary cortisol metabolites, such as THF and THE, are quantified and from the ratio of labelled to unlabelled metabolites and with a knowledge of the labelled dose of cortisol administered, the cortisol production rate can be calculated. When correctly performed, this is the 'gold standard' for quantitative assessment of cortisol production [7]. (The normal range for 24-hour isotopic cortisol production rate is 23–84 μmol.) However, it is expensive and time-consuming to perform, and is therefore a research tool rather than a routine diagnostic aid.

4.3.4 PLASMA CORTISOL

The first reliable means of measuring plasma glucocorticoids (cortisol and cortisone) was the 17-OHCS assay [8]. Fluorometric assays measure cortisol and corticosterone but not the tetrahydro metabolites of steroids [9]. Interference from cholesterol and various drugs such as spironolactone makes steroid measurement by fluorometry unreliable at lower levels, so this technique has been superseded by specific RIAs for plasma cortisol and other steroids.

Whereas measurement of a 9 a.m. serum cortisol alone is of little value in the investigation of suspected Cushing's syndrome (as it can fall within the normal range (200–700 nmol l^{-1}) and an elevated cortisol may be an appropriate stress response), demonstration of loss of circadian rhythm is of value.

4.3.5 CIRCADIAN RHYTHM

Procedure

Assessment of circadian rhythm is the most difficult test of the hypothalamo-pituitary-adrenal axis to perform, and requires hospitalization. Blood is taken for ACTH and cortisol at 9 a.m., 6 p.m. and midnight.

Interpretation

Non-endocrine illness, such as heart failure or infection, causes an entirely appropriate increase in cortisol production and consequent loss of the normal circadian rhythm. The manner in which the circadian rhythm is assessed is crucial if meaningful results are to be obtained; stress accompanying the anticipation of venepuncture, unfamiliar surroundings or intercurrent illness can result in elevated levels, especially at night. The patient must have been hospitalized for a least 48 hours and be asleep prior to midnight blood taking. Circadian rhythm is lost in depression and alcoholism, and is therefore of limited use as a diagnostic procedure, but rather a confirmatory test when the diagnosis is strongly suspected.

Once excessive cortisol production has been established, the next step is to demonstrate an abnormal regulation of the hypothalamo-pituitary-adrenal axis.

4.3.6 LOW DOSE DEXAMETHASONE SUPPRESSION TEST

Dexamethasone should not cross-react with a good cortisol assay. Although originally applied to the investigation of suppressibility of urinary 17-OHCS [10], the low dose dexamethasone suppression (LDDS) test is currently performed in conjunction with serum cortisol measurement. Results show total concordance with UFC estimation in the diagnosis of Cushing's syndrome, and the test is much easier to perform [11,12].

Procedure

There are several versions of the LDDS test and all can be performed on an out-patient basis, requiring 9 a.m. venepuncture before and after dexamethasone administration. In normal individuals, RIA-measured serum cortisol post-dexamethasone should be undetectable.

The overnight dexamethasone suppression test has been described using different doses, each administered orally at midnight with measurement of serum cortisol 8 hours later. The classical 48-hour Liddle test involves administration of 0.5 mg of dexamethasone at precise 6-hour intervals, starting at 9 a.m. on day 1, for eight doses and measuring serum cortisol at 9 a.m. on day 3, exactly 6 hours after the last dose of dexamethasone.

Interpretation

The 48-hour test has been reported to have a true positive rate of 97%–100% [11,12]. In contrast, the overnight dexamethasone suppression test using either 1.5 mg or 2 mg has shown a 30% false positive rate [13]. Cronin and colleagues [14] have reported a false positive rate of 12.5% (i.e. specificity of 87.5%) using 1 mg at midnight, and a false negative rate of 2% (i.e. sensitivity of 98%). As the absorption of dexamethasone is shown to be variable [15], in the case of the overnight test it has been advocated that dexamethasone should also be measured to ensure an adequate plasma dexamethasone level [16]. However, this is expensive and requires availability of a dexamethasone assay. Under normal conditions and when properly performed, inadequate plasma dexamethasone levels do not present a problem during the 48-hour test. If the overnight test is positive, it is illogical to perform a 48-hour test afterwards.

Effect of enzyme-inducing drugs

Phenytoin, rifampicin, phenobarbitone and other drugs inducing liver enzymes increase the clearance rate of dexamethasone, with consequent low plasma levels. This may result in false positives (i.e. failure of cortisol suppression). It has been claimed that the rate of cortisol clearance is little affected by phenytoin, and therefore hydrocortisone can be used in place of dexamethasone. This is performed by oral administration of 50 mg of hydrocortisone at midnight and measurement of serum corticosterone at 8 a.m. [17]. We have no experience of this test, and it is based on a dubious premise: it requires access to a corticosterone assay and is only indicated when a patient receiving relevant drug therapy has an unexpectedly positive result.

4.3.7 INSULIN TOLERANCE TEST

Procedure

Due to insulin resistance of Cushing's syndrome, hypoglycaemia is induced by administering intravenously $0.3\,u\,kg^{-1}$ of short acting insulin, and sampling for cortisol and blood sugar at 0, 30, 45, 60, 90 and 120 minutes. For an adequate stimulus to be delivered, blood sugar must fall below $2.2\,mmol\,l^{-1}$ with accompanying symptoms of neuroglycopaenia, including sweating and palpitations. Hypothyroidism, hypoadrenalism, and a history of epilepsy or cardiac disease are all contraindications to this test. It must be ensured that patients remain conscious and able to answer simple questions throughout the test, and 50 ml of 50% dextrose must be available for treatment of hypoglycaemia in an emergency. If the patient does lose consciousness, dexamethasone in preference to hydrocortisone should be administered, as that allows continuation of measurement of serum cortisol.

Interpretation

The cortisol response to hypoglycaemia is lost in Cushing's syndrome due to the disturbed dynamics of the hypothalamo-pituitary-adrenal axis [18]. However, patients suffering from depression retain their cortisol response to hypoglycaemia, and this is the most useful parameter in distinguishing between the two conditions [19].

As 18% of patients with Cushing's syndrome do not have a cortisol response to hypoglycaemia, this limits the value of hypoglycaemia as a diagnostic feature [3]. It is, however, of confirmatory value in certain cases, especially where depression is suspected.

4.4 CONDITIONS MIMICKING CUSHING'S SYNDROME

4.4.1 DEPRESSION

Depression is a common symptom of Cushing's syndrome and also part of the differential diagnosis [20]. Butler and Besser reported loss of circadian rhythm, elevated plasma cortisol and urinary 17-oxogenic corticosteroids in association with a failure of suppression of plasma cortisol during the 48-hour dexamethasone suppression test in patients with severe depression [21].

However, in depression, the cortisol response to hypoglycaemia is intact and this may be of value in clinical differentiation. Occasionally, it can be very difficult to distinguish between the two conditions, and Cushing's syndrome may be excluded only after the depression has been treated.

4.4.2 OBESITY

Obesity may be associated with diabetes mellitus and hypertension, and Cushing's syndrome often needs to be excluded. On clinical examination, centripetal distribution of fat, pigmentation of striae and proximal myopathy support Cushing's syndrome; the 'buffalo hump' is common to both disorders.

Increased cortisol production has been documented in obesity, although when corrected for excretion it is normal [22], measured by the radiolabel dilution technique. The UFC and plasma cortisol response to dexamethasone suppression are normal [6]. A recent study involving our department demonstrated the cortisol response to CRH to be slightly subnormal in obese individuals and exaggerated in Cushing's syndrome, allowing discrimination between the two conditions [23].

4.4.3 ALCOHOLISM

Alcoholism can produce a clinical and biochemical picture indistinguishable from Cushing's syndrome. It has been shown that urinary 17-OHCS, 17-oxosteroid levels as well as plasma cortisol may be elevated and fail to suppress with dexamethasone [24]. Normal or undetectable plasma ACTH has been recorded. The underlying pathogenesis of alcoholic pseudo-Cushing's is ill-understood, but the biochemical abnormalities revert to normal on cessation of alcohol consumption, sometimes within days (typically on admission to hospital). A high YGT and raised MCV should suggest the diagnosis. Measurement of alcohol levels is occasionally warranted.

4.4.4 CYCLICAL CUSHING'S SYNDROME

A further potential diagnostic pitfall is the cyclical activity of the disease exhibited in some patients, with periods of spontaneous remission when all investigations are normal, lasting days or even years [25,26].

Conclusion

No single test has adequate sensitivity and specificity to allow its use in isolation when investigating a patient with suspected Cushing's syndrome. This is especially true

Table 4.2 Recommendations for the investigation of a patient with suspected Cushing's syndrome

First line: out-patient
1. 24-hour UFC collections ×3
2. Low dose dexamethasone test

Second line: in-patient
1. Circadian rhythms ×2
2. Insulin tolerance test

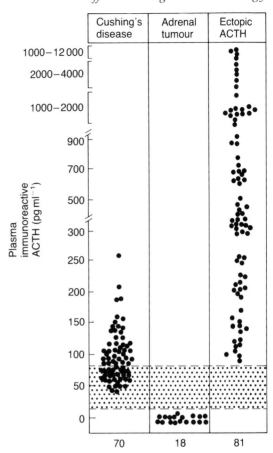

Fig. 4.3 9 a.m. plasma immunoreactive ACTH in 169 consecutive patients with Cushing's syndrome. (Reproduced by kind permission of Churchill-Livingstone).

when Cushing's needs to be differentiated from one of the conditions mentioned above. A strategy to screen patients for possible Cushing's syndrome would be to perform three 24-hour UFC collections plus a 48-hour LDDS test measuring plasma cortisol. If the results are suggestive of Cushing's syndrome, an insulin tolerance test and cortisol circadian rhythms should be performed to confirm the diagnosis, before proceeding to establishing the precise aetiology (Table 4.2).

4.5 DIFFERENTIAL DIAGNOSIS AND AETIOLOGY

The precise aetiology of Cushing's syndrome should be investigated once the diagnosis is confirmed, and the first step is to establish whether it is ACTH-dependent or not. In our experience, all patients with adrenal tumours have undetectable plasma ACTH levels. Adrenal computerized tomography (CT) will rapidly confirm the diagnosis of a cortisol secreting adrenal adenoma (Fig. 4.3).

The major difficulty in clinical practice is distinguishing between a pituitary and an ectopic source of ACTH secretion, a problem necessitating the use of combined biochemical and radiological techniques. No single investigation is infallible, hence diagnosis usually relies on the accumulated results of several investigations.

Cushing's disease is three to four times more common in women than men, while, due to the greater incidence of small cell carcinoma of the lung, ectopic ACTH secretion is more frequently seen in men. Therefore if a man has ACTH-dependent Cushing's syndrome it is relatively less likely to be due to Cushing's disease.

4.5.1 ECTOPIC ACTH SYNDROME

The classical ectopic ACTH syndrome [27] may be clinically distinguishable from

73

Table 4.3 The features of the ectopic ACTH syndrome

Short history
Weight loss
Severe myopathy
Pigmentation
Hypokalaemic alkalosis
Very high plasma ACTH
Overt neoplasm, usually small cell lung carcinoma

Cushing's disease by a short history, weight loss, severe myopathy, pigmentation and hypokalaemia, and is associated with overt neoplasms and very high ACTH levels (Table 4.3).

However, the small 'occult' ectopic ACTH-secreting tumours may present with a clinical picture identical to that of Cushing's disease, making a biochemical distinction very difficult. On occasion, although the biochemical evidence indicates ectopic ACTH secretion, it may not be possible to identify a tumour.

4.5.2 ACTH DETERMINATION

ACTH is of limited value in differentiating pituitary from ectopic ACTH secretion, as there is a large overlap and it may well be in the normal range [28]. However, very high levels of ACTH are usually indicative of ectopic production and may be associated with hyperpigmentation. ACTH secreted from the pituitary is normally a 39-residue peptide derived from the precursor pro-opiomelanocortin (POMC) (Fig. 4.4).

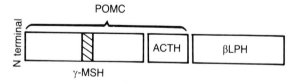

Fig. 4.4 The ACTH precursor molecule pro-opiomelanocortin (POMC).

Abnormal processing of POMC due to incomplete glycosylation can result in secretion of various ACTH precursors ('big ACTH'). RIAs for ACTH can fail to detect this, resulting in apparently inappropriately low levels when compared to cortisol.

Chromatography has been used to characterize abnormal forms of ACTH [29,30]; more recently, the development of immuno-radiometric assays (IRMA) with monoclonal antibodies for the various precursors of ACTH has simplified their identification and quantification [31]. However, commercial IRMAs, in which both antibodies are to the N-terminal 1-39 amino acids of the ACTH molecule, may fail to detect aberrant large forms of ACTH, resulting in the reporting of misleadingly low levels [32]. Detection of 'big ACTH' in plasma is usually indicative of ectopic secretion, although rarely it can be pituitary in origin [33].

4.5.3 SERUM POTASSIUM

Plasma potassium is low in 72%–100% of patients with ectopic ACTH secretion and in only 10% of patients with Cushing's disease [34,35]. Great care must be taken in the handling of specimens to avoid haemolysis and consequent spuriously high values. Blood must be drawn with care, promptly spun and separated. Potassium should be interpreted in conjunction with the bicarbonate, which is not affected by haemolysis, and should be high in the presence of hypokalaemia. The discriminatory power of potassium is lost in patients on diuretics, in which case the primary physician should be contacted to enquire about the availability of a prediuretic potassium estimation.

4.5.4 GLUCOSE INTOLERANCE

Glucose intolerance and diabetes mellitus are more common with ectopic ACTH.

4.5.5 HIGH DOSE DEXAMETHASONE SUPPRESSION TESTS

Historically, this has been the principal test in differentiating between the various causes of Cushing's syndrome [10].

Procedure

The test is performed in an identical manner to the 48-hour LDDS, except that a dose of 2 mg of dexamethasone is administered instead of 0.5 mg. The original method of measuring urinary 17-hydrocorticoids has been superseded by the availability of plasma cortisol assays.

Interpretation

In Cushing's disease, a fall in plasma cortisol of greater than 50% is expected, which is in contrast to adrenal tumours or ectopic ACTH secretion where suppression is generally absent. Published data indicate that approximately 90% of patients with Cushing's disease show the expected suppression of plasma cortisol. A similar suppression is seen in approximately 10% of patients with the ectopic ACTH syndrome [3,36,37].

4.5.6 INTRAVENOUS DEXAMETHASONE SUPPRESSION TEST

Failure of suppression of plasma cortisol during an HDDS can occur due to inadequate plasma levels because of non-compliance, malabsorption or increased liver metabolism. To circumvent this potential problem, the intravenous approach has been advocated.

Procedure

The test entails a 5-hour infusion of dexamethasone at a rate of 1 mg per hour, and has the advantage that it can be performed on an out-patient basis.

Interpretation

The same criteria apply as for a high dose 48-hour dexamethasone suppression test. Suppression greater than 50% is indicative of Cushing's disease, and the intravenous approach is capable of differentiating Cushing's disease from an adrenal tumour [38]. It has recently been reported that, using the same infusion protocol, a fall of $>190 \, nmol \, l^{-1}$ was seen in all patients with Cushing's disease, compared with two out of seven with the ectopic ACTH syndrome [39].

The intravenous dexamethasone suppression test may be a useful and simple aid in differentiating pituitary from ectopic ACTH secretion, but further work and data are required to validate this view fully and to establish the value of the test.

4.5.7 METYRAPONE TEST

This was originally described to distinguish between adrenal tumour-induced Cushing's syndrome and Cushing's disease. The principal action of metyrapone is to block the final step in cortisol synthesis, i.e. the conversion of 11-deoxycortisol to cortisol, and thus stimulate ACTH secretion by negative feedback.

Procedure

As originally described [40], 750 mg of metyrapone are administered every 6 hours for 24 hours, although alternative regimens such as intravenous metyrapone have been used [41].

With the evolution of assays, it is now normal practice to measure plasma cortisol, 11-deoxycortisol and ACTH at 0, 1, 2, 3, 4 and 24 hours; 24-hour urinary 17-oxogenic steroid excretion is measured on the day before, the day of and the day after administration of metyrapone.

Interpretation

In response to metyrapone, plasma cortisol falls, confirming the blockade of synthesis; a doubling of plasma ACTH and urinary 17-oxogenic steroids is taken as evidence of Cushing's disease, and no change is seen with adrenal tumours. Although the test can distinguish between Cushing's and adrenal tumours, it is poor at differentiating between ectopic and pituitary ACTH secretion [36], which, in fact, is the greatest clinical challenge. Plasma ACTH and urinary 17-oxogenic steroids typically rise in response to metyrapone in patients with ectopic ACTH secretion.

The metyrapone test is complicated, involving three days of urine collection. It should be abandoned in favour of the CRH test, which can be conducted on an outpatient basis.

4.5.8 CRH TEST

This has become a powerful tool in the investigation of Cushing's syndrome.

Procedure

The test involves intravenous administration of 100 mcg and measurement of cortisol and ACTH every 15 minutes for 2 hours.

Interpretation

ACTH and cortisol are secreted in response to CRH in healthy subjects, while an exaggerated increment occurs in patients with Cushing's disease. In the ectopic ACTH syndrome, ACTH and cortisol fail to respond to CRH [42]. Obese individuals are reported to have a subnormal response [23].

The principal role of the test is in differentiating between pituitary and ectopic ACTH secretion once Cushing's syndrome has been established and adrenal adenoma excluded by an undetectable plasma ACTH. In reviewing published data, Hermus and colleagues [43] concluded that of 83 patients with Cushing's disease approximately 90% responded to CRH testing. Cortisol levels can fluctuate widely in patients with Cushing's syndrome [44], and an apparent response to CRH testing may be no more than spontaneous variation in ACTH and cortisol secretion. An ectopic ACTH 'responder' and macronodular adrenal hyperplasia (see below) are two causes of false positive CRH tests [43], and these possibilities must be considered in difficult cases. There is, however, only one well documented case of an ectopic ACTH secreting tumour responding to CRH [45].

4.5.9 CRH AND DEXAMETHASONE SUPPRESSION TESTS

The combination of these two tests has been shown to increase the accuracy of differentiation of ACTH-dependent Cushing's syndrome [37,46]. In Cushing's disease, approximately 90% of patients showed the expected response to an HDDS test alone, and approximately 80% responded to CRH stimulation; when both are performed, a 100% sensitivity is achieved. The 10% of patients with ectopic ACTH secretion who show suppression following dexamethasone and have an appropriately absent CRH response remain a diagnostic difficulty.

4.5.10 HUMAN VERSUS OVINE CRH

Nieman and colleagues [47] compared human CRH (hCRH) and ovine CRH (oCRH) in the differential diagnosis of Cushing's syndrome. They concluded that oCRH resulted in a greater cortisol response and was of more value in distinguishing ectopic ACTH from Cushing's disease. However, our own recent study reached rather different conclusions: it was confirmed that oCRH results in a greater peak plasma cortisol, but by establishing separate normal ranges in our laboratory for oCRH and hCRH we found hCRH to be more sensitive in diagnosing Cushing's syndrome [48]. Further larger studies are required to clarify the situation, although it seems likely that, for commercial reasons, hCRH will become the more widely available.

4.5.11 TUMOUR MARKERS

Ectopic ACTH secreting tumours may be very difficult to visualize radiologically, as in the occult ectopic ACTH syndrome [49]. It is also well recognized that they can secrete one or more additional peptides [34]. It is therefore advisable to screen all patients with ACTH-dependent Cushing's syndrome, in whom the diagnosis is not absolutely clear, for tumour markers. These include plasma carcinoembryonic antigen (CEA), somatostatin, gastrin, calcitonin, pancreatic polypeptide, vasoactive intestinal peptide (VIP), glucagon, and human chorionic gonadotropin (hCG-beta). Other peptides to consider are alpha-fetoprotein, alpha-subunit, growth hormone releasing hormone (GHRH) and CRH. The demonstration of additional ectopic peptide secretion is helpful in the differentiation of ACTH-dependent Cushing's syndrome as it is evidence of extrapituitary ACTH production, and it is also of value when performing whole body venous sampling in an attempt to localize a tumour. Subsequently, it can be used as a tumour marker to monitor the efficacy of treatment, whether by surgery, radiotherapy or chemotherapy.

4.5.12 CRH SECRETING TUMOURS

A rare diagnostic pitfall is pituitary ACTH-dependent Cushing's syndrome due to ectopic secretion from a non-pituitary tumour of a corticotropin-releasing factor [50].

Nephro-blastomas, bronchial carcinoids, medullary cell carcinomas of thyroid, pancreatic islet cell, phaeochromocytomas and pituitary carcinoma have all been documented to secrete CRH-41 [51–55], as has a hypothalamic metastasis of a prostatic carcinoma [56]. In 1985, Howlett and colleagues described a bombesin-like peptide secreted by a medullary cell carcinoma of thyroid as a cause of Cushing's syndrome [36]. The clinical and biochemical features are that of the ectopic ACTH syndrome.

4.5.13 NODULAR HYPERPLASIA

Adrenocortical macronodular hyperplasia is a rare cause of Cushing's syndrome, which, if not appreciated, can result in inappropriate transsphenoidal hypophysectomy. The underlying pathophysiology is poorly understood, but it is believed that patients initially have a pituitary ACTH-secreting adenoma and go on to develop autonomous adenomas within the hyperplastic adrenal glands, with subsequent regression of the pituitary adenoma [57].

Patients typically have adrenal nodules coexisting with varying degrees of bilateral adrenal hyperplasia, ACTH levels tend to be low and intermittently undetectable and there is a failure to show 50% suppression of serum cortisol during an HDDS test. An excessive response to CRH has been documented.

4.5.14 CARNEY'S SYNDROME

Carney's syndrome is an autosomal dominant condition characterized by mesenchymal tumours, particularly atrial myxomas, spotty skin pigmentation, endocrine disorders and peripheral nerve tumours. Cushing's syndrome can occur, with the pathological finding of normal or small adrenal glands with multiple, small, deeply pigmented adrenal nodules. The biochemical features are the same as in macronodular hyperplasia. Recent evidence suggests that the adreno-cortical hyperfunction is the result of ACTH-receptor autoantibodies [58].

4.5.15 IMAGING

Radiology plays an important role in the investigation of Cushing's syndrome, especially if ectopic ACTH secretion is suspected, as the tumours may be as small as 0.4 cm in diameter, and the biochemical evidence can be equivocal or misleading. Therefore, it the aetiology of the Cushing's syndrome is not readily identifiable, a systematic radiological search is required to localize the tumour, which may involve CT of the chest, abdomen and pituitary, in addition to venous sampling.

Pituitary imaging

The majority of ACTH-secreting pituitary adenomas are less than 1 cm in diameter and enhance in the same manner as normal pituitary tissue following intravenous contrast medium. Modern CT scanners are capable of producing high resolution images of the pituitary. However, care must be taken in the interpretation of possible micro-adenomas, as the pituitary can be hetero-geneous (the distribution of contrast within the gland may not be uniform) in normal individuals; the biochemical evidence must also be considered before making a diagnosis of Cushing's disease.

Following intravenous contrast medium, ACTH-secreting tumours enhance and may be indistinguishable from the normal pituitary, so that the gland appears normal. Moreover, as the pituitary is heterogeneous, in post-mortem studies pituitary micro-adenomas have been identified in 27% of specimens [59]. It cannot, therefore, be assumed that a microadenoma detected on a scan is secreting ACTH. Biochemical data must also be considered.

Comparison of the relative merits of pituitary CT and magnetic resonance imaging (MRI) is fraught with the difficulty of ensuring that scanners are 'state-of-the-art'. CT is reported as having a sensitivity of about 47% [60] in the detection of ACTH-secreting microadenomas, and, although with the best equipment this figure may be improved, MRI does seem to have an advantage: with a 1.5 T machine and gadolinium enhancement, it has been reported as having 71%–83% sensitivity [61,62].

Whole body imaging

Indication

CT scanning of the chest and abdomen is essential if any doubt exists as to the aetiology of ACTH-dependent Cushing's syndrome, or if an adrenal tumour is suspected, as identification of metastases clearly alters the management [49,63].

Interpretation

In view of the very small size of some ectopic ACTH-secreting tumours, when performing CT scans it is necessary to make 0.5-cm slices through the chest and abdomen. We have recently reported a 0.5-cm lung carcinoid tumour not identified by thicker, non-contiguous slices [64]. Adrenal tumours greater than 6 cm in diameter, corresponding to a weight of approximately 100 g, must be regarded as malignant.

Whole body venous sampling

Indication

In ACTH-dependent Cushing's syndrome, when either the diagnosis is uncertain or ectopic ACTH secretion is suspected, but no tumour has been identified by radiological imaging, or if an ambiguous abnormality has been demonstrated on CT, it is vital to undertake selective venous sampling for ACTH. Specimens for ACTH and any additional peptides that may have been identified on screening should be obtained in an attempt to localize the site of ACTH secretion [65].

Interpretation

Samples should be obtained from the jugular veins and other major vessels and their tributaries, paying particular attention to any areas of radiological abnormality, bearing in mind that a tumour may have anomalous venous drainage. Simultaneous peripheral samples are required to ensure that vari-

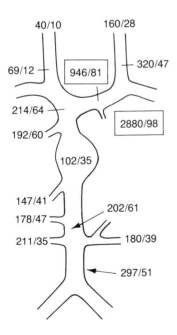

Fig. 4.5 A schematic representation of whole body venous sampling, demonstrating a mediastinal tumour secreting both ACTH (ng l^{-1}) and alpha-fetoprotein (µg ml^{-1}).

ations in plasma ACTH do not simply reflect the pulsatile nature of its secretion (Fig. 4.5).

Transseptal pulmonary venous sampling, in our experience, has failed to provide any useful information.

Meta-iodobenzyl guanidine scanning

Meta-iodobenzyl guanidine (MIBG) is an isotope principally used in the diagnosis and treatment of phaeochromocytoma, but is also taken up by a proportion of carcinoid tumours. Unfortunately, we have never found it to be of value in identifying an ectopic ACTH-secreting tumour.

Bronchoscopy

Doppman and colleagues [66] have failed to demonstrate any value in bronchial lavage and ACTH measurement in patients with suspected bronchial tumours.

Simultaneous bilateral inferior petrosal sinus sampling

Indication

Inferior petrosal sinus sampling is a powerful aid in differentiating the aetiology of ACTH-dependent Cushing's syndrome. It should be performed if doubt persists concerning the diagnosis after an HDDS test and a CRH stimulation test. It is also of value in pre-operative localization of an ACTH-secreting pituitary tumour within the fossa if trans-sphenoidal microadenomectomy is planned. Findling and colleagues [67] reported the value of unilateral inferior petrosal sinus sampling in differentiating pituitary from ectopic ACTH secretion, although subsequently Oldfield and colleagues [68] demonstrated that if samples were taken only from the petrosal sinus contralateral to a lateral tumour, a false negative result could be obtained.

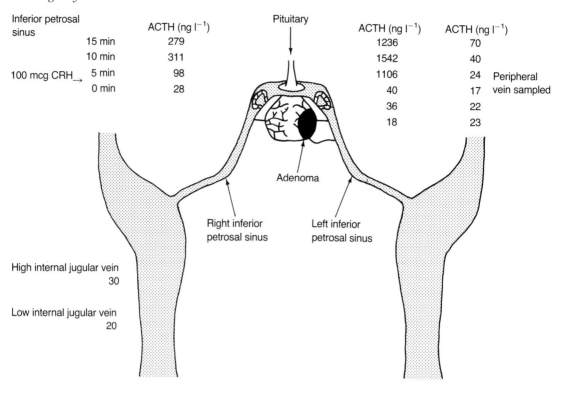

| Inferior petrosal sinus | | ACTH (ng l⁻¹) | Pituitary | ACTH (ng l⁻¹) | ACTH (ng l⁻¹) | |

Inferior petrosal sinus

	ACTH (ng l⁻¹)
15 min	279
10 min	311
100 mcg CRH → 5 min	98
0 min	28

Pituitary

ACTH (ng l⁻¹)	ACTH (ng l⁻¹)	
1236	70	
1542	40	
1106	24	Peripheral
40	17	vein sampled
36	22	
18	23	

Adenoma

Right inferior petrosal sinus

Left inferior petrosal sinus

High internal jugular vein 30

Low internal jugular vein 20

Fig. 4.6 A schematic representation of simultaneous bilateral inferior petrosal sinus sampling with CRH (100 mcg), confirming the diagnosis of Cushing's disease due to a left-sided adenoma.

Technique

The technique of simultaneous bilateral inferior petrosal sinus sampling is still evolving. It is currently our practice to introduce two catheters into the right femoral vein using the Seldinger technique and, under radiological control, guide them into the inferior petrosal sinuses. Plasma samples for ACTH are obtained simultaneously from the right and left catheters as well as a peripheral vein. In this way, samples are obtained from the low and high internal jugular vein, inferior petrosal sinus and peripheral vein, before CRH (100 mcg) is administered via the peripheral cannula (Fig. 4.6).

Interpretation

The ACTH gradient between the petrosal sinuses and peripheral vein samples, which can be taken as indicative of Cushing's disease, has been variously reported at between 1.4 and ⩾1.5 [68–71]. However, we have seen spontaneous variation between the highest and lowest value of three peripheral vein samples of up to 1.8 (mean 1.3). Tabarin and colleagues [72] have documented a peripheral to petrosal ratio of 1.7 in a case of ectopic ACTH secretion, and we believe that a ratio of >2 is necessary to diagnose Cushing's disease with confidence.

The measurement of other peptides in addition to ACTH has increased the efficacy of inferior petrosal sinus sampling, particularly prolactin [70,73,74]. Vasopressin secretion has been shown to lateralize to the site of ACTH-secreting tumours, which is of interest in understanding the aetiology of Cushing's disease [75]. However, its diagnostic value has yet to be assessed, particularly the vasopressin response to CRH during catheterization.

Lateralization of tumour

The value of inferior petrosal sinus sampling in the lateralization of ACTH-secreting tumours is complicated by the fact that tumours may be midline or have anomalous venous drainage. Furthermore, although the patient may be cured by surgery, the surgeon may fail to identify the tumour, or the specimen may have been lost in the process of removal. For these reasons, surgery may fail to confirm the findings. Oldfield and colleagues [68] reported accurate lateralization in all ten of their patients with micro-adenomas, assuming a gradient between the petrosal sinuses of >1.4 as significant. In our series, taking a gradient of >2 as significant and using CRH stimulation, localization of the adenoma within the fossa was confirmed at surgery in 66% of patients [76].

Indeterminate ACTH source

Despite extensive biochemical and radiological investigations, in approximately 5% of patients with ACTH-dependent Cushing's

syndrome it is not possible to decide if the ACTH is of pituitary origin, or to identify a tumour if it is believed to be extrapituitary in origin. In these circumstances, the hypercortisolaemia is treated by inhibiting adrenal cortisol synthesis with drugs such as metyrapone, *o,p'*DDD and ketoconazole. The patient may then be maintained in a eucorticoid state, and after an interval the relevant investigations can be repeated. When hypercortisolaemia is cyclical, it may be necessary to wait until there is evidence of hypersecretion before performing detailed biochemical investigation.

4.6 RECOMMENDATIONS

The diagnosis of Cushing's syndrome should be based on clinical suspicion, elevated UFC and suppression of cortisol following an

Table 4.4 Recommendations for the investigation of a patient with proven Cushing's syndrome. The choice of second line investigations must depend on the outcome of the first line tests

First line
Serum potassium
Glucose tolerance test
Plasma ACTH
PA and lateral chest X-ray
Skull X-ray
CRH test
High dose dexamethasone suppression test

Second line
CT or MRI of pituitary
Whole body CT scan
Whole body venous sampling
Simultaneous bilateral inferior petrosal sinus
  sampling

Third line
Treat medically and repeat appropriate
  investigations after an interval

LDDS. The loss of circadian rhythm and the cortisol response to hypoglycaemia are confirmatory investigations.

The measurement of plasma ACTH and a CT scan of the adrenals allow the diagnosis of an adrenal tumour with confidence.

The major challenge is in the differential diagnosis of ACTH-dependent Cushing's syndrome. Hypokalaemia and glucose intolerance are suggestive of ectopic ACTH secretion. The combination of HDDS and CRH tests allows an accurate diagnosis of Cushing's disease in 90% of patients. The metyrapone test, which is complicated and expensive to perform, adds nothing to the information available from the combined HDDS test and CRH test, and should be abandoned. CT scans, or MRI if available, of the pituitary, chest and abdomen may identify a tumour in cases where the biochemistry has failed to distinguish the source of ACTH secretion. In confusing cases, whole body venous sampling and inferior petrosal sinus with CRH stimulation should be undertaken, in order to confirm the diagnosis of Cushing's disease or to identify an occult extrapituitary tumour (Table 4.4).

Despite the most thorough and exhaustive series of investigations, it may still prove impossible to establish a precise diagnosis. In that case the hypercortisolaemia should be controlled with appropriate drugs and the investigations repeated in due course.

REFERENCES

1. Ross, E.J. and Lynch, D.C. (1982) Cushing's syndrome-killing disease; discriminatory value of signs and symptoms aiding early diagnosis. *Lancet*, **ii**, 646–9.
2. Brien, T.G. (1981) Human corticosteroid binding globulin. *Clin. Endocrinol.*, **14**, 193–212.
3. Crapo, L. (1979) Cushing's syndrome: a review of diagnostic tests. *Metabolism*, **28**, 955–77.
4. Nieman, L.K. and Cutler, G.B. (1990) The sensitivity of the urine free cortisol measurement as a screening test for Cushing's syndrome. In *72nd Annual Meeting of the Endocrine Society*, Atlanta, Georgia. Abstract 822.
5. Burke, C.W. and Beardswell, G.G. (1973) Cushing's syndrome. *Q. J. Med.*, **42**, 175–204.
6. Eddy, R.L., Jones, A.L., Gilliland, P.F., Ibarra, Jr, J.D., Thompson, J.Q. and McMurry, J.F. (1973) Cushing's syndrome: a prospective study of diagnostic methods. *Am. J. Med.*, **55**, 621–30.
7. Cope, C.L. and Black, E. (1958) The production rate of cortisol in man. *Br. Med. J.*, **i**, 1020–4.
8. Nelson, D.H. and Samuels, L.T. (1952) A method for the determination of 17-hydroxycorticosteroids in blood: 17-hydroxycorticosterone in the peripheral circulation. *J. Clin. Endocrinol. Metab.*, **12**, 519–26.
9. Mattingly, D. (1962) A simple fluorometric method for the estimation of free 11-hydroxycorticoids in human plasma. *J. Clin. Path.*, **15**, 374–9.
10. Liddle, G.W. (1960) Tests of pituitary-adrenal suppressibility in the diagnosis of Cushing's syndrome. *J. Clin. Endocrinol. Metab.*, **20**, 1539–60.
11. Kennedy, L., Atkinson, A.B., Johnston, H., Sheridan, B. and Hadden, D.R. (1984) Serum cortisol concentration during low dose dexamethasone suppression test to screen for Cushing's syndrome. *Br. Med. J.*, **289**, 1188–91.
12. Hankin, M.E., Theile, H.M. and Steinbeck, A.W. (1977) An evaluation of laboratory tests for the detection and differential diagnosis of Cushing's syndrome. *Clin. Endocrinol.*, **6**, 185–96.
13. Connolly, C.K., Gore, M.B.R., Stanley, N. and Wills, M.R. (1968) Single-dose dexamethasone in normal subjects and hospital patients. *Br. Med. J.*, **1**, 1020–4.
14. Cronin, C., Igoe, D., Duffy, M.J., Cunningham, S.K. and McKenna, T.J. (1990) The overnight dexamethasone test is a worthwhile screening procedure. *Clin. Endocrinol.*, **33**, 27–33.
15. Meikle, A.W., Lagerquist, L.G. and Tyler, F.H. (1975) Apparently normal pituitary-adrenal

suppressibility in Cushing's syndrome: dexamethasone metabolism and plasma levels. *J. Lab. Clin. Med.*, **86**, 472–8.

16. Meikle, A.W. (1982) Dexamethasone suppression tests: usefulness of simultaneous measurement of plasma cortisol and dexamethasone. *Clin. Endocrinol.*, **16**, 401–8.

17. Meikle, A.W., Stanchfield, J.B., West, C.D. and Tyler, F.H. (1974) Hydrocortisone suppression test for Cushing's syndrome: therapy with anticonvulsants. *Archs Intern. Med.*, **134**, 1068–71.

18. James, V.H.T., Landon, J., Wynn, V. and Greenwood, F.C. (1968) A fundamental defect of adrenocortical control in Cushing's disease. *J. Endocrinol.*, **40**, 15–28.

19. Besser, G.M. and Edwards, C.R.W. (1972) Cushing's syndrome. *Clin. Endocrinol. Metab.*, **1**, 451–90.

20. Jeffcoate, W.J., Silverstone, J.T., Edwards, C.R.W. and Besser, G.M. (1979) Psychiatric manifestations of Cushing's syndrome: response to initial lowering of plasma cortisol. *Q. J. Med.*, **48**, 465–72.

21. Butler, P.W.P. and Besser, G.M. (1968) Pituitary-adrenal function in severe depressive illness. *Lancet*, **i**, 1234–6.

22. Strain, G.W, Zumoff, B., Strain, J.J., Levin, J. and Fukushima, D.K. (1980) Cortisol production in obesity. *Metabolism*, **29**, 980–5.

23. Kopelman, P.G., Grossman, A., Lavender, P., Besser, G.M., Rees, L.H. and Coy, D. (1988) The cortisol response to corticotrophin-releasing factor is blunted in obesity. *Clin. Endocrinol.*, **28**, 15–18.

24. Rees, L.H., Besser, G.M., Jeffcoate, W.J., Goldie, D.J. and Marks, V. (1977) Alcohol-induced pseudo-Cushing's syndrome. *Lancet*, **i**, 726–8.

25. Bailey, R.E. (1971) Periodic hormonogenesis – a new phenomenon. Periodicity in function of a hormone-producing tumour in man. *J. Clin. Endocrinol. Metab.*, **32**, 317.

26. Atkinson, A.B., Kennedy, A.L., Carson, D.J., Hadden, D.R., Weaver, J.A. and Sheridan, B. (1985) Five cyclical cases of Cushing's syndrome. *Br. Med. J.*, **291**, 1453–7.

27. Meador, C.K., Liddle, G.W., Island, D.P., Nicholson, W.E., Lucas, C.P., Nuckton, J.G. and Leutscher, J.A. (1962) Cause of Cushing's syndrome in patients with tumors arising from 'nonendocrine' tissue. *J. Clin. Endocrinol. Metab.*, **22**, 693.

28. Howlett, T.A., Drury, P.L., Perry, L., Doniach, I., Rees, L.H. and Besser, G.M. (1986) Diagnosis and management of ACTH-dependent Cushing's syndrome: comparison of the features in ectopic and pituitary ACTH production. *Clin. Endocrinol.*, **24**, 699–713.

29. Himsworth, R.L., Bloomfield, G.A., Coombes, R.C., Ellison, M., Gilkes, J.J.H., Lowry, P.J., Setchell, K.D.R., Slavin, G. and Rees, L.H. (1977) 'Big ACTH' and calcitonin in an ectopic hormone secreting tumour of the liver. *Clin. Endocrinol.*, **7**, 45–62.

30. Ratter, S.J., Lowry, P.J., Besser, G.M. and Rees, L.H. (1980) Chromatographic characterisation of adrenocorticotrophin in human plasma. *J. Endocrinol.*, **85**, 359–69.

31. Crosby, S.R., Stewart, M.F., Ratclife, J.G. and White, A. (1988) Direct measurement of the precursors of adrenocorticotropin in human plasma by two-site immunoradiometric assay. *J. Clin. Endocrinol. Metab.*, **67**, 1272–7.

32. Findling, J.W., Engeland, W.C. and Raff, H. (1990) The use of immunoradiometric assay for the measurement of ACTH in human plasma. *Trends Endocrinol. Metab.*, **1**, 283–7.

33. Fuller, P.J., Lim, A.T.W., Barlow, J.W., White, E.L., Khalid, B.A.K., Coplov, D.L., Lolait, S., Funder, J.W. and Stockit, J.R. (1984) A pituitary tumour producing high molecular weight adrenocorticotrophin related peptides. Clinical and cell culture studies. *J. Clin. Endocrinol. Metab.*, **58**, 134–42.

34. Howlett, T.A. and Rees, L.H. (1985) Is it possible to diagnose pituitary-dependent Cushing's disease? *Ann. Clin. Biochem.*, **22**, 550–8.

35. Blunt, S.B., Sandler, L.M., Burnin, J.M. and Joplin, G.F. (1990) An evaluation of the distinction of ectopic and pituitary ACTH dependent Cushing's syndrome by clinical features, biochemical tests and radiological findings. *Q. J. Med.*, **77**(282), 1113–33.

36. Howlett, T.A., Price, J., Hale, A.C., Doniach, I., Rees, L.H., Wass, J.A.H. and Besser, G.M. (1985) Pituitary ACTH-dependent Cushing's syndrome due to ectopic production of a bombesin-like peptide by a medullary carcinoma

of the thyroid. *Clin. Endocrinol.*, **22**, 91–101.

37. Nieman, L.K., Chrousos, G.P., Oldfield, E.H., Averinos, P.C., Cutler, G.B. and Loriaux, D.L. (1986) The ovine corticotrophin-releasing hormone stimulation test and the dexamethasone suppression test in the differential diagnosis of Cushing's syndrome. *Ann. Intern. Med.*, **105**, 862–7.

38. Croughs, R.J.M., Docter, R. and De Jong, F.H. (1973) Comparison of oral and intravenous dexamethasone suppression tests in the differential diagnosis of Cushing's syndrome. *Acta Endocrinol.*, **72**, 54–62.

39. Biemond, P., De Jong, F.H. and Lamberts, F.W.J. (1990) Continuous dexamethasone infusion for seven hours in patients with the Cushing syndrome. *Ann. Intern. Med.*, **112**, 738–41.

40. Liddle, G.W., Estep, H.L., Kendall, J.W., Williams, W.C. and Townes, A.W. (1959) Clinical application of a new test of pituitary reserve. *J. Clin. Endocrinol. Metab.*, **19**, 875–94.38.

41. Strott, C.A., West, C.A., Nakagawa, K., Kondo, T. and Tyler, F.H. (1969) Plasma 11-deoxycortisol and ACTH response to metyrapone (plasma metyrapone assay). *J. Clin. Endocrinol.*, **29**, 6–11.'

42. Gillies, G. and Grossman, A.B. (1985) The CRFs and their control: chemistry, physiology and clinical implications. In *Clinics in Endocrinology and Metabolism: Pituitary Adrenocortical Axis.* (ed. G.M. Besser and L.H. Rees), W.B. Saunders, Philadelphia, pp. 821–43.

43. Hermus, A.R., Pieters, G.F., Benraad, T.J., Smals, A.G. and Kloppenborg, P.W. (1989) The CRH test and the high-dose dexamethasone test in the differential diagnosis of Cushing's syndrome. In *Recent Advances in Basic and Clinical Neuroendocrinology.* (ed. F.F. Casanueva and C. Dieguez), Elsevier, Amsterdam, pp. 351–4.

44. Hale, A.C., Coates, P.J., Doniach, I., Howlett, T.A., Grossman, A.B., Rees, L.H. and Besser, G.M. (1988) A bromocriptine-responsive adenoma secreting alpha-MSH in a patient with Cushing's disease. *Clin. Endocrinol.*, **28**, 215–23.

45. Malchoff, C.D., Orth, D.N., Abboud, C., Carney, J.A., Pairolero, P.C. and Carey, R.M. (1988) Ectopic ACTH syndrome caused by a bronchial carcinoid tumour responsive to dexamethasone, metyrapone and corticotrophin-releasing hormone. *Am. J. Med.*, **84**, 760–4.

46. Grossman, A.B., Howlett, T.A., Perry, L., Coy, H., Savage, M.O., Lavender, P., Rees, L.H. and Besser, G.M. (1988) CRF in the differential diagnosis of Cushing's syndrome: a comparison with the dexamethasone suppression test. *Clin. Endocrinol.*, **29**, 167–78.

47. Nieman, L.K., Cutler, G.B., Oldfield, R.H., Loriaux, D.L. and Chrouson, G.P. (1989) The ovine corticotropin-releasing hormone (CRH) stimulation test is superior to the human CRH stimulation test for the diagnosis of Cushing's disease. *J. Clin. Endocrinol. Metab.*, **69**, 165–9.

48. Faria, M.S., Kopelman, P.G., Besser, G.M. and Grossman, A.B. (1990) A comparison of the effects of human and ovine corticotrophin-releasing hormone-41 on the pituitary adrenal axis. *Neuroendocrinology*, **52**, 4.6 (abstract).

49. White, F.E., White, M.C., Drury, P.L., Kelsey Fry, I. and Besser, G.M. (1982) Value of computed tomography of the abdomen and chest in investigation of Cushing's syndrome. *Br. Med. J.*, **284**, 771–4.

50. Upton, G.V. and Amatruda, T.T. (1971) Evidence for the presence of tumour peptides with corticotrophin-releasing-factor-like activity in the ectopic ACTH syndrome. *New Engl. J. Med.*, **285**, 419–24.

51. Schteingard, D.E., Lloyd, R.V., Akil, H., Chandler, W.F., Ibarra-Perez, P., Rosen, S.G. and Ogletree, R. (1986) Cushing's syndrome secondary to ectopic corticotropin-releasing hormone-adrenocorticotropin secretion. *J. Clin. Endocrinol. Metab.*, **63**, 770–5.

52. Zarate, A., Kovacs, K., Flores, M., Moran, C and Felix, I (1986) ACTH and CRF-producing bronchial carcinoid associated with Cushing's syndrome. *Clin. Endocrinol.*, **24**, 523–9.

53. Belsky, J.L., Cuello, B., Swandon, L.W., Simmons, D.M., Jarrett, R.M. and Braza, F. (1985) Cushing's syndrome due to ectopic production of corticotropin-releasing factor. *J. Clin. Endocrinol. Metab.*, **60**, 496–500.

54. Jessop, D.S., Cunnah, D., Millar, J.G.B., Neville, E., Coates, P., Doniach, I., Besser, G.M. and Rees, L.H. (1987) A phaeochromo-

cytoma presenting with Cushing's syndrome associated with increased concentrations of circulating corticotrophin-releasing factor. *J. Endocrinol.*, **113**, 133–8.

55. Nawata, H., Higuchi, K., Ikuyama, S., Kato, K., Ibayashi, H., Mimura, K., Sueishi, K., Zingami, H. and Imura, H. (1990) Corticotropin-releasing hormone- and adrenocorticotropin-producing pituitary carcinoma with metastases to the liver and lung in a patient with Cushing's disease. *J. Clin. Endocrinol. Metab.*, **71**, 1068–73.

56. Carey, R.M., Varma, S.K., Drake, C.R., Thorner, M.O., Kovacs, K., Rivier, C. and Vale, W. (1984) Ectopic secretion of corticotropin-releasing factor as a cause of Cushing's syndrome. A clinical, morphologic, and biochemical study. *New Engl. J. Med.*, **311**, 13–20.

57. Anonymous editorial (1988) Nodular hyperplasia and Cushing's syndrome. *Lancet*, **ii**, 434.

58. Young, F.W., Carney, J.A., Musa, B.U., Wulffraat, N.M., Lens, J.W. and Drexhage, H.A. (1989) Familial Cushing's syndrome due to primary pigmented nodular adrenocortical disease. *New Engl. J. Med.*, **321**, 1659–64.

59. Burrow, G.N., Wortzman, G., Rewcastle, N.B., Holgate, R.C. and Kovacs, K. (1981) Microadenomas of the pituitary and abnormal sellar tomograms in an unselected autopsy series. *New Engl. J. Med.*, **304**, 156–8.

60. Kaye, T.B. and Crapo, L. (1990) The Cushing's syndrome: an update on diagnostic tests. *Ann. Intern. Med.*, **112**, 434–44.

61. Dwyer, A.J., Frank, J.A., Doppman, J.L., Oldfield, E.H., Hickey, A.M., Cutler, G.B., Loriaux, D.L. and Schiable, T.F. (1987) Pituitary adenomas in patients with Cushing disease: initial experience with Gd-DTPA-enhanced MR imaging. *Radiology*, **163**, 421–6.

62. Peck, W.W., Dillon, W.P., Norman, D., Newton, T.H. and Wilson, C.B. (1989) High-resolution MR imaging of pituitary microadenomas at 1.5 T: experience with Cushing disease. *Am. J. Radiol.*, **152**, 145–51.

63. Doppman, J.L., Nieman, L.K., Miller, D.L., Pass, H.I., Chang, R., Cutler, G.P., Schaaf, M., Chrousos, G.P., Norton, J.A., Ziessman, H.A., Oldfield, E.H. and Loriaux, D.L. (1989)

Ectopic adrenocorticotropic hormone syndrome: localisation studies in 28 patients. *Radiology*, **172**, 115–24.

64. Trainer, P.J. and Besser, G.M. (1990) Cushing's syndrome: difficulties in diagnosis. *Trends Endocrinol. Metab.*, **1**, 292–5.

65. Drury, P.L., Ratter, S., Tomlin, S., Williams, J., Dacie, J.E., Rees, L.H. and Besser, G.M. (1982) Experience with selective venous sampling in diagnosis of ACTH-dependent Cushing's syndrome. *Br. Med. J.*, **284**, 9–12.

66. Doppman, J.L., Pass, H.I., Nieman, L., Cutler, G.B., Chrousos, G.P. and Loriaux, D.L. (1989) Failure of bronchial lavage to detect elevated levels of adrenocorticotrophin (ACTH) in patients with ACTH-producing bronchial carcinoids. *J. Clin. Endocrinol. Metab.*, **69**, 1302–4.

67. Findling, J.W., Aron, D.C., Tyrrell, J.B., Shinsako, J.H., Fitzgerald, P.A., Norman, D., Wilson, C.B. and Forsham, P.H. (1981) Selective venous sampling for ACTH in Cushing's syndrome. *Ann. Intern. Med.*, **94**, 647–52.

68. Oldfield, E.H., Chrousos, G.P., Schulte, H.M., Schaaf, M., McKeever, P.E., Krudy, A.G., Cutler, G.B., Loriaux, D.L. and Doppman, J.L. (1985) Pre-operative lateralization of ACTH-secreting pituitary microadenomas by bilateral and simultaneous inferior petrosal venous sinus sampling. *New Engl. J. Med.*, **312**, 100–3.

69. Schulte, H.M., Allolio, B., Gunther, R.W., Benker, G., Windeck, R., Winkelmann, W. and Reinwein, D. (1987) Bilateral and simultaneous sinus petrosus inferior catheterisation in patients with Cushing's syndrome: plasma-immunoreactive-ACTH-concentrations before and after administration of CRF. *Horm. Metab. Res.* (suppl), **166**, 66–7.

70. Crook, P.A., Pestell, R.G., Calenti, A.J., Gilford, E.J., Henderson, K.J., Best, J.D. and Alford, F.P. (1988) Multiple pituitary hormone gradients from inferior petrosal sinus sampling in Cushing's disease. *Acta Endocrinol.*, **119**, 75–80.

71. McCance, D.R., McIlrath, E., McNeil, A., Gordon, D.S., Hadden, D.R., Kennedy, L., Sheridan, B. and Atkinson, A.B. (1989) Bilateral inferior petrosal sinus sampling as a

routine procedure in ACTH-dependent Cushing's syndrome. *Clin. Endocrinol.*, **30**, 157–66.

72. Tabarin, A., Greselle, J.F., Sangalli, F., Leprat, F., Angibeau, R.M., Latapie, J.L., Guerin, J., Caille, J.M. and Roger, P. (1990) The CRF test during bilateral inferior petrosal sinus sampling in the diagnosis of Cushing's disease. *Neuroendocrinology*, **52**, 4.38 (abstract).

73. Schulte, H.M., Allolio, B., Gunther, R.W., Benker, G., Winkelmann, W., Ohnhaus, E.E. and Reinwein, D. (1988) Selective bilateral and simultaneous catheterization of the inferior petrosal sinus: CRF stimulates prolactin secretion from ACTH-producing micro-adenomas in Cushing's disease. *Clin. Endocrinol.*, **28**, 289–95.

74. Allolio, B., Gunther, R.W., Benker, G., Reinwein, D., Winkelmann, W. and Schulte, H.M. (1990) A multihormonal response to corticotropin-releasing hormone in inferior petrosal sinus blood of patients with Cushing's disease. *J. Clin. Endocrinol. Metab.*, **71**, 1195–1201.

75. Wittert, G.A., Crock, P.A., Donald, R.A., Gilford, E.J., Boolel, M., Alford, F.P. and Espiner, E.A. (1990) Arginine vasopressin in Cushing's disease. *Lancet*, **i**, 991–4.

76. Trainer, P.J., Howlett, T.A., Dacie, J.E. and Besser, G.M. (1990) Simultaneous bilateral inferior petrosal sinus sampling with 100 mcg of corticotrophin-releasing hormone (CRH-41) for ACTH in 32 patients with ACTH-dependent Cushing's syndrome. *Neuroendocrinology*, **52**, 4.18 (abstract).

5

Hypothalamic pituitary ovarian axis

D.M. WHITE and S. FRANKS

5.1 INTRODUCTION

The physiology of the hypothalamic pituitary ovarian axis is integrated by feedback loops acting at several levels. In addition, at ovarian level, there are a number of paracrine factors that have the capacity to modulate gonadotropin action and contribute to the normal development of the dominant follicle, culminating in the release of a mature egg. Ovarian steroid hormones, in addition to their effect on the hypothalamus, pituitary and ovaries, also control the function of the endometrium. The endometrium has no direct hormonal feedback on the hypothalamus, pituitary or ovary, but is responsive to the hormone environment. The obvious manifestation of the cyclical hormonal changes is menstruation.

The menstrual cycle is divided into the follicular (proliferative) phase and, following ovulation, the luteal or secretory phase. Towards the end of the luteal phase, as sex steroid secretion diminishes, the negative feedback effect of these combined hormones is reduced, leading to a rise in gonadotropin concentrations, in particular follicle stimulating hormone (FSH). This stimulates development of early tertiary or antral follicles which have been recruited and attained the size of 1–4.5 mm in diameter. Recruitment of primordial follicles occurs continuously during prenatal life until the menopause. The factors that control this initial recruitment of follicles are uncertain. Histologically, granulosa cells group around the oocyte to form the primary follicle. The primary follicle develops into a secondary follicle as the granulosa cells surrounding the oocyte multiply and further cells migrate to the outer layer of the follicle. These cells will develop into the theca interstitial cells. With the development of the theca, the follicle acquires a blood supply, and the thecal cells mature and acquire luteinizing hormone (LH) receptors. Within the granulosa cell layer the antrum develops, forming an early tertiary follicle. The events up to the stage of antrum formation are independent of pituitary gonadotropin secretion, and are probably controlled by the follicle itself. The later stages of follicle development do, however, require both LH and FSH. The whole process takes about 3 months and finally ends either in ovulation or, in the majority of follicles recruited, atresia.

The subsequent development of antral follicles, culminating in ovulation of a single dominant follicle, depends on coordinated control by cyclical changes in LH and FSH. The rise in FSH in the early follicular phase of the cycle induces aromatase activity in the granulosa cells of the most advanced follicle and thereby the production of oestradiol from

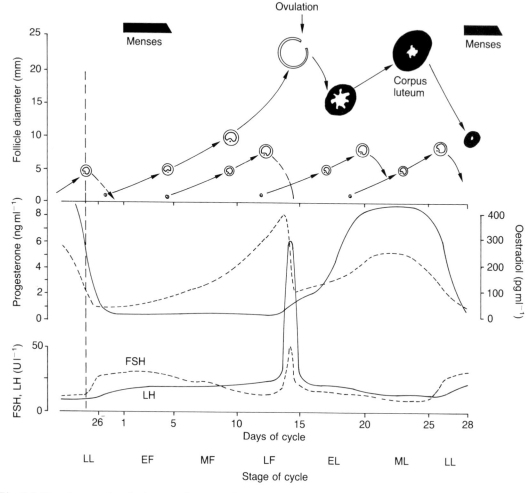

Fig. 5.1 The changes in pituitary and ovarian hormone concentration and follicle growth throughout the ovarian cycle. In the follicular phase of the cycle only a single follicle acquires dominance over the other follicles to proceed through to ovulation. The vertical dotted line indicates the onset of luteal regression. (---) progesterone; (- - - -) oestradiol. (Reproduced from Jeffcoat, S.L. (ed.) (1983) *Ovulation: Methods for its Prediction and Detection*. John Wiley and Sons, London.)

androgen substrate. Androgens are secreted by theca cells in response to LH and the slight but progressive increase in LH in the early to mid-follicular phase of the cycle ensures adequate substrate for FSH-induced activity of aromatase, the enzyme controlling conversion of androgen to oestrogen. There is a critical point where one follicle reaches

sufficient size to become independent of continued FSH stimulation. Oestradiol production increases to a peak of around 10–12 days following the onset of menstruation. The rise of oestradiol levels in the mid-follicular phase cause a fall in FSH levels due to negative feedback on the pituitary and hypothalamus. Later in the follicular phase, the rapidly rising oestradiol levels have positive feedback at pituitary level (and perhaps also at hypothalamic level), causing a surge of LH release. This surge in LH then triggers ovulation. Following the release of the ovum the ruptured follicle forms a corpus luteum. This LH surge which triggers ovulation also acts by an unknown mechanism on the theca interstitial cells to stop the 17-hydroxylase step in the steroid hormone pathway and returns these cells from androgen to progesterone producing cells. The luteinized granulosa cells also produce progesterone in response to LH; oestradiol and progesterone combine to suppress gonadotropin release (Fig. 5.1).

The effect of oestradiol and progesterone is enhanced by inhibin, which shows a progressive rise in the luteal phase of menstrual cycle and also has a negative feedback effect on FSH release. *In vitro* experiments have not shown any effect of inhibin on LH. Results from studies of granulosa cells in culture

suggest that inhibin is also likely to have local effects at ovarian level and cause suppression of oestradiol production by interaction with FSH.

If fertilization does not occur, the corpus luteum degenerates, the level of sex steroids fall and a new cycle is initiated by removal of negative feedback on FSH and LH. Figure 5.2 shows the cyclical changes which occur in the endometrium, cervix and vagina secondary to the hormonal changes occurring throughout the menstrual cycle.

The adrenal glands also produce sex steroids. Therefore, peripheral hormone measurements reflect adrenal and ovarian sex steroid hormone production. The adrenal gland contains the same enzymatic pathway for steroid production as the ovary (see Fig. 5.3). However, the final step in the pathway, converting testosterone to oestradiol, is not present in the adrenal, so the adrenal produces only androgenic sex steroids. This pathway is under the control of adreno-

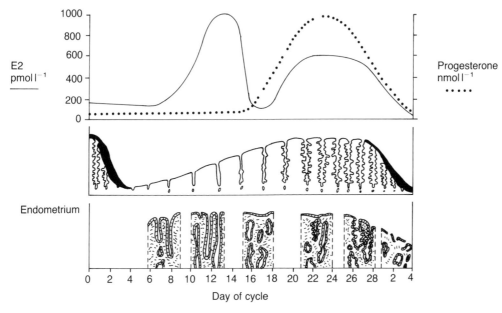

Fig. 5.2 Cyclical changes in the endometrium occurring throughout the menstrual cycle.

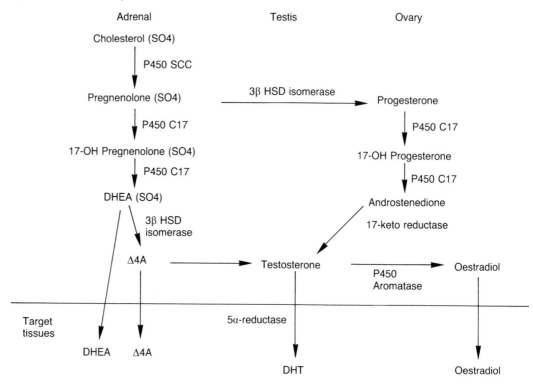

Fig. 5.3 The three major pathways of steroid metabolism in the adrenal, ovary and testis overlap. The main products from each organ are released into the circulation and act on specific target tissues. Of the androgens released, further metabolism to DHT can occur from DHEA, Δ4A or testosterone.

corticotropic hormone (ACTH). The major site of action of ACTH is the conversion of cholesterol to pregnenolone. The majority of substrate is channelled to produce cortisol, which provides negative feedback control of ACTH, but androgens are also major products of the adrenal. In normal women, some 50% of circulating peripheral concentration of androstenedione is derived from adrenal secretion.

Women who present with dysfunction of the hypothalamic pituitary ovarian axis do so in three major ways: (i) concern because of hirsutism, (ii) menstrual cycle dysfunction, or (iii) infertility. Investigation and, particularly, subsequent management is in a major way determined by whether fertility is a prime concern of the patient.

5.2 INVESTIGATION OF ANDROGEN EXCESS

5.2.1 CLINICAL PRESENTATION

Patients who present with androgen excess, i.e. hirsutism and/or frontal balding and acne, can have additional virilizing features of change of body shape, clitoromegaly and deepening of voice. Hirsutism can usefully be described semiquantitatively using the Ferriman–Gallwey (FG) score. Table 5.1 lists the most common causes of androgen excess.

Table 5.1 Causes of androgen excess

Ovarian
  Polycystic ovaries
  Virilizing tumours

Adrenal
  Congenital adrenal hyperplasia
  Cushing's syndrome
  Virilizing tumours

Idiopathic

Clinical information about the duration and severity of hirsutism and any accompanying derangement of the menstrual cycle provides a guide to the diagnosis and extent of investigation required (Table 5.2).

However, the majority of patients with androgen excess will have polycystic ovary syndrome (PCOS). The initial investigation of androgen excess is therefore an investigation of PCOS.

5.2.2 INVESTIGATION OF PCOS

Ultrasound scanning

The most frequently used method of diagnosing PCOS is by measurement of gonadotropins and testosterone. Characteristically, PCOS is associated with an elevated LH but with a normal FSH, resulting in an increase in the LH/FSH ratio as well as an increase in testosterone levels. However, ultrasound scanning via the abdominal or vaginal route using a real-time scanner enables the ovarian morphology to be assessed accurately and has had a major impact on the diagnosis of PCOS.

The normal ovarian appearance is distinct from that of polycystic ovaries, which have an increase in stroma, a thickened ovarian capsule and peripheral cysts (Fig. 5.4). This pattern needs to be distinguished from that which characterizes multifollicular ovaries (MFO), in which the multiple cysts are not associated with an increased stroma of the ovary (Fig. 5.5). MFO is characteristic of women with weight-loss-related amenorrhoea and is also seen in adolescent girls going through puberty. In contrast to the polycystic ovary, it represents the response of the normal ovary to an impaired gonadotropin signal. Although experience is important in assessing ovarian appearance by ultrasonography, with the abdominal and vaginal means of assessment, morphology can be clearly defined in 95% of patients [1].

The high prevalence of polycystic ovaries in hirsute and anovulatory patients prompted a study designed to examine the prevalence in the normal population. Polson and colleagues scanned 257 volunteers, of whom 56 had polycystic ovaries on scanning; 158 of the total were not on the contraceptive pill [2]. Taking a detailed menstrual history from

Table 5.2 Investigation of androgen excess

1. Longstanding hirsutism Normal menses	Testosterone Ovarian ultrasound
2. Hirsutism (short history) Cycle disturbance (oligo/amenorrhoea)	As above with LH/FSH Progesterone challenge
3. Hirsutism and virilization Serum testosterone 5 nmol l^{-1}	As above with DHEAS Consider adrenal CT scan Venous catheterization

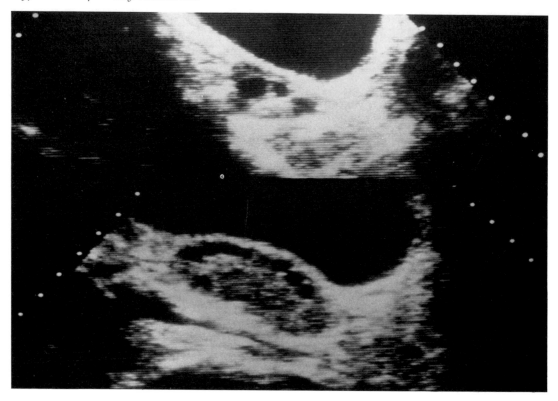

Fig. 5.4 Normal ovary (top) and polycystic ovary (bottom), at the same magnification. The polycystic ovary has increased central stroma, and multiple peripherally arranged small follicules (2–6 mm in size).

these women, it was found that in the 33 women who had polycystic ovaries, 76% had irregular cycles (as defined by menstrual cycles which vary from <21 days to >35 days in four consecutive cycles). Of the 8 women with polycystic ovaries and normal cycles, 6 had noted hirsutism (FG scale 6–14) but this was not sufficient for them to seek medical advice. Thus, the spectrum of clinical presentation of women with polycystic ovaries extends from the classic picture of the obese hirsute women with amenorrhoea as described by Stein and Leventhal, to the woman with polycystic ovary appearance on ultrasound scan with a regular menstrual cycle and mild hirsutism, or to the nonhirsute women with a slightly irregular cycle.

Biochemical tests: LH, FSH, testosterone

The accuracy of biochemical testing in the diagnosis of PCOS has been assessed by Hull using patients who were symptomatic (that is, those who had presented to a gynaecological endocrine clinic with irregular cycles and/or hirsutism) and had polycystic ovaries on ultrasound [1]. The commonly used biochemical indices of LH, FSH and testosterone were measured in these patients. Because of the wide fluctuation in LH and FSH levels throughout the menstrual cycle, early follicular phase levels of gonadotropins were used for assessment. An LH level of $>10\,IU\,l^{-1}$ was 96% accurate for a positive test, and 44% accurate for a negative test, giving a high

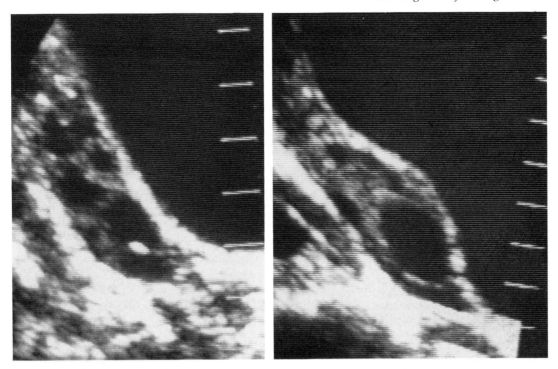

Fig. 5.5 Multifollicular ovary, with normal stromal volume, but multiple (2–10 mm) follicules scattered throughout the ovary.

sensitivity but low specificity and an overall diagnostic accuracy of 67%. The LH/FSH ratios were less accurate (using an LH/FSH ratio of 2.0, 2.5 and 3.0, the overall accuracy was 70%, 58% and 51%, respectively). However, a testosterone level of above $2.5\,\mathrm{nmol\,l^{-1}}$ gave a better overall accuracy of 83%, with 100% accuracy for positive tests and an accuracy of 60% with a negative test. Thus, testosterone remains the most useful of all biochemical indicators of PCOS in patients presenting with menstrual disturbance or hirsutism.

Progesterone challenge test

Because of the very high prevalence of polycystic ovaries in patients with clinical androgen excess and the wide range of bio-

chemical results in this group, all biochemical indicators can be normal with PCOS still being the correct diagnosis. Without access to ultrasonography for assessment of ovarian appearance, Hull has shown that a similarly high diagnostic accuracy can be achieved by the simple approach of the progesterone challenge test to assess oestrogen status in women with oligoamenorrhoea [3]. This applies to both hirsute and non-hirsute women with PCOS. Over 95% had a positive progesterone challenge test.

Other biochemical tests

Additional tests to assess androgen excess and PCOS have included measurement of androstenedione, 5α-reduced androgens, sex hormone binding globulin (SHBG) and the calculation of the free androgen index (testosterone × 100/SHBG). SHBG levels are decreased in obesity and in insulin resistance, irrespective of the presence of polycystic ovaries, and are therefore not a reliable indicator of PCOS. A number of different androgens have been used in the diagnosis of PCOS but none is very specific. The calculation of the free androgen index is more specific than a single androgen measurement. However, calculation of the free androgen index does not give additional diagnostic help when added to clinical information, assessment of oestrogen status or ovarian ultrasound and testosterone measurement.

Recommendation

In summary, the diagnosis of PCOS is confirmed by an ultrasound scan and measurement of testosterone and LH. In our experience almost all anovulatory women with PCOS have at least one biochemical abnormality, i.e. a raised LH or testosterone. In hirsute *ovulatory* women with PCOS, the LH level is frequently normal but the serum testosterone is significantly raised in the majority of cases.

The high prevalence of polycystic ovaries in the female population means this diagnosis does not exclude additional pathology. The decision for additional investigation is determined by clinical assessment and testosterone measurement. This applies to investigating androgen excess and is also applicable to the discussion below when investigating amenorrhoea and infertility.

5.3 INVESTIGATION OF CONGENITAL ADRENAL HYPERPLASIA

Steroid hormone synthesis in the adrenal gland proceeds along one of three major pathways to produce either aldosterone, cortisol or androgens. Enzyme dysfunction in the cortisol or aldosterone pathway has two major effects: (i) lack of the adrenal hormone distal to the enzyme block and (ii) overproduction of steroid metabolites in the unaffected enzyme pathway because of lack of negative feedback which increases ACTH drive. Any enzyme block to cortisol production will increase adrenal androgens.

5.3.1 BIOCHEMICAL TESTS

Classical congenital adrenal hyperplasia (CAH) with a complete enzyme block is discussed in detail elsewhere, but in the differential diagnosis of hirsutism and androgen excess, late onset (also called acquired or non-classical) CAH needs to be considered. Over 95% of patients with CAH have 21-hydroxylase deficiency with high levels of 17-hydroxyprogesterone (17-OHP), which is the metabolite prior to the enzyme block in the cortisol pathway.

Diagnosis of the disorder depends on finding an elevated 17-OHP concentration, either basal levels or post-stimulation with ACTH. Reference data from New and colleagues using 17-OHP concentrations 60 minutes after an ACTH bolus or after 360 minutes of an ACTH infusion clearly differentiated patients with classical, late onset and cryptic CAH (asymptomatic family members of classical CAH patients detected on genetic and hormonal studies) from the 'normal population' [4]. These three groups of patients are homozygotes for different genetic abnormalities of the 21-hydroxylase gene complex. Obligate heterozygotes from the three groups (obtained from genotyping family members of patients) underwent similar testing. There was no overlap with the three types of homozygote patients on 60-minute bolus or 360-minute infusion 17-OHP measurements but there was overlap of heterozygotes from the three groups with the normal population. Seventeen of 123 heterozygotes had ACTH-stimulated 17-

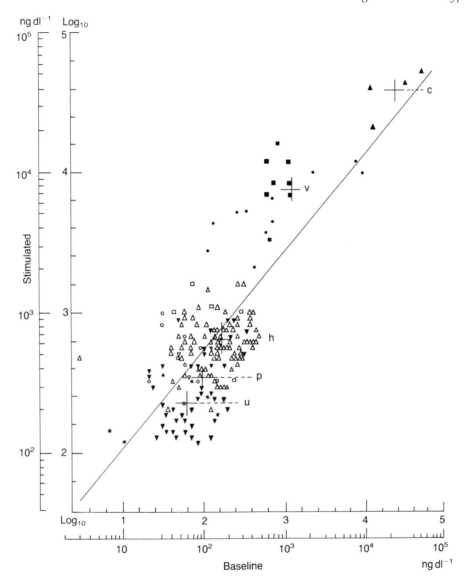

Fig. 5.6 Nonogram relating baseline and 60 min ACTH-stimulated serum 17-OHP concentrations. C, CAH; v, patients with non-classical symptomatic or asymptomatic (cryptic, acquired or late-onset) 21-OH deficiency; h, heterozygotes for classical CAH, non-classical symptomatic CAH (acquired or late-onset adrenal hyperplasia) and non-classical asymptomatic CAH (cryptic 21-OH deficiency); u, family members predicted by HLA genotyping to be unaffected; p, general population (not HLA genotyped). (▼), general population; (*), genetically unaffected; patients with (▲), CAH; (●), acquired adrenal hyperplasia; (■), cryptic 21-OH deficiency; heterozygotes for (△), CAH; (○), acquired adrenal hyperplasia; (□), cryptic 21-OH deficiency. (From *J. Clin. Endocrinol. Metab.*, **57**, 320–6 (1983)).

OHP measurement within the normal range (Fig. 5.6).

There was no advantage of ACTH infusion over a bolus, nor was measurement of androstenedione, the androgen metabolite distal to 17-OHP on the androgen pathway, superior to 17-OHP measurements. Therefore, an i.v. bolus of ACTH and a 60-minute 17-OHP is the simplest method of diagnosing CAH.

5.3.2 SELECTION OF PATIENTS FOR CAH SCREENING

The gene frequency for CAH varies widely between populations, with the highest rates in Ashkenaze Jews of 3.7%, 1.6% in Hispanics and decreasing to only 0.1% in a 'diverse white population'. This variation in gene frequency will influence whether the test should be performed routinely in androgen excess. At St Mary's Hospital 112 consecutive patients who presented with hirsutism and/or menstrual irregularity all had normal stimulated 17-OHP levels. The majority had polycystic ovaries. Therefore, in a population where CAH is uncommon there is no necessity for routine testing in the investigation of androgen excess. The only patient with CAH (cryptic) identified had been recruited as a normal control. She had an elevated testosterone and normal ovaries on ultrasound scan. So in this small subgroup (8 out of a total of 127 normal and PCOS women tested) we would advocate screening to exclude CAH.

5.4 INVESTIGATION OF CUSHING'S SYNDROME

Cushing's syndrome also produces hirsutism and virilization, but it is usually clearly associated with other features of cortisol excess. The diagnosis and investigation are discussed in Chapter 4.

5.5 INVESTIGATION OF VIRILIZING TUMOURS

The other important differential diagnosis of women presenting with androgen excess are virilizing tumours of adrenal or ovarian origin. These tumours are rare and careful selection of patients for further investigation to rule out a tumour is required. Meldrum and Guy reviewed published case reports in the British literature of women with ovarian tumours [5]. Of the 43 women described there was adequate information given on 41 cases: 41 (98%) had virilizing features in addition to hirsutism, and only 5 (11%) women had testosterone levels less than $5 \, \text{nmol} \, l^{-1}$, but in this subgroup all women were virilized. The diagnosis was by identification of an ovarian mass in the majority of cases. Twenty-five (58%) of the patients underwent catheter studies prior to surgery, 23 of whom had a testosterone ovarian/peripheral gradient (OPG) of greater than $2 \, \text{ng} \, l^{-1}$. The histological classification of hormone secreting tumours is complex because these tumours are not easily divided into distinct groups. Clinical presentation or biochemical abnormalities do not help in predicting histological type or prognosis. Ireland and Woodruff reviewed and reclassified 194 cases on the Novak Ovarian Tumour Registry [6]. The clinical presentation was very variable, with the age of presentation reported from prepubertal to postmenopausal. Overall 60% of the patients were virilized and 69% had a palpable mass. Only 30% of the patients had any endocrine investigation but, again, results were not consistent with histological type or subsequent progress. An elevated testosterone level can be of ovarian or adrenal origin. However, dehydroepiandrosterone (DHEAS) is a steroid hormone produced by the adrenal alone, so it is used in screening for adrenal virilizing tumours.

With the widespread availability of biochemical testing and non-invasive radiology, particularly ovarian ultrasound and computerized tomography (CT) scanning of adrenal, diagnosis of virilizing tumours should be possible earlier. The corollary of this is that patients who present with the common problem of hirsutism may coincidentally be found to have a mass on radiological investigations. These patients can then be considered for exploratory laparotomy or selective venous catheterization with further hormonal investigation. Moltz and colleagues [7] investigated eight normal ovulatory women in the early follicular phase of their cycles, measuring peripheral as well as ovarian and adrenal hormone levels of seven steroids to define the normal range. They then investigated women with clinical evidence of andro-

gen excess, 43 of whom had been diagnosed as having polycystic ovaries on laparoscopy. In this group 83% had hypersecretion of testosterone with elevated peripheral venous testosterone levels, but in all subjects these concentrations were less than $5.2\,\mathrm{nmol\,l^{-1}}$. The subsequent series of ten women with androgen secreting tumours all had peripheral testosterone levels of $>5\,\mathrm{nmol\,l^{-1}}$, and venous catheterization defined the site of the tumour. This confirms the work of other investigators, nine out of the ten patients of Surrey and colleagues [8] had elevated peripheral testosterone levels of $>5.0\,\mathrm{nmol\,l^{-1}}$.

Figure 5.7 summarizes the strategy for investigation of androgen excess.

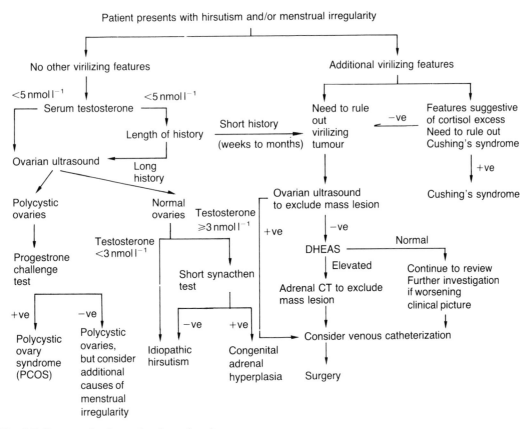

Fig. 5.7 Strategy for investigation of androgen excess.

Selection of tests for investigation depend primarily on the length of history, whether additional virilizing features are present and the serum testosterone. The majority of patients presenting with hirsutism have PCOS and unless there are additional clinical reasons for concern or a significantly elevated testosterone of $>5.0 \, \text{nmol} \, l^{-1}$, no further investigations are required in such cases.

5.6 INVESTIGATION OF FEMALE INFERTILITY

The three major areas of investigation in couples with infertility are: (i) confirmation of ovulation and investigation of its disorders, (ii) adequacy of spermatogenesis, and (iii) whether there is a mechanical barrier to conception, i.e. tubal disease.

5.6.1 OVULATION AND ITS DISORDERS

Confirmation of ovulation

Basal temperature charts, which are often difficult to interpret, have been superseded by more accurate means of determining ovulation. Progesterone measurement in the mid-luteal phase is the most reliable and frequently used test to confirm ovulation. Serum progesterone measurement in 20 menstrual cycles in normal women with regular cycles, 9 of whom had proven fertility [9], indicated that the peak of progesterone secretion occurred 6–9 days after the preovulatory peak of oestradiol. In all conception cycles the minimum level of progesterone 6 days after ovulation was $30 \, \text{nmol} \, l^{-1}$ (95% confidence interval $28–53 \, \text{nmol} \, l^{-1}$). The range of progesterone measurements in the 196 non-conception cycles studied (113 women) was $3–93 \, \text{nmol} \, l^{-1}$. This suggests that anovulatory cycles occur in women who later prove to be fertile. A progesterone concentration of greater than $30 \, \text{nmol} \, l^{-1}$ has therefore been accepted as confirmation of ovulation but a result cannot be interpreted unless timed accurately to the mid-luteal phase of the cycle, i.e. retrospective analysis according to the day of the subsequent menstrual period. Similarly, a negative result should be confirmed before anovulation is accepted. The accuracy of a single measurement is enhanced if associated with ultrasound scanning. Serial scans will monitor follicular growth, confirm when ovulation has occurred, and allow the correct timing of progesterone measurement, i.e. 5–10 days after ovulation. In normal women, a linear increase in the size of the dominant follicle can be observed by serial ultrasound scans. The maximum follicular diameter is usually between 20 mm and 25 mm, but the normal range at the time of ovulation is wide, 18–31 mm. Ovulation can be confirmed on scanning only if a follow-up scan shows that the follicle has collapsed. The presence of free fluid in the pouch of Douglas is additional evidence that ovulation has occurred. Ultrasound scanning in the diagnosis of ovulation has been compared with basal body temperature (BBT) charts, serial LH and oestradiol measurements. The rise in BBT, oestradiol peak and LH peak occurs 48–24 hours before ultrasound evidence of ovulation in the majority of cycles. The beginning of the progesterone rise coincides with these peaks. In approximately 15% of the spontaneous cycles monitored by Adams and colleagues [10] follicular rupture did not occur. As with progesterone measurements, one abnormal cycle in a woman with a history of regular cycles does not diagnose anovulation.

5.6.2 ANOVULATION

Causes and presentation

Women with disordered ovulation may present with irregular menses, oligomenorrhoea or amenorrhoea (greater than 6 months without menstrual bleeding). Table 5.3 gives a

Table 5.3 Classification of anovulation

1. Primary ovarian failure
2. Disorders of gonadotropin regulation
   Specific disorders:
      Hyperprolactinaemia
      Other pituitary endocrinopathies
      Non-functioning tumours of the
        hypothalamus or pituitary
      Kallmann's syndrome
   Functional disorders
      Weight loss and exercise
      Psychological
      Chronic illness
      Idiopathic hypogonadotropic hypogonadism
3. Polycystic ovary syndrome

functional classification of anovulation which broadly divides causes of anovulation into those associated with primary ovarian failure and those due to deficiency or disordered hypothalamic regulation of gonadotropin secretion.

5.6.3 PRIMARY OVARIAN FAILURE

Women presenting with primary ovarian failure may or may not have associated menopausal symptoms signifying oestrogen deficiency, such as hot flushes or vaginal dryness. The histology of the ovary in women with ovarian failure is similar to the post-menopausal ovary, with very few or absent primordial follicles. The 'resistant ovary syndrome' probably represents the opposite end of the spectrum of abnormal folliculogenesis. On histology of the ovaries in this group, follicles are still present but are unresponsive to FSH stimulation. This condition is almost always irreversible, and although pregnancy has been reported in women with resistant ovary syndrome and premature menopause, including one women reported as having streak ovaries at laparoscopy, these reports are extremely rare. The causes of primary ovarian failure include:

Chromosomal abnormalities (most commonly due to an XO genotype)
External radiation or cytotoxic chemotherapy
Autoimmune disorders of the ovary.

This last is diagnosed by detection of positive ovarian antibodies. However, limitation of techniques to detect the antibodies means that the diagnosis is difficult to confirm.

5.6.4 DISORDERS OF GONADOTROPIN REGULATION

Specific disorders

Hyperprolactinaemia

This is one of the most common causes of amenorrhoea. Patients present with oestrogen deficient amenorrhoea with or without galactorrhoea. The prevalence of galactorrhoea associated with hyperprolactinaemia is variable; the range reported in different series is from 30%–90%. Therefore, the presence or absence of galactorrhoea does not exclude or confirm hyperprolactinaemia as the cause of amenorrhoea. The excessive prolactin secretion disrupts the hypothalamic control of gonadotropin releasing hormone (GnRH), leading to abnormal pulsatile secretion of gonadotropins and inadequate ovarian stimulation. There are several mechanisms whereby prolactin interferes with gonadotropin secretion; they include interference with normal GnRH release, as well as probable peripheral action, impairing the responsiveness of the ovary to LH and FSH.

The single most common cause of hyperprolactinaemia is a prolactin secreting pituitary tumour, but hyperprolactinaemia can be due to a pituitary or hypothalamic lesion disrupting dopamine release. However, despite using sophisticated radiological techniques significant hyperprolactinaemia may be associated with normal radiology.

Other pituitary endocrinopathies

Acromegaly and pituitary dependent Cushing's disease are frequently associated with anovulation. The mechanism is unclear, but may be due to gonadotropin deficiency caused by the tumour mass, concurrent hyperprolactinaemia or, as in the case of Cushing's disease, hypersecretion of adrenal androgens.

Non-functioning tumours of the hypothalamus and pituitary

Destructive pituitary lesions can lead to gonadotropin deficiency and anovulation.

Kallmann's syndrome

Congenital deficiency of GnRH has a wide spectrum of presentation, from isolated deficiency presenting as secondary amenorrhoea with normal pubertal development to classical Kallmann's syndrome associated with anosmia and other congenital abnormalities.

5.6.5 FUNCTIONAL DISORDERS OF GONADOTROPIN REGULATION

Weight loss and exercise
Psychogenic
Chronic illness
Idiopathic

The most common cause of functional disorders of gonadotropin regulation is weight loss and/or exercise-induced amenorrhoea. Patients who are severely underweight [less than 66% of ideal body weight or a body mass index (BMI) of $<16\,kg\,m^2$] have a marked suppression of gonadotropin pulsatility which is reminiscent of a prepubertal pulse pattern. Characteristically, as weight is regained, the sequence of changes in LH and FSH pulsatility are similar to those that occur during puberty. These patients are biochemically and often clinically oestrogen deficient.

Return of menses usually accompanies recovery of weight but there can be a lag of several months before menstruation is resumed.

In addition to weight and exercise, both psychological stress and chronic illness can cause amenorrhoea by affecting hypothalamic control of gonadotropins. These stresses work through the same final common pathway causing hypothalamic dysfunction. In more profound causes of psychological disturbances such as schizophrenia, development of anovulation may be in part due to stress but also due to use of psychotropic drugs, e.g. phenothiazines, which stimulate prolactin secretion.

Idiopathic hypogonadotropic hypogonadism is the final category of disordered functional gonadotropin regulation. This group includes women who develop secondary amenorrhoea without any clearly defined aetiology but who manifest the same abnormalities of gonadotropin secretion as seen in the specific disorders described above.

5.6.6 POLYCYSTIC OVARY SYNDROME

This is the most common cause of anovulation. The mechanism of anovulation is unclear in this group, but there is a failure of FSH-dependent follicular maturation. Characteristically, women with PCOS have clinical and/or biochemical evidence of androgen excess. There is evidence, in the marmoset, that androgen excess may interfere with the oestrogen response of granulosa cells to stimulation by FSH. Additional experimental evidence has shown that other paracrine factors, for example epidermal growth factor or transforming growth factor alpha, are very potent inhibitors of oestradiol production although the precise role of these factors in ovarian physiology and in the pathogenesis of anovulation are not yet fully understood.

5.6.7 INVESTIGATION OF ANOVULATION

The investigation of anovulation requires a small number of investigations in the majority of women to reach a diagnosis. Women who are anovulatory and amenorrhoeic usually present with secondary amenorrhoea. The investigation and differentials diagnosis of primary amenorrhoea may require additional investigations because 60% of women with primary amenorrhoea will have developmental abnormalities of the ovaries and/or genital tract. The essential investigations are a measurement of serum FSH, prolactin and, in amenorrhoeic subjects, assessment of androgenous oestrogen production.

FSH

Women with ovarian failure will have elevated FSH levels in the menopausal range, i.e. $>20 \, \text{IU} \, \text{l}^{-1}$.

Ovarian biopsy is the only method of distinguishing primary ovarian failure from resistant ovary syndrome, but as the clinical presentation and management are the same this distinction is not necessary for clinical purposes.

LH measurements are also elevated in ovarian failure, but as LH can be increased in PCOS, LH measurement alone is not diagnostic. An elevated FSH however, is specific to primary ovarian failure.

Prolactin

There is no 'threshold' of serum prolactin concentration about which gonadotropin secretion sufficient to cause anovulation and amenorrhoea predictably occurs. The finding of a raised prolactin in the presence of amenorrhoea necessitates further evaluation with (i) measurement of thyroid function (thyroid stimulating hormone; TSH), because primary hypothyroidism can be associated with hyperprolactinaemic amenorrhoea and in this case specific treatment for the thyroid condition is necessary, and (ii) radiological assessment, i.e. CT scanning, to define the presence or absence of a structural pituitary abnormality.

Assessment of oestrogen production

Women who have biological evidence of oestrogen deficiency have a wide range of oestradiol levels which are often within the 'normal range' for oestradiol in the early to mid-follicular phase of the cycle. The progestogen challenge test provides an *in vivo* bioassay of oestradiol production. The test can be done in a number of ways, but one of the simplest strategies is to give medroxy-progesterone 5 mg daily orally for five days. The response can be categorized as positive (with a normal withdraw bleed), impaired (with minimal vaginal bleeding lasting less than two days), or negative (no response).

The usefulness of the response to progestogen to predict responsiveness to clomiphene has been compared to clinical assessment of oestrogen deficiency (assessment of the appearance of the lower genital tract) and to measurement of serum oestradiol levels [11]. As would be expected, oestradiol levels were lower in those women with the clinical appearance of oestrogen deficiency or impaired or negative progestogen response. However, with the wide overlap of oestradiol values between the groups a single oestradiol value did not prove a good discriminator in predicting the clomiphene response. In contrast, a positive progestogen challenge test indicated a 75% chance of ovulation following clomiphene given over three cycles.

Oestrogen deficiency may occur in a number of disorders, including primary ovarian failure and disorders of gonadotropin secretion. It distinguishes these patients from the other major group, i.e. those with PCOS, who maintain adequate oestrogen production.

A number of dynamic tests have been developed in an attempt to separate hypothalamic from pituitary causes of anovulation and to diagnose PCOS. These tests will be briefly described but they are no longer in widespread clinical practice as the diagnosis in most women can be made from clinical assessment and the investigations described above. In women with PCOS, in addition to a positive progesterone test, an ultrasound scan will confirm the diagnosis.

The clomiphene test, i.e. giving a standard course of clomiphene and monitoring whether ovulation has occurred, gives a positive response in 60%–80% of women with PCOS, and a small minority of patients with mild or partially recovered weight related amenorrhoea. It is therefore not helpful in diagnosis, nor does it differentiate hypothalamic from pituitary causes of anovulation.

The luteinizing hormone releasing hormone (LHRH) test, involving measurement of the gonadotropin response to a bolus injection of 100 µg of LHRH has been suggested as an alternative to the clomiphene test to assess hypothalamic pituitary function. A flat or impaired LH response may, however, be seen in patients with either hypothalamic or pituitary disorders, and there is a wide range of individual responses which overlaps with the response of normal women. In addition, the response to the LHRH test does not predict the response of an individual patient to treatment with pulsatile LHRH or gonadotropins. Similarly, although women with PCOS as a group have higher LH responses to LHRH than normal controls, the heterogeneous nature of responses in PCOS women ensures that there is overlap with normal controls and so gives no additional diagnostic information to a baseline measurement of LH.

Figure 5.8 outlines the strategy for investigation of anovulation. The figures in brackets indicate the frequency of diagnosis in 100

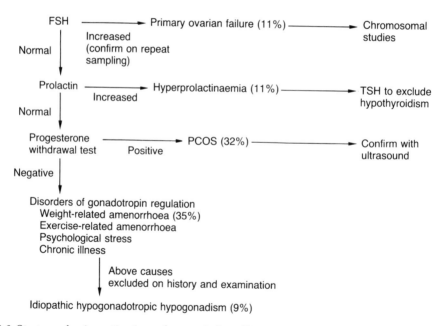

Fig. 5.8 Strategy for investigation of anovulation. Figures in parentheses indicate the frequency of diagnosis in patients presenting with secondary amenorrhoea to the gynaecological endocrine clinic at the Samaritan Hospital for Women (St Mary's Hospital group).

consecutive women presenting with secondary amenorrhoea [12]. Ninety-eight per cent of patients fell into five diagnostic categories, which were diagnosed on clinical presentation, FSH, prolactin and progesterone withdrawal test to determine oestrogen status. Therefore, unless there are features in the history or examination to suggest other endocrinopathies no further investigations need be routinely undertaken.

The investigation of patients with primary amenorrhoea has a different emphasis because abnormal gonadal, Mullerian duct or genital development account for 60% of cases. Therefore assessment of pubertal development and the genital tract are of particular importance.

5.6.8 LUTEAL PHASE DEFICIENCY

The diagnosis of anovulation in patients who present with oligomenorrhoea or amenorrhoea is straightforward but the investigation of patients who have more regular cycles and present with reduced fertility is more difficult. Luteal phase deficiency has been used to describe any abnormality of luteinization with inadequate progesterone production. Many causes have been postulated for luteal phase deficiency, including inadequate pulsatile gonadotropin release, an inadequate ovarian response to gonadotropin stimulation leading to abnormal folliculogenesis and an abnormal endometrial response to progesterone. The lack of a clear definition of luteal phase deficiency has lead to difficulties in assessing the accuracy of proposed diagnostic tests.

5.6.9 INVESTIGATION OF LUTEAL PHASE DEFICIENCY

Progesterone measurements

A single mid-luteal phase progesterone measurement of $>30\,\text{nmol}\,\text{l}^{-1}$ has been accepted as indicating ovulation. But as it is known that women of normal fertility have variable progesterone measurements in sequential cycles, serial cycle measurements are necessary to confirm an abnormality. In an attempt to improve diagnostic accuracy, investigators have used the sum of three mid-luteal progesterone measurements (normal $>45\,\text{nmol}\,\text{l}^{-1}$) or, in a research setting, daily progesterones (an area under the curve of $>320\,\text{nmol}\,\text{l}^{-1}$ is defined as normal). Although a group of subfertile women can be identified by these tests there are no controlled studies to see if the various treatments proposed for luteal phase deficiency significantly improve conception rates.

Endometrial biopsy

The sequential endometrial changes in the luteal phase of the cycle have been described by Noyes and colleagues [13]. If an endometrial biopsy is out of phase by two or more days with the expected day of the cycle, it has been proposed that this is diagnostic of luteal phase deficiency. Out-of-phase endometrial biopsies have been reported in 8%–31% of infertile women. Observer variation has been assessed by Scott and colleagues [14] and is small (0.9 ± 0.08 days). The problem in diagnosis is that the number of cycles that need to be biopsied to confirm the diagnosis has not been determined. Nor is the relationship to progesterone measurements clear. A progesterone of $>9\,\text{nmol}\,\text{l}^{-1}$ is sufficient to cause secretory changes in the endometrium but this level is clearly indicative of abnormal luteal function. A discrepancy between histological and endocrine data has been reported in up to 55% of samples.

The place of endometrial biopsy and serial progesterone measurements in infertility investigation cannot be defined adequately until the range of results in women with normal fertility is established and the fertility of women with abnormal results defined.

5.6.10 INVESTIGATION OF SPERM/CERVICAL MUCUS INTERACTION

The second major area of investigation in infertility is to assess the quality of spermatogenesis, i.e. sperm motility and number. The details of assessment of sperm function are discussed elsewhere. However cervical mucus is an important factor contributing to the adequacy of sperm function and fertility. The changes that occur in cervical mucus at mid-cycle, allowing it to become easily penetrable by sperm, are dependent on a normal preovulatory rise in oestradiol. Clinical assessment of cervical mucus alone is a poor predictor of fertility. Although the changes in cervical mucus that allow easy penetration of sperm are dependent on the preovulatory rise in oestradiol, serum oestradiol measurements are not a reliable guide to mucus quality in individual subjects. The post-coital test (PCT) looks at the interaction of cervical mucus with sperm. The PCT can be scored in a number of different ways but Hull and colleagues [15] interpreted a PCT as positive if there were >1 normally progressive sperm per high power field regardless of the cervical mucus score. This interpretation of the PCT predicted subsequent fertility. The two-year conception rate in couples with a positive PCT was 84% compared with 16% cumulative conception rate in couples with a negative PCT (defined as no forwardly progressive sperm despite adequate mucus).

Couples with a borderline or negative PCT require further investigation of adequacy of cervical mucus and sperm function. As the characteristics of cervical mucus are not predictive of fertility, a series of tests have been devised to assess sperm function in mucus.

Cross hostility testing

Cross hostility testing is an *in vitro* test using a sample of the patient's cervical mucus in the preovulatory phase of the cycle. The ability of the partner's semen to penetrate the mucus is assessed. After a fixed time interval (usually 1 hour) the number of sperm per high power field at various points from the edge of the mucus are counted and scored. The test is then repeated using the patient's mucus and donor semen. Donor mucus can also be used and the interaction of donor semen and donor mucus provides a control.

Sperm–mucus contact testing

Sperm–mucus contact testing (SCMC) assesses sperm function in mucus. The number of motile sperm that show shaking movements and are non-progressive in mucus are counted. A result is regarded as showing a significant abnormality if >50% of motile sperm shake and do not progress. It has been suggested that a positive SCMC indicates the presence of sperm antibodies. Although most patients (>90%) with a positive SCMC have sperm antibodies the titres vary widely, so the clinical significance cannot be predicted by this test.

Despite the various methods developed to assess sperm–mucus interaction, there is general agreement that a positive (i.e. abnormal) result is more likely to indicate a problem of sperm function. Poor sperm function in mucus has been shown by different groups to have a positive correlation with low sperm numbers, low sperm motility and to a lesser extent increased numbers of abnormally formed sperm. The degree of correlation varies with the different methods used.

5.6.11 TUBAL INFERTILITY

The final major area of infertility investigation is to determine whether there is any mechanical barrier to conception. This affects between 30% and 40% of infertile couples and is usually due to tubal dysfunction but occasionally to uterine abnormalities.

Laparoscopy and hysterosalpingography

are the most commonly used investigations to assess tubal function. The two procedures give good correlation when confirming tubal patency or diagnosing the site of tubal blockage [16]. The hysterosalpingogram is significantly worse at diagnosing peritubular and ovarian adhesions but gives a better assessment of the uterine cavity. It is our practice to use a laparoscopy as the initial investigation of tubal function unless history or examination suggests a uterine abnormality.

REFERENCES

1. Hull, M.G.R. (1989) Polycystic ovarian disease: clinical aspects and prevalence. In *Current Understanding of Polycystic Ovarian Disease. Research and Clinical Forums*, vol. 11, no. 4, Royal Wells Medical Press, UK.

2. Polson, D.W., Adam, J., Wadsworth, J. and Franks, S. (1988) Polycystic ovaries – a common finding in normal women. *Lancet*, 16 April, pp. 870–2.

3. Hull, M.G.R. (1987) Epidemiology of infertility and polycystic ovarian disease: endocrinological and demographic studies. *Gynecol. Endocrinol.*, **1**, 235–45.

4. New, M.I., Lorenzen, F., Lerner, A.J., Kohn, B., Oberfield, S.E., Pollack, M.S., Dupont, B., Stoner, E., Levy, D.J., Pang, S. and Levine, L.S. (1983) Genotyping steroid 21-hydroxylase deficiency: hormonal reference data. *J. Clin. Endocrinol. Metab.*, **57**, 320–6.

5. Meldrum, D.R. and Guy, E.A. (1979) Peripheral and ovarian venous concentrations of various steroid hormones in virilizing ovarian tumors. *Obstet. Gynec.*, **53**, 36–43.

6. Ireland, K. and Woodruff, J.D. (1976) Masculinizing ovarian tumors. *Obstet. Gynec. Surv.*, **31**, 83–111.

7. Moltz, L., Sorensen, R., Schwartz, U. and Hammerstein, J. (1984) Ovarian and adrenal vein steroids in healthy women with ovulatory cycles – selective catheterization findings. *J. Steroid Biochem.*, **20**, 901–5.

8. Surrey, E.M., de Ziegler, D., Gambone, J.C. and Judd, H.L. (1988) Preoperative localization of androgen-secreting tumors: clinical, endocrinologic, and radiologic evaluation of ten patients. *Am. J. Obstet. Gynec.*, **158**, 1313–22.

9. Hull, M.G.R., Savage, P.E., Bromham, D.R., Ismail, A.A.A. and Morris, A.F. (1982) The value of a single serum progesterone measurement in the midluteal phase as a criterion of a potentially fertile cycle ('ovulation') derived from treated and untreated conception cycles. *Fertil. Steril.*, **37**, 355–60.

10. Adams, J., Franks, S., Polson, D.W., Mason, H.D., Abdulwahid, N., Tucker, M., Morris, D.V., Price, J. and Jacobs, H.S. (1985) Multifollicular ovaries: clinical and endocrine features and response to pulsatile gonadotropin releasing hormone. *Lancet*, 21/28 December.

11. Hull, M.G.R., Knuth, U.A., Murray, M.A.F. and Jacobs, H.S. (1979) The practical value of the progestogen challenge test, serum oestradiol estimation or clinical examination in assessment of the oestrogen state and response to clomiphene in amenorrhoea. *Br. J. Obstet. Gynaec.*, **86**, 799–805.

12. Franks, S. (1987) Primary and secondary amenorrhoea. *Br. Med. J.*, **294**, 815–9.

13. Noyes, R.W., Hertig, A.T. and Rock, J. (1950) Dating the endometrial biopsy. *Fertil. Steril.*, **1**, 3.

14. Scott, R.T., Bagnall, J.A., Snyder, R.R., Reed, K.R., Strickland, D.M., Adair, C.A., Tyburski, C.C. and Hensley, S.B. (1988) The effect of interobserver variation in dating endometrial histology on the diagnosis of luteal phase defects. *Fertil. Steril.*, **50**, 888–92.

15. Hull, M.G.R., Savage, P.E. and Bromham, D.R. (1982) Prognostic value of the postcoital test: prospective study based on time-specific conception rates. *Br. J. Obstet. Gynaec.*, **89**, 299–305.

16. Fayez, J.A., Mutie, G. and Schneider, P.J. (1988) The diagnostic value of hysterosalpingography and laparoscopy in infertility investigation. *Int. J. Fertil.*, **33**, 98–101.

6

Disorders of sexual differentiation

M.O. SAVAGE and J.W. HONOUR

6.1 INTRODUCTION

Disorders of sexual differentiation are usually congenital abnormalities leading to ambiguous genitalia. Classification of patients with ambiguous genitalia (Table 6.1) depends upon karyotype and the formation and differentiation of the foetal gonads. Most patients with ambiguous genitalia can be included in one of these three categories.

6.2 PHYSIOLOGY OF FOETAL SEXUAL DIFFERENTIATION

A knowledge of normal sexual differentiation will provide a theoretical basis for the investigation of patients with ambiguous genitalia. In 1953, Jost established that the castrated male embryo develops as a female, indicating that the foetal testis is essential for male development [1]. The chromosomal sex of the embryo, established at conception, directs the development of either ovaries or testes. In the male, specific genes on the short arm of the Y-chromosome code for testis determination [2], and hence contribute to testicular differentiation. Testicular Leydig cells synthesize and secrete testosterone from 8 weeks of gestation, aided by stimulation with placental human chorionic gonadotropin (HCG). Testosterone diffuses locally to maintain and vir-

ilize the Wolffian ducts, which become the vas deferens, seminal vesicles and epididymis. Anti-mullerian hormone (AMH) or mullerian-inhibitory factor (MIF) is a glycoprotein member of the TGF-beta family which is secreted during the same time period by testicular Sertoli cells to inhibit the formation of the uterus, fallopian tubes and upper vagina from the mullerian structures.

In androgen dependent tissues testosterone is converted to dihydrotestosterone (DHT), which virilizes the external genitalia. Peripheral androgen action depends on the binding of the androgen in the target tissues to an X-chromosome controlled receptor (Fig. 6.1).

In the female, ovarian development occurs in the presence of two X-chromosomes and external gonadal development occurs spontaneously. Genital development in both sexes is completed by 20 weeks of foetal life. In the male, growth of the formed penis is dependent upon continued testicular testosterone secretion under stimulation by pituitary gonadotropins.

6.3 DIFFERENTIAL DIAGNOSIS OF AMBIGUOUS EXTERNAL GENITALIA

The causes of virilization of a female, inadequate development of the male genitalia and

Table 6.1 Classification of patients with ambiguous genitalia

1. Virilized female – virilization of genetic female with normal ovaries
2. Incomplete male – incomplete virilization of genetic male with differentiated testes
3. Abnormal gonadal differentiation

abnormal gonadal differentiation are given in Tables 6.2, 6.3 and 6.4, respectively.

The clinical picture affords some assessment of the time in development when sexual differentiation was disturbed. Individual disorders will be discussed in this chapter to illustrate the value of specific diagnostic tests. Genetic links are emerging for several of the conditions.

6.3.1 CLINICAL ASSESSMENT OF PATIENTS WITH AMBIGUOUS GENITALIA

The general appearance of the genitalia, while important when deciding the appropriate gender for the child, is of very little help in defining the aetiology of the primary disorder. Clitoral hypertrophy is a sign of androgen exposure after the twelfth week of gestation. Exposure at progressively earlier stages of differentiation leads to retention of the urogenital sinus and labioscrotal fusion which may appear rugose. If androgen exposure occurs sufficiently early in female foetal development the labia fuse to form a penile structure. An opening through which urine escapes, usually the exit of the urogenital sinus, is often sited near the base of the enlarged clitoris. In severe masculinization a more distal urethral orifice may be located ventrally between the phallic tip and

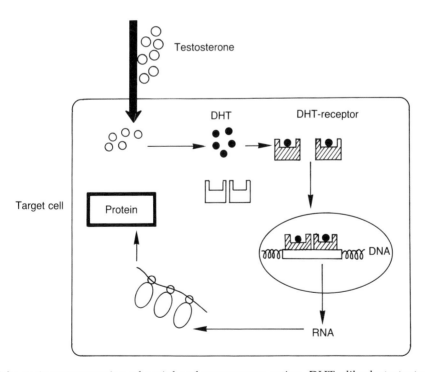

Fig. 6.1 Schematic representation of peripheral testosterone action. DHT, dihydrotestosterone.

107

Table 6.2 Causes of female pseudohermaphroditism

1. *Virilization by foetal androgens*
   Congenital adrenal hyperplasia
   21-Hydroxylase deficiency
   *11*β-Hydroxylase deficiency
   3β-Hydroxysteroid dehydrogenase deficiency
   Other causes of foetal androgen overproduction
   Foetal adrenal adenoma [3]
   Nodular adrenal hyperplasia [4]
   Persistent foetal adrenal in preterm infants [5]
2. *Foetal virilization by maternal hormones*
   Ovarian tumours [6,7]
   Adrenal tumours [8]
3. *Iatrogenic foetal virilization*
   Progestins [9]
4. *Female pseudohermaphroditism with associated congenital malformations* [10,11,12]
5. *Unexplained female pseudohermaphroditism* [13,14]
6. *Local lesions simulating female pseudohermaphroditism*
   Lipoma/haemangioma due to neurofibromatosis [15]

Table 6.3 Causes of male pseudohermaphroditism

1. Impaired Leydig cell activity
   Inborn errors of testosterone biosynthesis
   Deficient formation of pregnenolone
   3β-hydroxysteroid dehydrogenase defect
   17α-hydroxylase defect
   17,20-desmolase defect
   17β-hydroxysteroid dehydrogenase defect
   Leydig cell hypoplasia [16]
2. Impaired processing of androgens by peripheral tissues
   5α-reductase defect
   Androgen receptor defects
   Complete testicular feminization
   Incomplete testicular feminization
   Reinfenstein syndrome [17]
   Infertile male syndrome
   Post receptor resistance [18]
3. Other forms
   Iatrogenic male pseudohermaphroditism [19]
   Persistent mullerian structures [20]

Table 6.4 Causes of abnormal gonadal differentiation with ambiguous genitalia

Mixed gonadal dysgenesis [21]
Dysgenetic male pseudohermaphroditism [22]
Agonadism – micropenis with rudimentary testes [23]
Dysmorphic syndromes with hypogonadism [10]
True hermaphroditism [24]
XX male [25]
Drash syndrome [26,27]

the perineum. In males, micropenis is a sign of androgen withdrawal late in pregnancy. Pseudohermaphroditism is associated with a number of dysmorphic syndromes (Tables 6.2 and 6.3). In some cases the genital ambiguity remains unexplained or is the result of some local lesion.

Diagnostic tests are performed in the context of the clinical presentation of the patient. The principles of clinical assessment are shown in Table 6.5. Radiological investiga-

Table 6.5 Clinical assessment of a patient with ambiguous genitalia

---

Family history
Examination of external genitalia
General examination for dysmorphic features

1. No gonads palpable
   Female pseudohermaphroditism
   Male pseudohermaphrodite with intra-
       abdominal testes
2. One gonad palpable
   Abnormal gonadal differentiation
   Mixed gonadal dysgenesis (XO/XY)
   True hermaphroditism
3. Two gonads palpable
   Male pseudohermaphrodite
   True hermaphrodite with bilateral ovotestes

---

tions such as pelvic ultrasound and urethrogram may help to define the anatomy of the internal genitalia and the urethra, which may be seen to communicate posteriorly with a vaginal cavity.

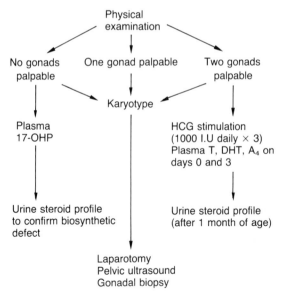

Fig. 6.2 Laboratory investigation of patients with ambiguous genitalia. T, testosterone; DHT, dihydrotestosterone; 17-OHP, 17-hydroxyprogesterone; HCG, human chorionic gonadotropin; A_4, androstenedione.

The most important part of the clinical examination is careful palpation for gonads. If no gonads are palpable a male may have intra-abdominal gonads, but the most likely diagnosis is female pseudohermaphroditism, commonly due to congenital adrenal hyperplasia (CAH). The diagnosis of CAH is virtually certain if symptoms of salt-loss develop over the ensuing 10 days after birth, though this can be normal in a preterm baby. If one gonad is palpable or there is asymmetry of the perineum, the likely diagnoses are mixed gonadal dysgenesis, characterized by a streak on one side and a testis on the other, or true hermaphroditism with asymmetrical gonads. When both gonads are palpable in the scrotum or labial folds, the patient is probably a male pseudohermaphrodite or conceivably a true hermaphrodite with bilateral ovotestes.

6.3.2 LABORATORY ASSESSMENT OF PATIENTS WITH AMBIGUOUS GENITALIA

In all patients a karyotype analysis is essential. A general scheme for further laboratory assessment based on clinical findings is shown in Fig. 6.2. This will now be described briefly, followed by a more detailed discussion of the important diagnosis procedures.

If no gonads are palpable and the karyotype is 46XX a raised 17-hydroxyprogesterone (17-OHP) will support the diagnosis of 21-hydroxylase deficiency. In 11β-hydroxylase deficiency plasma 11-deoxycortisol is elevated. Gas chromatography (GC) and mass spectrometry (MS) of urinary steroid metabolites (steroid profile analysis) may be helpful. In the patient with one palpable gonad an exploratory laparotomy will probably be necessary to define the anatomy of internal genitalia, i.e. possible mullerian structures. An intra-abdominal gonad should be biopsied to exclude an ovotestis. The patient with two palpable gonads requires an HCG stimulation test to assess testicular androgen secretion.

Basal and post-HCG levels of androgens are needed to distinguish a disorder of testosterone biosynthesis from a peripheral androgen resistance.

Urinary steroid profile analysis is not helpful in a newborn male with ambiguous genitalia and a likely biosynthetic defect of testosterone. If the child is aged 1 month or older a steroid profile may reveal evidence for 5α-reductase deficiency [28], thus avoiding an HCG injection and blood tests. The interpretation of a urine steroid profile based on ratios of steroid isometric metabolites must consider other factors, particularly thyroid function, which might affect steroid metabolism. In the very young infant GC/MS analysis of the urine steroids will be needed to be certain of the identity of steroids defining the defect.

Studies of *in vitro* androgen binding and determination of 5α-reductase activity in fibroblast cultures from genital skin may reveal evidence for defects of peripheral androgen action. A number of mutations have been found in the genes coding for androgen receptors on the X-chromosome [29] and type 2 5α-reductase [30].

6.3.3 INDIVIDUAL DIAGNOSTIC PROCEDURES

Karyotype analysis

Karyotype analysis from peripheral blood lymphocyte culture, using banding techniques, is essential in the investigation of all intersex patients. Analysis of fibroblasts cultured from gonadal tissue may also be helpful, sometimes identifying cell lines not detected in the peripheral blood. The child's management must be planned with the knowledge of the patient's genotype. Whereas the karyotype should not dictate gender assignment, certain abnormalities of sex chromosomes indicate a likely aetiology. For example, an XO/XY mosaic is usually seen in mixed gon-

adal dysgenesis [22]. Most true hermaphrodites are 46XX, although 13% are 46XX/46XY [24].

Determination of plasma steroid concentrations

The development of radioimmunoassay (RIA) methods for determination of plasma steroids has made a major contribution to the investigation of intersex disorders. Occasionally it has been possible to detect increased plasma steroid concentrations by high pressure liquid chromatography (HPLC) analysis with ultraviolet (UV) detection [31,32]. Three groups of steroid disorder are principally involved: (i) CAH [33], (ii) testosterone biosynthetic defects (Fig. 6.3) and (iii) disorders of peripheral androgen action [34].

The specificity of steroid assays by RIA is judged by cross-reactivity studies, which should demonstrate in the assay for one steroid low interference by related androgenic steroids. Ideally steroids should be separated by a chromatographic step prior to the RIA. A neat method for measuring DHT involves chemical oxidation of testosterone in the sample prior to RIA of the DHT with an antiserum to testosterone, which has a high cross-reaction for DHT [35].

When investigating the neonate it is important that steroids from the foetal adrenal zone are tested for cross-reactivity in any assay to measure plasma concentrations of steroids. Since the foetal adrenal steroids are conjugated with sulphuric acid these conjugates are not extracted into organic solvents, and this provides a means of separating the free steroid hormones from the foetal steroids. Even specialist laboratories offering measurements of 17-hydroxyprogesterone may be unable to distinguish the results from affected cases from normal values in the first few days of life. Thereafter there may still be difficulties in interpreting results in low birth weight and preterm infants [36].

110

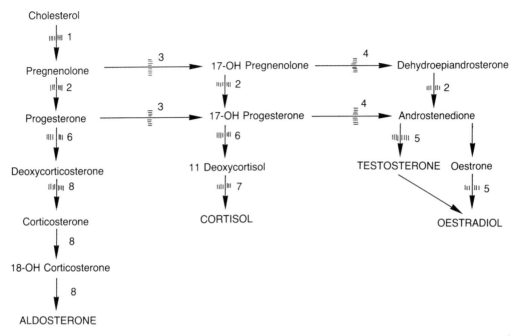

Fig. 6.3 Enzyme defects in steroid biosynthesis. 1, 20α-hydroxylase; 22α-hydroxylase, 20,22-desmolase; 2, 3β-hydroxysteroid dehydrogenase; 3, 17α-hydroxylase; 4, 17,20-desmolase; 5, 17β-hydroxysteroid dehydrogenase; 6, 21-hydroxylase; 7, 11β-hydroxylase; 8, 11β-hydroxylase, aldosterone synthase.

Determination of urinary steroid excretion

Androgen metabolites can be measured in urine by colorimetry as 17-oxosteroids, although many laboratories no longer offer this assay [37]. Androgen excretion rates will be raised in patients with CAH but this does not help the differential diagnosis of the causes of ambiguous genitalia. A more informative analysis of steroids in urine is obtained from an analysis which separates steroids using GC and detects the products with a flame ionization detector or by MS. The resulting steroid profile gives information about adrenal androgens and cortisol metabolism as well as revealing excess excretion of intermediates in the biosynthetic pathway from pregnenolone to the steroid hormones. The steroids are identified by their relative retention times in the chromatogram and by the fingerprint ob-

tained for each compound, which is given after analysis with a mass spectrometer [38].

Apart from the difficulties in collecting a 24-hour urine sample, a drawback of a steroid profile analysis is that several urine metabolites are produced from a given hormone (Table 6.6).

Catabolism of steroids takes place largely in the liver, where enzymes act on steroid hormones. These lead to:

1. Addition of four hydrogen atoms to saturate the A ring.
2. Reduction of the C-20 keto group.
3. Oxidation of the 17β-hydroxyl group.
4. Conjugation with glucuronic and sulphuric acid.

Some metabolites have names based on systematic nomenclature; others have trivial, even alphabetical, names. A number of factors

Table 6.6 Urine metabolites of steroid hormones

Testosterone	Androsterone (5α)
Androstenedione	Aetiocholanolone (5β)
Dehydroepiandrosterone (DHA)	
DHA-sulphate	DHA-S
17α-hydroxyprogesterone	17-hydroxypregnanolone
	Pregnanetriol
11-deoxycortisol (S)	Tetrahydro-S
Cortisol (F)	THF (5β)
	allo-THF (5α)
	Cortol
Cortisone (E)	THE
	Cortolone

have to be considered when making conclusions about the hormone from which urine products are derived.

In newborn children cortisol is actively oxidized to cortisone and most metabolites in the urine are of cortisone. Further hydroxylation of cortisone occurs at 1β and 6α positions to give extremely polar metabolites, which may be excreted as conjugates with glucuronic acid or without conjugation and which are often not extracted from urine into organic solvents [39,40]. Other steroids are likewise metabolized by the newborn infant in ways different from the adult.

The steroids from the definitive zone of the adrenal cortex are quantitatively less important than the androgens from the foetal adrenal cortex – mainly dehydroepiandrosterone sulphate (DHA-S). The different conjugation of the foetal steroids enables them to be extracted by chemical means, thus leaving the free and glucuronide conjugated products of the adult zone to be analysed separately. The sulphate fraction largely reflects the activity of the foetal adrenal cortex. An example of the profile from the glucuronide fraction of steroids obtained in this way from a normal infant is shown in Fig. 6.4a.

The steroid profiles from neonates are very much more complicated than the total steroid analysis of urine from an adult (Fig. 6.4b). Over the first 3–6 months, the foetal adrenal zone regresses and the excretion rates of the sulphated steroids diminish in most infants except those born before 30 weeks gestation. In many circumstances the excretion rates of steroids by normal children need to be corrected for body size and judged against normal ranges on this basis [41]. The diagnosis of CAH can usually be made on the basis of the grossly elevated excretion of precursor metabolites. A diagnosis of 5α-reductase can be made by looking at the ratios of 5α- to 5β-reduced metabolites of androgens and cortisol metabolites [42]. The value of this test depends on the age of the child. Unfortunately this is not useful in a newborn and, in general, in the young child the analysis should be performed with GC/MS in a specialist centre.

HCG stimulation test

In the paediatric patient, basal gonadal steroids are frequently undetectable in plasma, and gonadal function can often be assessed only by Leydig cell stimulation using HCG. This test is particularly helpful in the child with bilateral undescended testes, but the timing is critical. Immediately after birth, the plasma testosterone concentrations

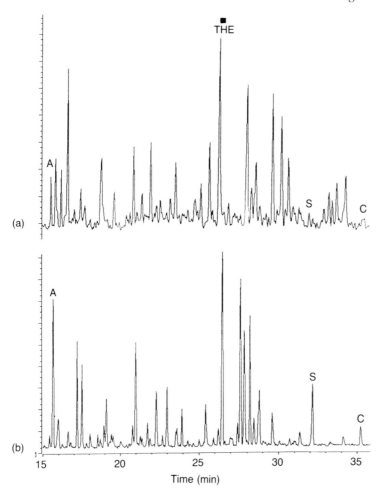

Fig. 6.4 Steroid analysis by capillary column gas chromatography: (a) glucuronide and free steroids in the urine of a newborn infant; (b) total steroids in the urine of an adult male. A, S and C are internal standards. After THE in the chromatogram of urinary steroids in the newborn there are a number of polar cortisone metabolites. In the adult, THE is followed by a series of cortisol metabolites, then cortolones and cortols.

of a normal male child can be up to 10 nmol l^{-1}. This level declines over the first week. A spontaneous rise of gonadotropins then occurs in males, such that plasma testosterone concentration is 3–12 nmol l^{-1} during the period from 10 to 60 days after birth [43]. This surge of testosterone may be helpful in defining the aetiology of male pseudohermaphroditism, as testosterone levels are normal or elevated in infants with androgen insensitivity and subnormal in testosterone biosynthetic defects [44].

Many different regimes exist for the HCG stimulation test. Samples for plasma androgens are taken basally then 24 or 48 hours after the last injection of HCG. Examples of regimes are 1000 IU × 3 at daily intervals, 2000 IU × 2 at 72-hour intervals and 1500 IU ×

113

7 at 48-hour intervals. Leydig cell desensitization occurs following multiple HCG injections [45], hence the rationale for alternate day administration. All these regimes induce significant elevation of plasma androgens with the amplitude of response increasing just before and during puberty. A two- to threefold increase in testosterone is seen in normal prepubertal males, with a more attenuated response expected during infancy and puberty [46].

Plasma gonadotropin levels

Determinations of plasma gonadotropins are unlikely to give diagnostic information in newborn infants with ambiguous genitalia. Luteinizing hormone (LH) measurements are justified at the time of expected puberty in patients with suspected androgen receptor defects where a characteristic pattern of LH and testosterone levels develops. LH secretion is elevated so that there is Leydig cell stimulation with high plasma levels of testosterone and oestradiol [17,47]. Some elevation of gonadotropins is seen in adult patients with 5α-reductase deficiency [48] but not to the same extent as in those with receptor defects. In primary gonadal defects such as gonadal dysgenesis, LH, and more especially follicle stimulating hormone (FSH), are elevated. Hypogonadotropic hypogonadism with inability to smell (Kallmann's syndrome) is caused by a defect of migration of the olfactory nerves and neurons producing gonadotropin releasing hormone. An intragenic deletion has been described [49].

In vitro studies of androgen binding and metabolism in genital skin fibroblasts

Simple androgen receptor binding studies have been developed for intact fibroblasts [34]. Testosterone and DHT are used as ligands. Synthetic steroids, methyltrienolone and mibolerone are also used, with the ad-

vantage of not being metabolized. Quantitative analysis of receptor binding has revealed three levels of activity in tissue from subjects with androgen insensitivity:

1. The majority, with undetectable binding.
2. The least common, with low receptor binding.
3. Receptor positive type, with normal or increased receptor number with qualitative defects of the androgen–receptor complex.

The 5α-reductase activity of skin fibroblasts of patients with defects of this enzyme is extremely variable, which undermines the reliability of the test. Three types of abnormality have been distinguished according to the binding affinity for:

1. Testosterone and nicotinamide adenine dinucleotide phosphate (NADPH).
2. NADPH.
3. Testosterone.

Laparotomy, pelvic ultrasound, gonadal biopsy and urethrogram

Laparotomy, pelvic ultrasound and gonadal biopsy are particularly helpful in investigating the patient with abnormal testicular differentiation. In this situation the anatomy and nature of any intra-abdominal genital structures may not be obvious from the external appearance of the genitalia. In males Mullerian remnants need to be identified and removed, as does ovarian tissue in a true hermaphrodite. Similarly, in a patient raised as a female all testicular tissue must be removed to prevent virilization. Intra-abdominal testicular tissue, when associated with gonadal dysgenesis, carries a high risk of malignancy [50] (Fig. 6.5).

A urethrogram can demonstrate the presence of a vaginal cavity communicating with the urethra and may also delineate Mullerian structures.

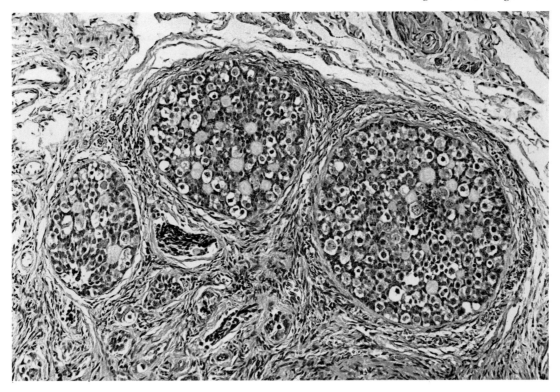

Fig. 6.5 Gonadoblastoma. A pre-malignant lesion in the intra-abdominal gonad of a patient with testicular dysgenesis.

Molecular biology

Genes encoding proteins involved in primary events of testicular differentiation appear to be located within the 60×10^6 base pairs on the Y-chromosome. Functional genes are localized in the proximal long arm and the short arm. Most of the chromosome comprises highly repeated sequences of DNA, so the preparation of specific probes for the Y-chromosome has been difficult. This is compounded by a possible evolutionary link with the X-chromosome and translocation with the autosomes. The application of molecular genetics to the study of single gene and chromosome defects is, however, revealing mutations which interfere with normal human sexual differentiation. Most 46XX males

have acquired a submicroscopic portion of the Y-chromosome with testis-determining material [51].

There is an increased risk of gonadal neoplasia in dysgenetic gonads when a Y-chromosome is present [50]. Y-chromosome DNA analysis may be useful in the search for part of the Y-chromosome [52].

Classical genetics was able to show that CAH due to steroid 21-hydroxylase deficiency is inherited as a monogenic autosomal recessive trait that is closely linked to the human leukocyte antigen (HLA) major histocompatibility complex on the short arm of chromosome 6 [33]. No such association was found for 11β-hydroxylase deficiency, which is coded separately in a region near chromosome 8q21. The genes for the enzymes in

Table 6.7 Location of genes encoding steroid bio-synthetic enzymes

	Chromosome
Mitochondrial	
20,22-desmolase (P450scc)	15
11β-hydroxylase	8
18-oxidase	8
Microsomal	
17α-hydroxylase/17,20-lyase	10
3β-hydroxysteroid dehydrogenase	1
21-hydroxylase	6

steroid biosynthesis have been cloned and localized throughout the genome (Table 6.7).

A number of techniques are now being used to study the molecular basis of CAH [53–56]. These methods include restriction fragment length polymorphisms, pulsed field gel electrophoresis and gene amplification with the polymerase chain reaction. Some of the defects ascribed to enzymes in steroid biosynthesis may prove to be due to abnormalities of the electron transport intermediates (e.g. adrenoxin, adrenodoxin reductase) [57,58].

Mutations in the X-linked androgen receptor gene in genetic males cause functional defects in the androgen receptor protein that result in the androgen insensitivity syndrome. Mutations have been found within the steroid binding domain and at points which affect the interactions with zinc fingers [59,60].

6.4 DIAGNOSIS OF SPECIFIC CAUSES OF AMBIGUOUS GENITALIA

6.4.1 THE VIRILIZED FEMALE

Congenital adrenal hyperplasia

The commonest causes of ambiguous genitalia in the newborn female are enzyme defects of cortisol synthesis with diversion of intermediates to androgen production [61]. A reduction in steroid 21-hydroxylase or absence of 11β-hydroxylase or 3β-hydroxysteroid dehydrogenase can be the cause of CAH. These enzymes are normally part of the steroid metabolic pathways which link intermediates between cholesterol and cortisol, and aldosterone and androgens (see Fig. 6.3). The division of steroid synthesis to these products reflects the functional activities of the zones of the adrenal cortex. The outer zona glomerulosa principally secretes aldosterone, the zona fasciculata is the site of cortisol production and the zona reticularis secretes androgens. In the absence of, or lowered potential for, cortisol production there are high adrenocorticotropic hormone (ACTH) concentrations, leading to adrenal hyperplasia and excess androgen production.

21-Hydroxylase deficiency

A defect of the steroid 21-hydroxylase deficiency accounts for 90% of cases of female pseudohermaphroditism and should be excluded before proceeding to assign other causes for ambiguous genitalia. CAH due to 21-hydroxylase deficiency causes variable virilization. In Europe 60% of all cases of steroid 21-hydroxylase deficiency will present in the first 10 days with a salt-losing crisis due to low production of aldosterone.

17-OHP is a biosynthetic precursor of cortisol and in patients with deficiency of 21-hydroxylase the production of 17-OHP increases and plasma levels are elevated. The measurement of 17-OHP in serum, plasma, saliva and blood spots is used to assist the diagnosis of this disorder. The timing of blood sampling is very important in order for the laboratory to interpret the findings. In all newborn infants 17-OHP concentrations in serum are above $100 \, \text{nmol} \, \text{l}^{-1}$ on the first day of life, and in term babies, but not necessarily in preterm babies, the levels fall over the first week to less than $5\,nmol\,l^{-1}$. After day 3 there is usually good discrimination of 17-OHP in affected cases $(100-800\,nmol\,l^{-1})$ from normal infants $(<15\,nmol\,l^{-1})$.

Differences in results of a directly measured 17-OHP compared with that measured in an organic extract of serum prior to the RIA suggest that steroids in blood (probably steroid sulphates from the foetal adrenal) interfere in the direct RIA, which gives an abnormally high result [36,62]. In normal neonates salivary concentrations of 17-OHP are $<1.5\,nmol\,l^{-1}$ and blood spot concentrations are $<70\,nmol\,l^{-1}$ [36,63]. A 17-OHP assay which involves solvent extraction before the RIA is essential.

Measurement of plasma renin activity (PRA) and aldosterone help to define the extent of enzyme blockage in the mineralocorticoid pathway and these tests can be used to monitor efficacy of treatment in CAH. Patients with the salt-losing rather than the simple virilizing form of 21-hydroxylase deficiency have high PRA and low aldosterone. The normal ranges for PRA and aldosterone are higher for newborn infants than for adults [64–66]. PRA falls to adult values by 3–5 years after birth.

The diagnosis of CAH needs to be confirmed or refuted as soon as possible in order to counsel parents anxious about the ambiguity of their newborn child. It used to be said that urine steroid analysis was unreliable. This is no longer true now that it is recognized that pregnanetriol is not an important metabolite of 17-OHP [67]. Also, with the help of MS, the structures of a number of unique metabolites have been elucidated [68], and a characteristic, very complicated urine steroid profile can be attributed to a number of steroids not having a 21-hydroxyl group [69]. (See Table 6.8 for other steroids in the profile). This diagnostic profile is recognized from day 3 after birth (Fig. 6.6). A result (including mass spectrometric analysis)

Table 6.8 Steroids in urine of newborn infant (not usually seen in urine of a normal neonate) characteristic of CAH due to 21-hydroxylase deficiency

17α-hydroxypregnanolone[a]
15β,17α-dihydroxypregnanolone
Pregnane-3α,17α,20α-triol[a]
3α,17α-dihydroxy-5β-pregnane-11,20-dione
3α,11β,17α-trihydroxy-5β-pregnan-20-one
16-hydroxypregnanolone
11-oxo-pregnanetriol[a]
3α,17α-dihydroxy-5α-pregnane-11,20-dione
5-pregnane-3,X,20,21-tetrol
3,X,Y-trihydroxy-5-pregnan-20-one

[a] Major steroids in adult with CAH (21-hydroxylase defect).

can be obtained within 30 hours of getting the sample to the laboratory.

The gene encoding 21-hydroxylase (CYP21B) has been characterized along with a 98% identical pseudogene (CYP21A). Located on the short arm of chromosome 6 in the midst of the class III HLA region, the gene is closely linked to the highly polymorphic genes encoding HLA-B and HLA-DR. Almost all of the mutations characterized so far in patients with 21-hydroxylase deficiency appear to result from recombinations between the CYP21B and CYP21A. These are either deletions caused by unequal crossing over during meiosis or apparent transfers of deleterious mutations as a result of a phenomenon called gene conversion [53,54,56,70]. Although molecular biology is not particularly useful as a diagnostic test in the newborn child with suspected CAH, the technology will have benefit for antenatal diagnosis in a family with an affected sibling. If the mutation is known, gene amplification techniques can be used with small amounts of tissue taken with chorionic villus biopsy. Tissue can be obtained around 10 weeks of the pregnancy and the tests can be completed within days [71]. Dexamethasone administration to

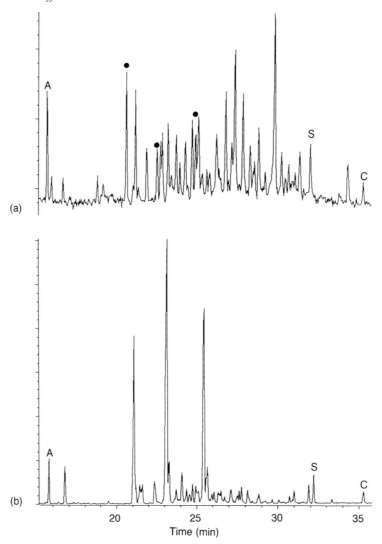

Fig. 6.6 Steroid profile of free and glucuronide steroids from the urine of a four-day-old baby with congenital adrenal hyperplasia due to 21-hydroxylase defect (a) compared with the profile in a 2-year-old (b). In the older child, there are only three main metabolites. Of these, the first peak (17-hydroxypregnanolone) is the most helpful for diagnosis in the newborn. The identities of other unusual steroids are given in Table 6.8.

the mother will lead to suppression of the foetal pituitary-adrenal axis and severe virilization may be prevented. This treatment must be started as early as possible in pregnancy, and if an affected female foetus is confirmed from the analysis on chorionic villi, then treatment must be continued to term. A full karyotype should be performed with the biopsy material to exclude chromosomal abnormalities such as Down's syndrome.

11β-Hydroxylase deficiency

In rare cases of CAH the defect is due to absence of the steroid 11β-hydroxylase and the serum concentration of 11-deoxycortisol (compound S) should be determined [72]. As with the interpretation of 17-OHP results in the newborn, care should be taken in assigning significance to a raised result for 11-deoxycortisol concentration in serum. In known cases of 11β-hydroxylase deficiency plasma S exceeds $1000 \, \text{nmol} \, l^{-1}$ [73]. A modestly elevated value by a direct RIA may be the result of interference in the assay and should be confirmed after extraction of steroids from plasma to an organic solvent. The urine steroid profile will show a relatively simple pattern with a high excretion of 6-hydroxytetrahydro-11-deoxycortisol as well as tetrahydro-S.

Androstenedione measurements may be helpful in the diagnosis and management of CAH due to 21-hydroxylase and 11β-hydroxylase defects [74,75]. In 11β-hydroxylase deficiency with a high production of deoxycorticosterone (a potent mineralo-corticoid) there is suppression of PRA with a rise on satisfactory adrenal suppression.

3β-Hydroxysteroid dehydrogenase (3β-OHSD) deficiency

This rare defect is difficult to confirm biochemically in a newborn child because the markers for the defect (dehydroepiandrosterone (DHA) and pregnenolone) are normal products of the adrenal in the newborn due to inactivity of this enzyme in the large foetal adrenal zone. The excretion rates of DHA metabolites may be elevated if corrected for body size and compared with appropriate normal data. Plasma DHA-S concentrations are high in preterm infants compared with infants delivered at term [76]. Infants with 3β-OHSD deficiency are usually very sick and a 24-hour steroid collection may not be possible before steroid treatment is necessary.

Plasma measurements of DHA and ACTH may help the diagnosis before steroids are given. In the short term dexamethasone or prednisolone are the preferred treatments because this allows measurements of endogenous steroids during an ACTH stimulation test. If a child suspected of having a 3β-OHSD defect is maintained with synthetic steroids (plus fludrocortisone if necessary for electrolyte balance) then given daily injections of depot ACTH (Synacthen) the markers for the defect (pregnenetriol, DHA) are clearly elevated in a urine steroid profile. The synthetic steroids have little effect on the steroid profile due to their lower excretion rate and different metabolism to the endogenous steroids. This approach was successful in one child maintained for several years on steroids [77]. Hydrocortisone ($15-20 \, \text{mg} \, M^{-2}$ per day) is the preferred long term treatment of a child with CAH. 3β-OHSD deficiency leads to low aldosterone production, consequently mineralo-corticoid replacement (fludrocortisone $150 \, \mu g \, m^{-2}$ per day) is needed. PRA is elevated prior to treatment but normalized with electrolyte control.

Clitoral hypertrophy in premature or low birth weight infants may suggest the diagnosis of CAH. The clinical appearance may be an artefact due to relative underdevelopment of the labia and often resolves as the infant gains weight. In very immature preterm babies (less than 30 weeks gestation) virilization has been attributed to androgen exposure (DHA) due to persistence of the foetal adrenal zone for months after birth. Some cases have required surgical clitoral reduction [5].

Other causes

Virilization of the genitalia has been attributed to maternal ingestion of progestogens and androgens. This is now less likely than the rare occasions in the past because most of the prescription drugs of this type are now much less potent. Other causes of a virilized female are the result of exposure to androgens from an adrenal or ovarian tumour. In these cases the child will have normal endocrinology after birth but will need corrective surgery on the external genitalia.

6.4.2 THE INCOMPLETE MALE

Incomplete virilization of a 46XY foetus is due to a failure of sex steroid production or to resistance to these hormones because of receptor defects [61]. Most laboratories will need the help of specialized centres to resolve such cases although certain investigations can be undertaken locally. Following confirmation of chromosomes, the serum concentrations of cortisol and testosterone should be checked. From these results some clear decisions can be made. Defects of sex steroid production with lack of testosterone synthesis during the critical period of gonadal development can be separated into:

1. Those affecting cortisol and androgen production (CAH).
2. Those affecting androgens alone.

Defects of cortisol and androgen production

Low steroid production in male pseudohermaphroditism can be attributed to rare forms of CAH due to defects of cholesterol 20,22-desmolase (side-chain cleavage), 17α-hydroxylase or 3β-OHSD. These enzymes affect the production of all important adrenal and gonadal steroids, and disorders of the enzymes can be fatal for the child, so few cases are documented in the literature.

Cholesterol 20,22-desmolase deficiency

20,22-Desmolase deficiency was initially called lipoid adrenal hyperplasia on account of the histological appearance of the large adrenals

at post-mortem [78]. This appearance reflects the ACTH stimulated adrenal, which cannot process cholesterol. When assessing whether there is a normal cortisol production it must be remembered that the circadian rhythm of cortisol does not emerge until a child is 6 months of age [79]. A single low result does not exclude normal cortisol production. To be certain, it may be necessary to perform an ACTH stimulation test. The laboratory should be clear of the extent to which cortisone is measured in the assay since this is more important in the newborn infant than cortisol itself. There is conflicting evidence about the nature of the lesion causing desmolase deficiency. Biochemically, P450scc protein may or may not be found in the tissue. Matteson and colleagues [80,81] were able to observe hybridization of DNA with oligonucleotide probes. The defects are therefore thought to be due to small deletions or point mutations. There are less than 40 cases in the literature. When reviewed in 1985, 56% were of Japanese heritage [82].

17α-Hydroxylase deficiency

17α-Hydroxylase deficiency is identified biochemically by demonstrating high serum levels and urine metabolites of progesterone and corticosterone [83]. 17α-Hydroxylase deficiency is associated with low PRA. The experience with urine steroid profile analysis in such cases in the newborn period is limited. The pattern of steroids in urine of one case, later confirmed to have 17α-hydroxylase deficiency, showed unusually high excretion rates of 16α-hydroxypregnenolone. At 15 months of age the child excreted excess corticosterone metabolites, just as is found in the urine of adults with this disease [84]. A 46XX foetus with this defect is phenotypically normal and most cases are not detected until hypertension or failure of puberty are investigated. Base deletions and duplications leading to stop and termination codons have explained several of the deficiencies in the enzyme in patients with 17α-hydroxylase deficiency [55,85,86].

3β-OHSD deficiency

3β-OHSD deficiency in a male is associated with poor masculinization. Pregnenetriol (metabolite of 17-hydroxypregnenolone) is the marker for the defect in urine [87]. DHA [88] and 16-hydroxy-DHA are also elevated. Males with defects of cortisol and androgen production can be reared as boys needing adrenal steroid replacement with the addition of androgens at puberty. In 3β-OHSD deficiency PRA is elevated. Treatment can be monitored to some extent by normalization of PRA.

Defects of androgen production

The HCG test will, in many cases, be necessary to unmask or accentuate an enzyme deficiency affecting testosterone production.

17-Ketosteroid reductase deficiency

Infants with this defect are born with female looking external genitalia and a phallus closely resembling a normal clitoris. On closer examination there may be mild posterior fusion of the labial–scrotal folds and a urogenital sinus. There is a high prevalence within the Arab population of the Gaza Strip. This defect is confirmed when the ratio of androstenedione to testosterone is elevated [89,90], particularly after HCG stimulation. Infants may present with swelling in the groin or labia. There is marked virilization at puberty.

5α-Reductase deficiency

The rare 5α-reductase deficiency seems to occur more frequently in consanguinous communities. There is failure of conversion of testosterone to DHT so that external genital virilization is impaired. An HCG test can contribute to the diagnosis, which is made by demonstrating elevated testosterone to DHT ratio in plasma [91,92] or an elevated ratio of 5β to 5α metabolites (aetiocholanolone to androsterone) in urine [42,93]. In a urine steroid profile there is evidence for this disorder also in the distribution of cortisol metabolites (high ratio of tetrahydrocortisol to allo-tetrahydrocortisol) [28]. In newborns, however, the majority of cortisol metabolites reflect the strong oxidation to cortisone for which there is no isomeric pair of metabolites to measure. A raised tetrahydrocortisol (THF) to α-THF ratio is nevertheless useful for assessing the defect in suspected cases aged 1 month to 4–7 years when the excretion of androgens may be too low to make an assessment from the ratio of aetiocholanolone to androsterone. The low ratio of 5α- to 5β-reduced cortisol metabolites can be detected around 1 month of age if GC/MS is used to look at the ratio of 5α-THF to THF, which are present at too low a level to be measured accurately by GC analysis alone. The ambiguity of genitalia may be so mild that the child may be reared as a female until puberty, when there is a striking development of male musculature and psychosexual orientation, reflecting the pubertal surge of testosterone.

17,20-Desmolase deficiency

To some extent the 17,20-desmolase defect [94] is related to the 17-hydroxylase defect. The association between the two defects is due to the fact that these enzyme activities are coded by the same gene [81]. The appearance of the external genitalia may vary from female through male with perineal hypospadias to hypoplastic male. At puberty there may be raised 17-hydroxyprogesterone, 17-hydroxypregnenolone and gonadotropins. HCG produces a marked rise in plasma levels of these steroids without change in the already low androgens. There is a similar response to ACTH, showing the absence of the defect in the adrenal as well as the gonads [95,96]. Testicular tissue fails to metabolize C_{21}-steroids to androgens.

REFERENCES

1. Jost, A. (1953) Hormonal and genetic factors affecting the development of the male genital system. *Recent Prog. Horm. Res.*, **8**, 379–413.
2. Page, D.C., Mosher, R., Simpson, E.M., Fisher, E.M.C., Mardon, G., Pollack, J., McGillivray, B., Chapelle, A. de la and Brown, L.G. (1987) The sex-determining region of the human Y chromosome encodes a finger protein. *Cell*, **51**, 1091–104.
3. Kenny, F.M., Nashida, Y. and Askari, A. (1968) Virilising adrenal tumors of the adrenal cortex. *Am. J. Dis. Childh.*, **115**, 445–51.
4. Donaldson, M.D.C., Grant, D.B., O'Hare, M.J. and Shackleton, C.H.L. (1981) Familial congenital Cushing's syndrome due to bilateral nodular hyperplasia. *Clin. Endocrinol.*, **14**, 519–26.
5. Midgley, P., Azzopardi, D., Oates, N., Shaw, J.C.L. and Honour, J.W. (1990) Virilisation of female preterm infants. *Archs Dis. Childh.*, **65**, 701–3.
6. Verhoeven, A.T.M., Mostblum, J.L., van Lonsden, H.A.I.M. and van der Velden, W.H.M. (1973) Virilisation in pregnancy coexisting with an ovarian mucinous cystadenoma; a case report and review of virilising ovarian tumours in pregnancy. *Obstet. Gynec. Surv.*, **28**, 597–622.
7. Hensleigh, P.A. and Woodruff, J.D. (1978) Differential maternal–fetal response to androgenising luteoma or hyperreaction luteinalis. *Obstet. Gynec. Surv.*, **33**, 262–7.
8. Kirk, J.M.W., Perry, L.A., Shand, W.S., Kirby, R.S., Besser, G.M. and Savage, M.O. (1990) Female pseudohermaphroditism due to a maternal adrenocortical tumor. *J. Clin. Endocrinol. Metab.*, **70**, 1280–4.
9. Grumbach, M.M., Ducharme, J.R. and Molokshok, R.E. (1959) On the fetal masculinising action of certain oral progestins. *J. Clin. Endocrinol. Metab.*, **19**, 1369–80.
10. Rimoin, D.L. and Schimke, R.N. (1971) *Genetic Disorders of the Endocrine Glands*, C.V. Mosby, St Louis.
11. Park, I.J., Jones, H.J.W and Melhem, R.E. (1972) Non adrenal familial female pseudo-hermaphroditism. *Am. J. Obstet. Gynec.*, **112**, 930–4.
12. Dubowitz, V. (1962) Virilisation and malformation of a female infant. *Lancet*, **ii**, 405–9.
13. Grumbach, M.M. and Ducharme, J.R. (1960) The effects of androgens on fetal sex and development. *Fertil. Steril.*, **11**, 157–80.
14. Gordon, L.S., Morillo-Gucci, G., Mulholland, G., Simpson, J.L. and German, J. (1981) Progressive idiopathic clitoral hypertrophy in a child. *Birth Defects*, ser. 10, 201–3.
15. Haddad, H.A. and Jones, H.W. (1960) Clitoral enlargement simulating pseudohermaphroditism. *Am. J. Dis. Child.*, **99**, 282–7.
16. Berthezene, F., Forest, M.G., Grimaud, J.A., Claustrat, B. and Mornex, R. (1976) Leydig cell agenesis. *New Engl. J. Med.*, **295**, 969–72.
17. Wilson, J.D., Harrod, M.J., Hemsell, D.L. and McDonald, P.C. (1974) Familial incomplete male pseudohermaphroditism type 1: evidence for androgen resistance and variable manifestation in a family with Reifenstein syndrome. *New Engl. J. Med.*, **290**, 1097–103.
18. Griffin, J.E. and Wilson, J.D. (1980) The syndromes of androgen resistance. *New Engl. J. Med.*, **302**, 198–209.
19. Aarskog, D. (1970) Clinical and cytogenic studies in hypospadias. *Acta Paediat. Scand.*, suppl. 203.
20. Brook, C.G.D., Wagner, H., Zachmann, M., Prader, A., Armendares, S., Frenk, S., Aleman, P., Najjar, S.S., Slim, M.S., Genton, N. and Bozic, C. (1973) Familial occurrence of persistent mullerian structures in otherwise normal males. *Br. Med. J.*, **1**, 771–3.
21. Donahue, P.K., Crawford, J.D. and Hendred, W.H. (1979) Mixed gonadal dysgenesis, pathogenesis and management. *J. Paediat. Surg.*, **14**, 287–300.
22. Rajfer, J. and Walsh, P.C. (1981) Mixed gonadal dysgenesis – dysgenic male pseudohermaphroditism. In *The Intersex Child: Paediatric and Adolescent Endocrinology*, **8**, 105–15.
23. Dewhurst, C.J., Paine, C.G. and Blank, C.E. (1963) An XY female with absent gonads and vestigial pelvic organs. *Br. J. Obstet. Gynaec.*, **70**, 675–84.

24. Niekerk, W.A. van (1981) True hermaphroditism. In *The Intersex Child: Paediatric and Adolescent Endocrinology*, **8**, 80–99.

25. Chapelle, A. de la (1972) Analytical review: nature and origin of males with XX sex chromosomes. *Am. J. Hum. Genet.*, **24D**, 71–105.

26. Habib, R., Loirat, C., Gubler, M.C., Niaudet, P., Bensman, A., Levy, M. and Broyer, M. (1985) The nephropathy associated with male pseudohermaphroditism and Wilms' tumour (Drash syndrome): a distinctive glomerular lesion – report of 10 cases. *Clin. Nephrol.*, **24**, 269–78.

27. Pelletier, J., Breuning, W., Kashtan, C.E., Mauer, S.M., Manivel, J.C., Striegel, J.E., Houghton, D.C., Junien, C., Habib, R., Fouser, L., Fine, R.N., Silverman, B.L., Haber, D.A. and Housman, D. (1991) Germline mutations in the Wilms' tumor suppressor gene are associated with abnormal urogenital development in Denys–Drash syndrome. *Cell*, **67**, 437–47.

28. Imperato-McGinley, J., Gautier, T., Pichardo, M. and Shackleton, C.H.L. (1986) The diagnosis of 5α-reductase deficiency in infancy. *J. Clin. Endocrinol. Metab.*, **63**, 1313–18.

29. Imperato-McGinley, J. and Canovatchel, W.J. (1992) Complete androgen insensitivity – pathophysiology, diagnosis and treatment. *Trends Endocrinol. Metab.*, **3**, 75–81.

30. Labrie, F., Sugimoto, Y., Luu-The, V., Simard, J., Lachance, Y., Bachvarov, D., Leblanc, G., Durocher, F. and Faquet, N. (1992) Structure of the human type II 5α-reductase gene. *Endocrinology*, **131**, 1571–3.

31. Canalis, E., Calderella, A.M. and Rearden, G.E. (1979) Serum cortisol and 11-deoxycortisol by liquid chromatography. Clinical studies and comparison with radioimmunoassay. *Clin. Chem.*, **25**, 1700–3.

32. Stoner, E., Loche, S., Mirth, A. and New, M.I. (1986) Clinical utility of adrenal steroid measurement by high performance liquid chromatography in pediatric endocrinology. *J. Chromat.*, **374**, 358–62.

33. New, M.I., White, P.C., Speiser, P.W., Crawford, C. and Dupont, B. (1989) Congenital adrenal hyperplasia. *Recent Adv. Endocrinol. Metab.*, **3**, 29–76.

34. Hughes, I.A. and Pinsky, L. (1989) Sexual differentiation. In *Paediatric Endocrinology* (ed.

R. Collu, J.R. Ducharme and H.J. Guyda), Raven, New York, pp. 251–93.

35. Puri, V., Puri, C. and Anand Kumar, T.C. (1981) Serum levels of dihydrotestosterone in male rhesus monkeys estimated by non-chromatographic radioimmunoassay method. *J. Steroid Biochem.*, **14**, 877–81.

36. Wallace, A.M., Beesley, J., Thomson, M., Giles, C.A., Ross, A.M. and Taylor, N.F. (1987) Adrenal status during the first month of life in mature and immature infants. *J. Endocrinol.*, **112**, 473–80.

37. Rudd, B.T. (1983) Urinary 17-oxogenic and 17-oxosteroids. A case for deletion from the clinical chemistry repertoire. *Ann. Clin. Biochem.*, **20**, 65–71.

38. Shackleton, C.H.L., Taylor, N.F. and Honour, J.W. (1980) *An Atlas of Gas Chromatographic Profiles of Neutral Steroids in Health and Disease*, Packard-Becker DV, Delft.

39. Derks, H.J.G. and Drayer, N.M. (1978) The identification and quantification of three new 6-hydroxylated corticosteroids in human neonatal urine. *Steroids*, **31**, 289–305.

40. Taylor, N.F., Curnow, D.H. and Shackleton, C.H.L. (1978) Analysis of glucocorticoid metabolites in the neonatal period: catabolism of cortisone acetate by an infant with 21-hydroxylase deficiency. *Clinica Chim. Acta*, **85**, 219–29.

41. Honour, J.W. (1989) The adrenal cortex. In *Clinical Paediatric Endocrinology*, 2nd edn (ed. C.G.D. Brook), Blackwell, Oxford, pp. 341–67.

42. Peterson, R.E., Imperato-McGinley, J., Gautier, T. and Shackleton, C.H.L. (1985) Urinary steroid metabolites in subjects with male pseudohermaphroditism secondary to 5α-reductase deficiency. *Clin. Endocrinol.*, **23**, 494–500.

43. Forest, M.G. and Cathiard, A.M. (1975) Patterns of plasma testosterone and androstenedione in normal newborns: evidence for testicular activity at birth. *J. Clin. Endocrinol. Metab.*, **41**, 977–80.

44. Chaussain, J.C., Gendrel, D., Roger, M., Boudailleiz, B. and Job, J.C. (1979) Longitudinal study of plasma testosterone in male pseudohermaphroditism during early infancy. *J. Clin. Endocrinol. Metab.*, **49**, 305–6.

45. Forest, M.G., David, M., Lecoq, A., Jeune, M.

and Bertrand, J. (1980) Kinetics of the HCG-induced steroidogenic response of the human testis III. Studies in children of the plasma levels of testosterone and HCG: rationale for testicular stimulation test. *Pediat. Res.*, **14**, 819–24.

46. Hughes, I.A. (1986) *Handbook of Endocrine Tests in Children*, Wright, Bristol.

47. Savage, M.O., Chaussain, J.L., Evain, D., Roger, M., Canlorbe, P. and Job, J.C. (1978) Endocrine studies in male pseudohermaphroditism in childhood and adolescence. *Clin. Endocrinol.*, **12**, 397–406.

48. Peterson, R.E., Imperato-McGinley, J., Gautier, T. and Sturla, E. (1977) Male pseudohermaphroditism due to steroid 5-alpha reductase deficiency. *Am. J. Med.*, **62**, 170–91.

49. Bick, D., Franco, B., Sherins, R.J., Heye, B., Maddalena, A., Incerti, B., Pragiola, A., Mettinger, T. and Ballabio, A. (1992) Intragenic deletion of KALIG-1 gene in Kallmann's syndrome. *New Engl. J. Med.*, **326**, 1752–5.

50. Savage, M.O. and Lowe, D.G. (1990) Gonadal neoplasia and abnormal sexual differentiation. *Clin. Endocrinol.*, **32**, 519–33.

51. Anderson, M., Page, D.C. and Chapelle, A. de la (1986) Chromosome Y-specific DNA is transferred to the short arm of the X-chromosome in human XX males. *Science*, **233**, 786–8.

52. Tho, S.P.T. and McDonough, P.G. (1987) Use of Y DNA probes to identify children at risk for dysgenetic gonadal tumors. *Clin. Obstet. Gynaec.*, **30**, 671–81.

53. Rumsby, G., Fielder, A.H.L., Hague, W.M. and Honour, J.W. (1988) Heterogeneity in the gene locus for steroid 21-hydroxylase deficiency. *J. Med. Genet.*, **25**, 596–9.

54. White, P.C. and New, M.I. (1988) Molecular genetics of congenital adrenal hyperplasia. *Clin. Endocrinol. Metab.*, **2**, 941–65.

55. Yanase, T., Kagimoto, M., Matsui, N., Simpson, E.R. and Waterman, M.R. (1989) Combined 17α-hydroxylase/17,20 lyase deficiency due to a stop codon in the N-terminal region of 17α-hydroxylase cytochrome P-450. *Molec. Cell. Endocrinol.*, **59**, 249–53.

56. Collier, S., Sinnott, P.J., Dyer, P.A., Price, D.A., Harris, R. and Strachan, T. (1989) Pulsed field gel electrophoresis identifies a high degree of variability in the number of tandem 21-hydroxylase and complement C4 gene repeats in 21-hydroxylase deficiency haplotypes. *EMBO J.*, **8**, 1393–1402.

57. Peterson, R.E., Imperato-McGinley, J., Gautier, T. and Shackleton, C.H.L. (1985) Male pseudohermaphroditism due to multiple defects in steroid-biosynthetic microsomal mixed-function oxidases. *New Engl. J. Med.*, **313**, 1182–91.

58. Miller, W.L. (1986) Congenital adrenal hyperplasia. *New Engl. J. Med.*, **314**, 1321–2.

59. Hughes, I.A. and Evans, B.A.J. (1986) Complete androgen insensitivity syndrome characterised by increased concentration of a normal androgen receptor in genital skin fibroblasts. *J. Clin. Endocrinol. Metab.*, **63**, 309–15.

60. Quigley, C.A., Evans, B.A., Simenthal, J.A., Marschke, K.B., Sar, M., Lubahn, D.B., Davies, P., Hughes, I.A., Wilson, E.M. and French, F.S. (1992) *Molec. Endocrinol.*, **6**, 1103–12.

61. New, M.I. and Josso, N. (1988) Disorders of gonadal differentiation and congenital adrenal hyperplasia. *Endocrinol. Metab. Clin. North Am.*, **17**, 339–66.

62. Makella, S.K. and Ellis, G. (1988) Non-specificity of a direct 17-hydroxyprogesterone radioimmunoassay kit when used with samples from neonates. *Clin. Chem.*, **34**, 2070–5.

63. Walker, R.F., Read, G.F., Hughes, I.A. and Riad-Fahmy, D. (1979) Radioimmunoassay of 17-hydroxyprogesterone in saliva, parotid fluid and plasma of congenital adrenal hyperplasia patients. *Clin. Chem.*, **25**, 542–5.

64. Sassard, J., Sann, L., Vincent, M., Francois, R. and Cier, J.F. (1975) Plasma renin activity in normal subjects from infancy to puberty. *J. Clin. Endocrinol. Metab.*, **40**, 524–5.

65. Dillon, M.J., Gillin, M.E.A., Ryness J.M. and de Swiet, M. (1976) Plasma renin activity and aldosterone concentration in the human newborn. *Archs Dis. Childh.*, **51**, 537–40.

66. Fiselier, T., Lijnen, P., Monnens, L., van Munster, P., Jansen, M. and Peer, P. (1983) Levels of renin, angiotensin I and II, angiotensin covering enzyme and aldosterone in

infancy and childhood. *Eur. J. Paediat.*, **141**, 3–7.

67. Holsboer, F. and Knorr, D. (1977) Determination of urinary 17-hydroxypregnanolone by gas chromatography – mass spectrometry in patients with congenital adrenal hyperplasia. *J. Steroid Biochem.*, **8**, 1197–9.

68. Joannou, G.E. (1981) Identification of 15β-hydroxylated C_{21} steroids in the neonatal period: the role of 3, 15β, 17-trihydroxy-5β-pregnan-20-one in the perinatal diagnosis of congenital adrenal hyperplasia (CAH) due to 21-hydroxylase deficiency. *J. Steroid Biochem.*, **14**, 901–12.

69. Honour, J.W. (1986) Biochemical aspects of congenital adrenal hyperplasia. *J. Inherited Metab. Dis.*, **9**, suppl. 1, 124–34.

70. Spieser, P.W., Dupont, J., Zhu, D., Serrat, J., Buegeleisen, M., Tusie-Luna, M.-T., Lesser, M., New, M.I. and White, P.C. (1992) Disease expression and molecular genotype in congenital adrenal hyperplasia due to 21-hydroxylase deficiency. *J. Clin. Invest.*, **90**, 584–95.

71. Rumsby, G. and Honour, J.W. (1990) *In vitro* gene amplification for antenatal diagnosis of congenital adrenal hyperplasia. *J. Med. Genet.*, **27**, 676–8.

72. Perry, L.A., Al-Dujaili, E.A.S. and Edwards, C.R.W. (1982) A direct radioimmunoassay for 11-deoxycortisol. *Steroids*, **9**, 115–28.

73. Hughes, I.A., Arisaka, O., Perry, L.A. and Honour, J.W. (1986) Early diagnosis of 11β-hydroxylase deficiency in two siblings confirmed by analysis of a novel steroid metabolite in newborn urine. *Acta Endocrinol., Copenhagen*, **111**, 349–54.

74. Besch, N.F., Buoy, E., Haller, W.S., Johnson, H.J. and Besch, P.K. (1986) Radioimmunoassay for 4-androsten-3,17-dione, including the synthesis, production and characterisation of the antiserum. *Clin. Chem.*, **32**, 1357-67.

75. Thomson, S., Wallace, A.M. and Cook, B. (1989) A ^{125}I radioimmunoassay for measuring androstenedione in serum and blood spot samples from neonates. *Clin. Chem.*, **35**, 1707–12.

76. Grueters, A. and Korth-Schutz, S. (1982) Longitudinal study of plasma dehydroepi-androsterone sulfate in preterm and fullterm infants. *J. Clin. Endocrinol. Metab.*, **55**, 314–20.

77. Taylor, N.F., Clymo, A.B. and Shackleton, C.H.L. (1978) Steroid excretion by an infant with 3β-hydroxysteroid dehydrogenase deficiency during conventional replacement therapy and following corticotrophin stimulation. *J.Endocrinol.*, **80**, 62.

78. Prader, A. and Gurtner, H.P. (1955) Das syndrom pseudohermaphroditus masculinus bei kongenitaler nebernieenrinden – hyperplasia ohne androgen uber produktion. *Helv. Paediat. Acta*, **10**, 397–412.

79. Price, D.A., Close, G.C. and Fielding, B.A. (1983) Age of appearance of circadian rhythm in salivary cortisol in infancy. *Archs Dis. Childh.*, **58**, 454–6.

80. Matteson, K.J., Chung, B.-C., Urdea, M.S. and Miller, W.L. (1986) Study of cholesterol side-chain cleavage (20,22 desmolase) deficiency causing congenital lipoid adrenal hyperplasia using bovine-sequence P450scc oligo-deoxynucleotide probes. *J. Clin. Endocrinol. Metab.*, **118**, 1296–1305.

81. Matteson, K.M.J., Picardo-Leonard, J., Chung, B.-C., Mohandas, T.K. and Miller, W.M. (1986) Assignment of the gene for adrenal P450c17 (steroid 17α-hydroxylase/17,20 lyase) to human chromosome 10. *J. Clin. Endocrinol. Metab.*, **63**, 789–91.

82. Haufa, B.P., Miller, W.L., Grumbach, M.M., Conte, F.A. and Kaplan, S.L. (1985) Congenital adrenal hyperplasia due to deficient cholesterol side-chain cleavage activity (20,22 desmolase) in a patient treated for 18 years. *Clin. Endocrinol.*, **23**, 481–93.

83. Tourniaire, J., Audi-Parera, L., Loras, B., Blum, J., Castelnovo, P. and Forest, M.G. (1976) Male pseudohermaphroditism with hypertension due to 17α-hydroxylase deficiency. *Clin. Endocrinol.*, **5**, 53–61.

84. Dean, H.J., Shackleton, C.H.L. and Winter, J.S.D. (1984) Diagnosis and natural history of 17α-hydroxylase deficiency in a newborn male. *J. Clin. Endocrinol. Metab.*, **59**, 513–20.

85. Kagimoto, M., Winter, J.S.D., Kagimoto, K., Simpson, E.R. and Waterman, M.R. (1988) Structural characterisation of normal and mutant human steroid 17α-hydroxylase genes: molecular basis of one example of combined 17α-hydroxylase/17,20 lyase deficiency. *Molec.*

Endocrinol., **2**, 564–70.

86. Kagimoto, K., Waterman, M.R., Kagimoto, M., Ferreira, P., Simpson, E.R. and Winter, J.S.D. (1989) Identification of a common molecular basis for combined 17α-hydroxylase/17,20 lyase deficiency. *Hum. Genet.*, **82**, 285–6.

87. Bongiovanni, A.M. (1962) The adrenogenital syndrome with deficiency of 3-beta hydroxysteroid dehydrogenase. *J. Clin. Invest.*, **41**, 2086–92.

88. Martin, F., Perheentupa, J. and Adlercreutz, H. (1980) Plasma and urinary androgens in a pubertal boy with 3β-hydroxysteroid dehydrogenase deficiency. *J. Steroid Biochem.*, **13**, 197–201.

89. Balducci, R., Toscano, V., Wright, F., Bozzalan, F., Dipiero, G., Maroder, M., Pauli, P., Sciara, F. and Boscherini, B. (1985) Familial male pseudohermaphroditism with gynaecomastia due to 17β-hydroxysteroid dehydrogenase deficiency – a report of 3 cases. *J. Clin. Endocrinol. Metab.*, **23**, 439–44.

90. Gross, D.J., Landau, H., Kohn, G., Farkas, A., Elrayyes, E., El-Shawwa, R., Lasch, R.R. and Rosler, A. (1986) Male pseudohermaphroditism due to 17β-hydroxysteroid dehydrogenase deficiency: gender assignment in early infancy. *Acta Endocrinol., Copenhagen*, **112**, 238–46.

91. Savage, M.O., Preece, M.A., Jeffcoate, S.L., Ransley, P.G., Rumsby, G., Mansfield, M.D. and Williams, D.I. (1980) Familial male pseudohermaphroditism due to deficiency of 5α-reductase. *Clin. Endocrinol.*, **12**, 397–406.

92. Greene, S., Zachmann, M., Manella, B., Hesse, V., Hoepffner, W., Willgerodt, H. and Prader, A. (1987) Comparison of two tests to recognize or exclude 5α-reductase deficiency in prepubertal children. *Acta Endocrinol., Copenhagen*, **114**, 114–17.

93. Corrall, R.J.M., Wakelin, K., O'Hare, J.P., O'Brian, I.A.D., Ismail, A.A.A. and Honour, J.W. (1984) 5α-reductase deficiency: diagnosis via abnormal plasma levels of reduced testosterone derivatives. *Acta Endocrinol., Copenhagen*, **107**, 538–43.

94. Kaufmann, F.R., Costin, G., Goebelsmann, A., Stancyk, F.Z. and Zachmann, M. (1983) Male pseudohermaphroditism due to 17,20-desmolase deficiency. *J. Clin. Endocrinol. Metab.*, **57**, 32–6.

95. Forest, M.G., Lecornu, M. and De Peretti, E. (1980) Familial male pseudohermaphroditism due to 17,20-desmolase deficiency I. In vivo endocrine studies. *J. Clin. Endocrinol. Metab.*, **50**, 826–33.

96. Zachmann, M., Werder, E.A. and Prader, A. (1982) Two types of male pseudohermaphroditism due to 17,20-desmolase deficiency. *J. Clin. Endocrinol. Metab.*, **55**, 487–90.

7

Diagnostic tests in calcium disorders

D.C. ANDERSON and P.C. RICHARDSON

7.1 INTRODUCTION

7.1.1 CALCIUM AND PHOSPHORUS METABOLISM (Fig. 7.1)

Most of the body's calcium (99%) and phosphorus (85%) are in bone. In the child, calcium and phosphorus are retained for skeletal growth. In the adult, only enough is retained to offset obligatory losses, normally in urine and faeces. During pregnancy and lactation, extra losses occur through transfer to the foetus and breast milk, respectively. Regulation of calcium excretion in the kidney is controlled by tubular reabsorption, and in the bowel, by endogenous secretion. Thus, calcium and phosphorus absorption need to be adapted to changing physiological requirements.

Serum calcium and phosphate also need to be controlled within narrow limits for normal neuromuscular function and other cell functions to occur. The hormones essential for control of calcium and phosphorus metabolism are parathyroid hormone (PTH), 1,25-dihydroxycholecalciferol (1,25-DHCC) and calcitonin. Growth hormone, prolactin, sex steroids, thyroxine (T4) and cortisol also play a modulating role in calcium homeostasis.

7.1.2 PARATHYROID HORMONE

PTH acts on specific cell membrane receptors linked to adenyl cyclase in kidney and bone. The renal action leads to an increased urinary excretion of cyclic adenosine 3',5'-monophosphate (cAMP).

Renal action

Calcium

In the absence of PTH, some 97% of the filtered calcium load is reabsorbed by the kidney. PTH acts on the proximal tubule to increase calcium reabsorption, and raise the renal calcium threshold and hence the plasma calcium.

Phosphate

In the absence of PTH, over 90% of phosphate is reabsorbed, and PTH acts to decrease its tubular reabsorption. It thus lowers the tubular threshold for excretion and thereby the same excretion of phosphate for a lower plasma phosphate concentration.

1,25-DHCC

PTH stimulates 1α-hydroxylase activity in the kidney, this enzyme catalysing the conver-

Daily throughput of calcium and phosphorus

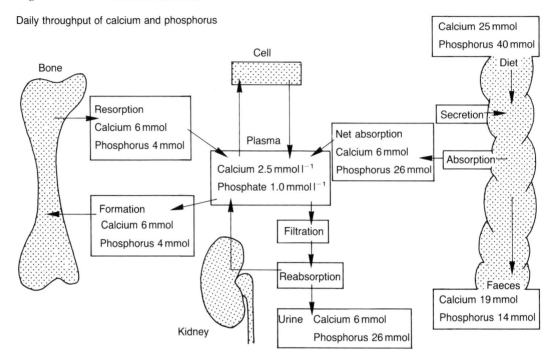

Fig. 7.1 General scheme of calcium and phosphate handling by the body.

sion of 25-hydroxycholecalciferol to the biologically active 1,25-DHCC.

Other tubular effects of PTH

PTH decreases tubular bicarbonate reabsorption, increasing the alkalinity of urine. Proximal reabsorption of sodium and magnesium are also enhanced.

Effects on bone

PTH stimulates the resorption of bone, with breakdown of both mineral and collagen. The hydroxyproline from bone is not reutilized, and urinary hydroxyproline reflects the effect of PTH on bone. Increased mineralization coupled to increased resorption is reflected in bone histology by excessive calcifying osteoid, and by a rise in bone alkaline phosphatase.

Intestinal effects

PTH enhances calcium and phosphate reabsorption from bone, an indirect effect consequent upon the action of 1,25-DHCC production and its effects on bone.

Control of PTH secretion

A fall in ionized calcium in plasma is the major stimulus to PTH production and secretion, and the negative feedback between ionized calcium and PTH secretion is the major mechanism responsible for maintenance of a constant calcium level [1]. A fall in ionized magnesium will also stimulate PTH secretion, but paradoxically, at low levels of magnesium, PTH secretion is diminished since the magnesium ion is essential for PTH secretion [2,3]. Prolonged hypocalcaemia stimulates parathyroid cell division and mass, with increased production of PTH. It takes months of normocalcaemia to return the parathyroid glands to their previous mass, during which time plasma calcium may overshoot into the hypercalcaemic range.

PTH is nowadays measured by immunoradiometric assay (IRMA), which does not measure the split degraded fragments of the PTH molecule.

7.1.3 1,25-DHCC

This is the biologically active form of vitamin D, although other metabolites (25-hydroxy, 24,25-dihydroxy, 25,26-dihydroxy) are also produced.

Effects on the intestine

In the absence of 1,25-DHCC, active absorption of calcium and phosphate from the gut is virtually zero. 1,25-DHCC also induces the production of a calcium binding protein within the gut [4].

Effect on bone

1,25-DHCC is required for the mineralization of bone. Excess vitamin D, however, is associated with bone resorption and intestinal calcium absorption, causing hypercalcaemia [5].

Renal actions

Given to hypoparathyroid patients, vitamin D stimulates absorption of calcium and renal excretion of phosphate.

Muscle action

Proximal muscle weakness is a striking feature of vitamin D deficiency.

Control of 1,25-DHCC production

In the short term, reduced calcium and phosphate, and a rise in PTH, will reduce 1,25-DHCC production. Conversely, increased calcium and phosphate, a rise in 1,25-DHCC and a reduced PTH reduce 1,25-DHCC synthesis.

7.1.4 CALCITONIN

Although its physiological role is obscure, exogenous calcitonin acts on bone to reduce bone turnover, and on the kidney to cause a generalized decrease in calcium, phosphate, sodium, magnesium, potassium and bicarbonate reabsorption [6].

7.2 THE DIAGNOSTIC METHODS

7.2.1 ROUTINE BIOCHEMISTRY
(Table 7.1)

Under this heading are included simple chemical diagnostic tests that are normally undertaken by a colorimetric method on a multichannel autoanalyser. The serum calcium level is generally regulated in any one individual between quite narrow limits of $2.1-2.6 \, mmol \, l^{-1}$. Three fractions make up the total: ionized (50%), protein bound (40%) and complexed, principally with citrate and phosphate (10%). The ionized fraction is that which is physiologically important [7]. This level can be measured quite readily now using a calcium electrode, purchased at relatively low cost. Few laboratories, however,

Table 7.1 Normal routine plasma values

Calcium	$2.2-2.60 \, mmol \, l^{-1}$
Phosphate	$0.7-1.25 \, mmol \, l^{-1}$
Albumin	$35-50 \, g \, l^{-1}$
Alkaline phosphatase	$35-130 \, U \, l^{-1}$ (adults)
Parathyroid hormone (PTH)	$10-55 \, pmol \, ml^{-1}$
25 OH vitamin D	$19-107 \, nmol \, l^{-1}$

do this, partly because it is so seldom clinically necessary, even though careful studies comparing free calcium levels with those derived from accepted algorithms have shown that the latter are inadequate for precise work. In general a simple 'correction' for the serum albumin concentration is sufficient to point to true (ionized) hypocalcaemia.

The serum phosphate level (normal adult range $0.8-1.6\,\mathrm{mmol\,l^{-1}}$) varies more widely than the calcium in response, for example, to changes in phosphate intake. Furthermore, levels are controlled by a wide range of factors acting at the renal tubular level. Only 10% is protein bound in serum, the remainder existing as free and complexed anions. Its level is considerably higher in children than in adults. The parathyroid glands exert a major effect at the renal level, on phosphate excretion, and levels of serum phosphate are high in hypoparathyroidism and low in primary hyperparathyroidism. The serum phosphate level exerts important secondary regulatory actions, both upon bone mineralization and upon renal production of vitamin D. Abnormalities of phosphate are of prime importance in some forms of (hypophosphataemic) rickets/osteomalacia and chronic parenchymal (hyperphosphataemic) renal failure.

Blood urea or creatinine measurements are essential, to indicate significant renal impairment. Sodium, potassium, chloride and bicarbonate together provide useful pointers to relevant metabolic disturbance, such as metabolic alkalosis or acidosis and mineralocorticoid deficiency.

The 'routine profile' would normally incorporate serum calcium, phosphate and alkaline phosphatase, plus one or more liver enzymes and bilirubin. If all of the above are normal, significant metabolic bone disease of any kind (other than osteoporosis) is unlikely and some, such as rickets or renal osteodystrophy, can be excluded. The relatively inexpensive tests utilize colorimetric assays, lending themselves to autoanalysis; there is

much to be said for retaining a relatively low threshold for a single 'screening profile', and certainly for block analyses (of, for example, phosphate, albumin and alkaline phosphatase whenever a calcium concentration is measured). There might also be arguments for carrying out subsidiary analyses, not requested by the clinician but triggered by an abnormal finding. For example, it would be sensible to assay routinely serum urea (or creatinine), sodium, potassium, chloride and bicarbonate the first time that an elevated serum phosphate is found, and to do this whether or not the clinician has requested them.

7.2.2 SERUM ALKALINE PHOSPHATASE

The total level of serum alkaline phosphatase, generally included in a 'routine' laboratory profile, is usually measured by the capacity of alkaline phosphatase to hydrolyse esters of phosphate in an alkaline medium. In the non-pregnant state alkaline phosphatase in serum generally consists of approximately 60% bone and 20% liver isoenzyme, the remainder being of intestinal origin. In pregnancy, levels are higher, with significant amounts coming from the placenta, and postpartum from the lactating breast.

The bone isoenzyme differs from the liver and placental isoenzymes originating from a differing gene, which is located on chromosome 1. The mRNA sequence predicts a 524 amino acid polypeptide that is 50% homologous to placental and intestinal forms. The tissue specific forms differ slightly in molecular weight and can be separated by gel electrophoresis and differing sensitivities to heat denaturation.

The precise role of alkaline phosphatase in bone is poorly understood. It has long been suggested that it plays an important role in bone mineral deposition. Current evidence suggests that its effect is prior to hydroxyapatite deposition, acting as a transport protein of inorganic phosphate or as an in-activator of localized phosphorylated inhibitors of mineralization.

Indication

This simple test is indicated in the routine assessment of any suspected metabolic bone disorder. The bone isoenzyme is produced characteristically by osteoblasts and to a lesser extent by osteocytes, and its production is raised in conditions of increased bone turn-over, notably during childhood and adolescence, and in the presence of rickets and osteomalacia, renal osteodystrophy, primary and secondary hyperparathyroidism, metastatic bone disease, healing fractures and Paget's disease of bone. In conditions where general calcium metabolism is disordered, this is associated with alterations in serum calcium and phosphate, whereas these are generally normal in primary bone disorders such as Paget's disease.

Although there are situations where it is useful to measure alkaline phosphatase isoenzymes, for routine clinical purposes it is generally unnecessary to do so, as the total level of alkaline phosphatase combined if necessary with gamma glutamyl transferase (GGT), is adequate.

Interpretation

The finding of an elevated level of the enzyme requires careful interpretation, usually being an indicator of liver or bone disease. In the case of the former other liver function tests, particularly the serum level of GGT, are raised.

Low levels of alkaline phosphatase are seldom of clinical importance – they may be due to enzyme deficiency (hypophosphatasia), a rare genetic disorder in which low or absent levels of bone alkaline phosphatase are associated with rickets and osteomalacia. When bone turnover is shut down by administration of bisphosphonate drugs, acquired hypophosphatasia may ensue. It is at present uncertain whether this phenomenon is associated with a long-term increased risk of bone fracture due to impaired healing of microfractures.

7.2.3 BONE SPECIFIC PROTEINS

Osteocalcin (bone GLA-protein) is the only protein thus far discovered that appears to be confined to bone and dentine. Its role is not clear but it is synthesized by osteoblasts and incorporated into bone matrix. The synthesis of osteocalcin is vitamin K-dependent.

Serum levels reflect rates of bone turnover measured by iliac-crest histomorphometry and this may allow its use in identification of groups at risk of osteoporosis and in the classification of established osteoporotics [8]. There is a wide variation in the levels of osteocalcin in patients with Paget's disease, with 40% of patients with other signs of disease activity showing normal levels. In other conditions osteocalcin seems to reflect bone matrix synthesis, and so is clearly increased in hyperparathyroidism and hyperthyroidism but may not be increased in patients with bone metastases until decoupling of resorption and formation occurs, in the situation of hypercalcaemia.

Osteonectin is increased in some patients with osteogenesis imperfecta and was hoped to have potential in assessment of bone turn-over in osteoporosis. Unfortunately, this has not proved to be possible thus far, as bone specific osteonectin cannot be identified separately from platelet-derived substance. Similarly, osteopontin and sialoprotein are potential but as yet unproven markers of bone turnover.

Indications

These tests are not as yet generally available and their application is as research tools until

131

specific advantages over cheaper established tests are demonstrated, and the tests become accessible to general laboratories.

7.2.4 BREAKDOWN PRODUCTS OF TYPE I COLLAGEN

During processing of type I collagen there is cleavage of the aminoterminal (procollagen-I-N) and carboxyterminal (procollagen-I-C) extension peptides, which can subsequently be measured in blood and may represent useful markers of bone turnover [9]. Values above normal have been reported in hyperparathyroidism and Paget's disease but their clinical use remains to be established and as such they are not generally clinically indicated.

7.2.5 PARATHYROID HORMONE

Recently an important development has been in the advent of two-site IRMA for PTH. PTH is secreted as an 84-amino acid peptide, of which residues 1–34 are necessary for biological activity. After secretion the molecule is degraded in the kidney and elsewhere, and C-terminal fragments are excreted in the urine. Hence, C-terminal fragments selectively accumulate in chronic renal failure. The main physiological role of the parathyroid glands, mediated via PTH, is to regulate the circulating level of ionized serum calcium. As levels of ionized calcium fall, PTH secretion is switched on; the hormone promotes an elevation of calcium by three mechanisms: (i) it promotes proximal tubular reabsorption of calcium; (ii) it promotes the action of 25-hydroxy vitamin D 1α-hydroxylase and 1,25(OH)2D3 synthesis, which in turn promotes gut calcium absorption; and (iii) it stimulates net bone resorption, indirectly by action on osteoblasts, whose function is inhibited while access of osteoclasts is increased. A fourth effect is to promote renal phosphate loss.

Indication

Assay of PTH is indicated in any patient with hypercalcaemia, and a rapid assay may be important in distinguishing primary hyperparathyroidism from malignant hypercalcaemia. Of less immediate diagnostic importance is its measurement in patients with hypocalcaemia or renal disease.

Interpretation

Knowledge of the local assay method and its specificity and sensitivity are important in the interpretation of results. In general, a significantly elevated level (>30%) of PTH is a strong indicator of hyperparathyroid disease. Failure to suppress PTH to subnormal levels does not exclude malignancy.

7.2.6 PARATHYROID HORMONE RELATED PEPTIDES (PTHrps)

These are polypeptides whose n-terminal sequence shares enough homology with PTH to bind to and activate PTH receptors. They are produced (as a family since there are several sites of cleavage) by squamous cell carcinomas that lead to hypercalcaemia of malignancy [10]. Since it is not the only cause of malignant hypercalcaemia PTHrp assays, when available, will be of interest in unravelling the pathophysiology of malignant hypercalcaemia. So far such assays have not become routinely available.

7.2.7 CALCITONIN

Calcitonin is a 32-amino acid polypeptide produced by the C-cells of the thyroid gland. Greatly elevated circulating levels of calcitonin are found in patients with medullary carcinoma of the thyroid (a tumour of C-cell origin), where they are of diagnostic importance, but do not seem to be associated with significant bone disease.

Indications

Dynamic tests of calcitonin secretion are particularly indicated in individuals suspected of having multiple endocrine adenomastosis (MEN) type 2 which is associated with C-cell hyperplasia. The possible role of low calcitonin in specific forms of osteoporosis (for example during pregnancy) clearly merits further research.

Interpretation

Assay is fraught with the same problems as that of PTH and reliable IRMAs are needed if this area is to progress.

7.2.8 VITAMIN D METABOLITES

Assay methodology has improved recently, but still relatively few laboratories offer a routine service. There are two principal problems. Firstly, separation of the metabolites of the endogenous form, vitamin D3 (cholecalciferol), from the predominantly dietary form, vitamin D2 (calciferol), requires high pressure liquid chromatography (HPLC) prior to radioimmunoassay (RIA). It may be important for clinical purposes, and certainly for research, to measure both separately, although this is not normally the case. Secondly, the active 1,25(OH)2D metabolites are greatly out-weighed by levels of the inactive metabolites 24,25(OH)2D (10- to 50-fold higher) and the precursor 25-ODH (50- to 100-fold higher). So far it has therefore proved necessary to include a separation step prior to the final assay system.

Indications

The clinical indications for these assays lie in the diagnosis of rickets and osteomalacia. In general, levels are relatively stable and a single measurement should suffice; 25-hydroxyvitamin D levels are of more value in diagnosing vitamin D deficiency, since hy-pocalcaemia leads to secondary hyperparathyroidism, which in turn promotes renal formation in the kidney of 1,25(OH)2D. Therefore 1,25(OH)2D3 levels remain relatively normal until stores of 25(OH)D run out; by the same token, brief exposure to sunlight or to dietary vitamin D may restore 1,25(OH)2D levels while 25(OH)D remains very low. There is clinically little indication to measure the levels of 24,25(OH)2D, which appears to be biologically inactive. Its principal interest is that its formation is switched on by 1,25(OH)2D in target tissues.

7.2.9 OTHER HORMONES

Thyrotoxicosis may present with hypercalcaemia or osteoporosis and is generally diagnosed by a single measurement of serum levels of triiodothyronine (T3), T4 and thyroid stimulating hormone (TSH). Cushing's syndrome commonly presents with osteoporosis and is readily diagnosed by measurement of 24-hour urinary free cortisol and failure of serum cortisol to suppress overnight by 1.5–2 mg dexamethasone (see Chapter 4).

7.3 URINARY MEASUREMENTS

7.3.1 AMINO ACID SCREEN

Indication

In patients with rickets or osteomalacia a urinary amino acid screen will help exclude Fanconi's syndrome, in which the primary defect is a generalized renal failure of tubular reabsorption of phosphate, glucose and amino acids.

7.3.2 CALCIUM EXCRETION

Indication

The 24-hour urinary excretion of calcium is low in nutritional/sunlight deprivational rickets.

It is very low in familial hypocalciuric hypercalcaemia. It is elevated in patients with idiopathic hypercalciuria. In general the 'poor man's' test is equally satisfactory: namely, to measure the urine calcium/creatinine ratio on a fasting morning sample. This obviates the need to hospitalize the patient with strict dietary control in order to get interpretable results.

7.3.3 HYDROXYPROLINE-CONTAINING BREAKDOWN PRODUCTS OF COLLAGEN

Indications

These are of value in the diagnosis and monitoring of states of increased bone turnover. Unfortunately, they are subject to dietary contributions resulting from gelatin in the diet. Therefore, if 24-hour urine measurements are to be made, this must be on a gelatin-free diet for 24 hours or more before the collection. This is, therefore, a relatively impractical outpatient method and a fasting urinary hydroxyproline/creatinine ratio is almost as good and much simpler to carry out. Hydroxyproline is not easy to assay, and probably the best method is to measure it colorimetrically after HPLC. Recently, more specific breakdown products of type 1 collagen have been advocated, cross-linkage of type 1 collagen leads to production of pyridinoline cross-linking amino acids. Whether the measurement of these compounds offers any advantage over hydroxyproline is not as yet determined: one problem is that non-bony sources (e.g. skin collagen) also contribute to the excretion of both hydroxyproline and pyridinoline.

7.3.4 CLEARANCE MEASUREMENTS

In general, clearances are expressed as a ratio to that of creatinine clearance. They are calculated as follows:

$$\frac{\text{Urine (calcium)} \times \text{Plasma (creatinine)}}{\text{Plasma (calcium)} \times \text{Urine (creatinine)}}$$

For calcium and phosphate these should be done on fasting 1- or 2-hour urine specimens, preferably with mid-point blood sampling. From these values, other derivations are possible. Evidently, the value of such calculations depends upon the question being asked and the clinical context. One source of error lies in the measurement of creatinine and the intrinsic assumption that creatinine clearance = glomerular filtration rate, which is not strictly correct.

For phosphate there have been a number of calculations made from this basic ratio of phosphate to creatinine clearance, related to serum phosphate, of which the phosphate excretion index of Nordin [2] and the TMPxP are examples.

7.4 IMAGING TECHNIQUES IN METABOLIC BONE DISEASES

7.4.1 PLAIN RADIOLOGY

Although there has been much new development in the field of diagnostic imaging of the skeleton, the plain radiograph is still of major importance in the evaluation and review of disorders of bone metabolism. Universal availability at relatively low cost means that in many cases the carefully taken radiograph will remain one of the cornerstones of the diagnosis of bone disorders. It is, however, the skill of the radiographer and standardization of protocols which lead to greater diagnostic accuracy, and utilization of serial radiographs to assess response to treatment or disease progression.

Indications

The choice of radiographs performed should be based on the nature of the condition to be evaluated. It is the authors' practice to rou-

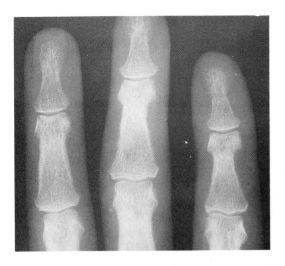

Fig. 7.2 X-ray of the fingers showing subperiosteal bone erosions in a case of primary hyperparathyroidism.

tinely X-ray only the hands (for sub-periosteal absorption, Fig. 7.2) and abdomen (for renal calculi and/or nephrocalcinosis) of patients with suspected hyperparathyroidism.

Patients investigated for osteoporosis normally undergo careful antero-posterior and lateral views of the thoracic and lumbar spine, and where there is a suspicion of osteomalacia the pelvis and proximal femora would be imaged in addition for pseudofractures (Fig. 7.3).

In general, the choice of radiographs is best determined by the site of lesions demonstrated by scintigraphy. The routine use of skeletal surveys is limited only to patients with multiple myelomatosis where the X-ray may yield useful information not indicated on the scan. It is well documented that in patients with sclerotic changes from Paget's disease the X-ray may be more sensitive in identifying such lesions, but the importance of this is limited as such areas are not generally suitable for assessing for therapeutic response.

7.4.2 ISOTOPE SCINTIGRAPHY

The use of ^{99m}Tc-labelled bisphosphonate bone scans provides a simple method of assessing metabolic processes throughout the skeleton and of localizing areas of abnormality. This highly sensitive imaging technique provides information which in many cases can be non-specific and must always be interpreted alongside other evidence, in particular radiology of the affected areas, before reaching a definitive diagnosis.

The technique is widely available at low cost and with low levels of exposure to ionizing radiation for the patient. The characteristic changes in some conditions of generalized skeletal abnormality can be difficult to differentiate from the appearances of normal patients. The use of computerized image analysis can improve sensitivity but is not yet routinely available. Quantification of disease extent and activity is also possible where these techniques are carefully employed. Use of measurements of whole body isotope retention, assessed by whole skeletal imaging or urinary excretion rates, has been used in the assessment of a variety of skeletal disorders, to provide a quantitative measure of disease extent and activity which does not rely on the interpretation of images produced by the gamma camera.

Indications

The main conditions where the isotope scan is of major value in metabolic bone disorders are in the evaluation of the patient with suspected bony invasion from tumour or in the assessment and follow up of patients with Paget's disease (Fig. 7.4a,b).

The isotope scan can also yield useful information in hyperparathyroidism and renal osteodystrophy osteomalacia, and will detect recent vertebral fracture in patients with osteoporosis.

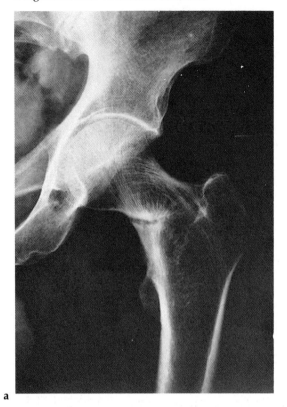
a

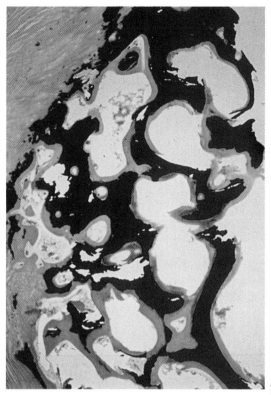
b

Fig. 7.3 (a) X-ray of the hip joint showing pseudofracture. (b) Bone biopsy from the same patient demonstrating widened osteoid seams typical of osteomalacia.

7.4.3 BONE DENSITY MEASUREMENT

Over the past two decades accurate and clinically useful techniques of quantification of bone density by non-invasive techniques have been developed and widely introduced [11]. They require equipment not routinely available in the general radiology departments and are therefore mainly applicable to those centres with a specialist interest in skeletal metabolism, though this may well rapidly change with public awareness of osteoporosis and as the precision of methods improves. The four main imaging techniques employed are: single-photon absorptiometry (SPA), dual-photon absorptiometry (DPA), dual X-ray absorptiometry (DPA-X) and quantitative computerized tomography (QCT).

SPA is performed with low radiation dose, and is accurate, precise and relatively inexpensive. It is, however, suitable only for the examination of the peripheral skeleton, the usual sites being the radius, femur, tibia or os calcis. It can accurately predict fracture risk and has been used to assess total body calcium measurements. The clinical usefulness is limited by its failure to give an assessment of axial skeletal density.

DPA has evolved from SPA. Measurement of axial bone density is possible and, indeed, the technique can be applied to bone at any

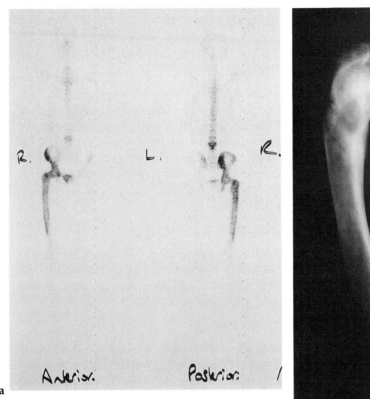
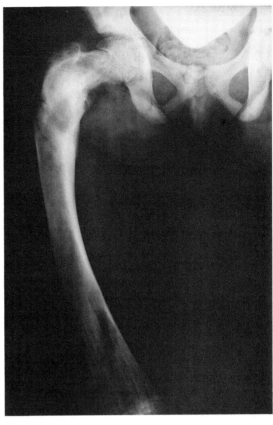

Fig. 7.4 (a) ⁹⁹Tc MDP bone scan showing increased radionuclide uptake in the femur of a patient with Paget's disease. (b) X-ray showing typical appearances of Pagetic bone.

site. It is, however, laborious and time consuming and as such has been used mainly as a research tool: a major problem here has also been the relative instability of the isotope source, which makes calibration over time and between machines very difficult.

The development of dual energy X-ray equipment (DPA-X or DEXA) has now largely superseded the DPA in clinical practice, and is a rapidly growing area of the imaging industry. The technique provides relatively inexpensive, sensitive and precise measurements of bone density, and refinements in scanning hardware and image analysis software have led to the increasing installation of several types of commercial machine. The same machine allows measurement of lumbar spine, femoral neck, and total body density and/or calcium.

QCT provides a measurement technique for spine trabecular bone density, separately from that of the cortex. The results with third and fourth generation CT scanners are precise and sensitive. The refinement of standardized 'phantoms' (against which bone density can be assessed) has led to the technique being used increasingly in both the initial assessment of the patient with osteoporosis and in the evaluation of therapeutic response.

Indications

All these techniques are rapidly passing from the stage of being pure research tools to being valuable aids in the assessment of patients with disorders of skeletal metabolism and their response to therapy. It is becoming clear that they will also be of value in the selection of those patients at risk of complications resulting from osteoporosis.

7.4.4 BONE HISTOLOGY

Transiliac bone biopsy (see below) is a safe and well tolerated procedure when done by those familiar with the technique [12]. It has a valuable place in the diagnosis, assessment and follow-up of patients with metabolic bone processes of bone resorption and formation. Standard bone histomorphometry, coupled with double tetracyclines labelling, greatly increases the value of the investigation.

Indications

It is our current practice to perform transiliac bone biopsy in the diagnosis of patients with idiopathic osteoporosis or suspected osteomalacia, and it is also used in the assessment of therapeutic effect in patients treated for osteoporosis. In patients with Paget's disease of the pelvis, bone biopsy, taken together with bone scans, provides the 'gold standard' in assessing therapeutic effect.

Interpretation

The interpretation of histomorphometric data requires a skilled osteopathologist with experience in the technique. The details of such techniques are not within the scope of this chapter.

7.5 DYNAMIC TESTS

7.5.1 PARATHYROID HORMONE INFUSION TEST

In the diagnosis of pseudo-hypoparathyroidism the demonstration of a blunted response of urinary cAMP and/or phosphate and calcium excretion to administered PTH is of diagnostic value. This condition should be considered in any case of non-surgical hypoparathyroidism.

Indications

With improvements in PTH assay this test is becoming obsolete but in the more difficult case there may still be a role for its application.

Procedure

Following an overnight fast, a standard intravenous infusion of PTH (100 units) is given, and urine is collected over a 3-hour period for cAMP measurement.

Interpretation

Careful criteria for the identification of type 1 pseudohypoparathyroidism using this test have been published elsewhere.

7.5.2 HYDROCORTISONE SUPPRESSION TEST

Indication

This test still has a limited role to play in the different diagnosis of mild hypercalcaemia.

Procedure

The original test of Dent described using 40 mg hydrocortisone daily for ten days, but it is now more common to use 100 mg daily or the equivalent dose of an alternative steroid.

Interpretation

Patients with primary hyperparathyroidism will almost never show a fall in serum calcium whereas those with vitamin D dependent causes (sarcoid and other granulomatous diseases and vitamin D intoxication) will do so, as will some cases of hypercalcaemia of malignancy.

7.6 INVESTIGATION OF SPECIFIC CALCIUM DISORDERS

The individual assessment must be tailored to the patient's history and physical examination. It is, however, often useful to have a framework of investigation to start with and to refine this to meet the individual situation. We here discuss our approach to the diagnosis of common diseases.

7.6.1 HYPERCALCAEMIA

The problem essentially is to distinguish between hypercalcaemia of malignancy, hyperparathyroidism and other less common causes. The first line investigations should therefore be aimed at distinguishing between these three groups.

1. Confirm persisting elevation of total Ca^{2+} and measure serum PO_4, albumin, creatinine and alkaline phosphatase; carry out measurement of immunoglobulins and protein electrophoresis. Thyroid function tests, full blood count and ESR. Fasting urinary Ca^{2+}/creatinine ratio. Check Na and K and remember Addison's disease – if in doubt, check ACTH and cortisol, carry out Synacthen test and treat with hydrocortisone while awaiting results.
2. Measure immunoreactive PTH.
3. Bone scintigraphy, chest and abdominal radiographs; X-ray one hand. Look for a neoplasm.

The results of these investigations should allocate the majority of patients clearly into one of the above groups. There are of course always difficult cases in whom all results are borderline. In those with high or 'normal' PTH levels attempts should be made to determine the location of any parathyroid adenoma by means of ultrasound and CT scanning of the neck and/or parathyroid isotope scan. Selective venous sampling or arteriography may sometimes be of value.

The once widely used steroid suppression test should be confined to the diagnosis of sarcoidosis and Addison's disease. The measurement of cAMP is of limited use, despite initially optimistic hopes for its use in separating hyperparathyroid patients from those with malignancy.

In a small number of patients where the diagnosis is difficult bone biopsy may be of help in differentiating the cause.

Finally, the modern management of the condition with bisphosphonates in itself provides a diagnostic test; patients with hypercalcaemia of malignancy invariably respond but those with hyperparathyroidism fail to do so.

7.6.2 THE INVESTIGATION OF THE PATIENT WITH OSTEOPAENIA

As increasing numbers of patients are being referred for investigation of osteopaenia, the purpose of any investigations done should be clear from the outset: namely, (i) to identify the underlying pathological process; (ii) to quantify the severity; and (iii) to monitor therapeutic intervention.

Our clinical practice is to evaluate all patients with these goals in mind, aiming for maximal information with minimal expense and inconvenience to the patient.

All patients have serum Ca^{2+}, PO_4, alkaline phosphatase, urea and electrolytes, including bicarbonate, albumin, liver and thyroid function, full blood profile, sedimentation rate and protein electrophoresis at outset. Fasting urinary calcium/creatinine ratio is measured.

Standard radiographs are taken of thoracic and lumbar spine to document collapse and evaluate possible malignant pathologies. Bone density is quantified by DPX in all cases and selectively by SPA and QCT in patients of particular interest. Bone biopsy is performed in any patient with unexplained osteoporosis and in those suspected of osteomalacia. Therapeutic success is monitored by serial bone density estimations and vertebral height measurement.

7.6.3 BONE BIOPSY

This can be performed as an out-patient procedure under local anaesthesia and patients are usually given a premedication sedative such as 50 mg pethidine and 25 mg phenergan intramuscularly 1 hour beforehand.

Procedure

The patient is placed on his back with the lower limbs flexed a little at the knees and hips. The biopsy is taken 2.5 cm behind and below the anterior superior iliac spine. Meunier's modification, or the Lalor version, of the Bordier drill are both widely used; we prefer an 8 mm internal diameter drill. The drill consists of a trocar, a stabilizing sleeve, a toothed drill and a metal rod for removing the specimen. To anaesthetize skin, soft tissues and the inner and outer periosteal surfaces, 1% xylocaine with 1/100 000 adrenaline (about 20 ml) is used. The drill takes a core containing both cortical surfaces and the joining trabecular bone. Following the procedure the skin is sutured and a pressure dressing applied.

7.6.4 DOUBLE TETRACYCLINE LABELLING

In this investigation tetracycline is deposited along the calcification front in bone as two distinct lines which can be visualized in bone sections under fluorescent microscopy. The technique gives useful information on bone mineralization and formation.

Procedure

This involves administering a course of 300 mg demethylchlortetracycline (DMCT) twice daily for 2 days followed by a gap of 10 days, followed by 300 mg DMCT twice a day for 4 days. The bone biopsy is carried out 4–8 days later.

Interpretation

The method allows an assessment of bone turnover to be made.

7.6.5 PAGET'S DISEASE OF BONE

The aims of investigation in this condition are to establish the diagnosis, to evaluate the extent and to assess therapeutic response. Serum alkaline phosphatase measurements are elevated in over 90% of patients at time of diagnosis and provide a useful marker of response, particularly in patients with extensive disease or a high level. The urinary hydroxyproline/creatinine ratio is more sensitive but also more variable and in most cases adds relatively little. The isotope bone scan provides diagnostic information and quantification/ semi-quantification of serial scans is an invaluable monitor of therapy. The differentiation from malignant disease can be difficult and careful radiographic assessment is necessary. A common situation is for a patient to present with disease in one (symptomatic) bone, which is obviously involved on X-ray. Before proceeding with further X-rays a bone scan is performed, with ^{99m}Tc-labelled bisphosphonate as imaging agent; affected bones are then X-rayed. A decision is then made at this time on which parameters (and bones) are most suitable for long term follow-up response.

REFERENCES

1. Engel, K., Pederson, S.O., Nielsen, S.P. *et al.* (1983) In: Ionized calcium workshop No. 1. *Scand. J. Clin. Lab. Invest.*, **43**, 1–126.
2. Nordin, B.E.C. (ed.) (1976) *Calcium, Phosphate and Magnesium Metabolism.* Churchill Livingstone, New York.
3. Brown, E.M. and Chen, J.C. (1989) Calcium, magnesium and the control of PTH secretion. *Bone Min. Res.*, **5**, 249–57.
4. Broner, F. (1982) Intestinal calcium absorption and transport. In *Membrane Transport of Calcium* (ed. E. Carafoli), pp. 237–62.
5. De Luca, H.T. (1983) Metabolism of action of vitamin D. In *Bone and Mineral Research Annual* (ed. W.A. Peck), Exertpa Medica, pp. 7–73.
6. Talmage, R.V., Cooper, C.W. and Tortrud, S.U. (1983) The physiological significance of calcitonin. *Bone Min Res.*, **1**, 74–143.
7. Potts, J.T., Jr, Kronnenberg, M. and Rosenblatt, M. (1982) Parathyroid hormone, chemistry biosynthesis and mode of action. *Adv. Prot. Chem.*, **35**, 323–96.
8. Delmas, P.D., Stenner, D., Wahlner, H. *et al.* (1983) Increase in bone γ-carboxyglutamic acid protein with ageing in women. *J. Clin. Invest.*, **71**, 1316.
9. Delmas, P.D. (1988) Biochemical markers of bone turnover. In *Osteoporosis: Etiology, Diagnosis and Management* (ed. B.B. Riggs and L.J. Melton III), Raven Press, New York, p. 297.
10. Sura, L.J., Winslow, G.A., Welternale, R. *et al.* (1987) A parathyroid hormone related protein implicated in malignant hypercalcaemia: cloning and expression. *Science*, **237**, 893–6.
11. Fogelman, I. (1988) Bone scanning and photon absorptiometry in metabolic bone disease. *J. Clin. Endocrinol. Metab.* **2**, 59–86.
12. Boyce, B.F. (1988) Uses and limitations of bone biopsy in management of metabolic bone disease. *J. Clin. Endocrinol. Metab.*, **2**, 31–57.

8

Diagnosis of multiple endocrine neoplasia syndromes

R.V. THAKKER

8.1 INTRODUCTION

Multiple endocrine neoplasia [1] is characterized by the occurrence of tumours involving two or more endocrine glands within a single patient. The disorder has previously been referred to as multiple endocrine adenopathy (MEA) or the pluriglandular syndrome. However, glandular hyperplasia and malignancy may also occur in some patients, and the term multiple endocrine neoplasia (MEN) is now preferred.

There are two major forms of MEN, referred to as type 1 and type 2, and each form is characterized by the development of tumours within specific endocrine glands (Table 8.1).

MEN type 1 (MEN1; Wermer's syndrome), is characterized by the combined occurrence of tumours of the parathyroid glands, pancreatic islet cells and anterior pituitary. MEN type 2 (MEN2; Sipple syndrome), describes the occurrence of medullary thyroid carcinoma (MTC) in association with phaeochromocytoma. Three clinical variants of MEN2 are recognized, and these are referred to as MEN2a, MEN2b and MTC-only.

In MEN2a, the most common variant, the development of MTC is associated with phaeochromocytoma and parathyroid tumours. However, in MEN2b parathyroid involvement is rare, and the occurrence of MTC and phaeochromocytoma is found in association with marfanoid habitus, mucosal neuromas, medullated corneal fibres and intestinal autonomic ganglion dysfunction (ganglioneuromatosis) leading to megacolon.

In the variant of MTC-only, medullary thyroid carcinoma appears to be the sole manifestation of the syndrome. Although MEN1 and MEN2 usually occur as distinct and separate syndromes as outlined above, some patients occasionally may develop tumours that are associated with both MEN1 and MEN2. For example, patients suffering from islet cell tumours of the pancreas and phaeochromocytomas, or from acromegaly and phaeochromocytoma, have been described, and these patients may represent an 'overlap' syndrome.

All these forms may either be inherited as autosomal dominant syndromes, or they may occur sporadically, i.e. without a family history. However, this distinction between sporadic and familial cases may sometimes be difficult, as in some sporadic cases the family history may be absent because the parent with the disease may have died before developing any symptoms.

The recognition of a MEN syndrome in a patient is important, as the management

142

Table 8.1 The multiple endocrine neoplasia (MEN) syndromes, their characteristic tumours and associated biochemical abnormalities. (↑), Increased; (PTH), parathyroid hormone; (VIP), vasoactive intestinal peptide; (WDHA), watery diarrhoea, hypokalaemia and achlorhydria; (PP), pancreatic polypeptide; (GH), growth hormone; (ACTH), adrenocorticotropin; (5-HIAA), 5-hydroxyindoleacetic acid

Type	Tumours	Biochemical features
MEN1	Parathyroids	Hypercalcaemia and ↑ PTH
	Pancreatic islets	
	Gastrinoma	↑ Gastrin and ↑ basal gastric acid output
	Insulinoma	Hypoglycaemia and ↑ insulin
	Glucagonoma	Glucose intolerance and ↑ glucagon
	Vipoma	↑ VIP and WDHA
	PPoma	↑ PP
	Pituitary (anterior)	
	Prolactinoma	Hyperprolactinaemia
	GH-secreting	↑ GH
	ACTH-secreting	Hypercortisolaemia and ↑ ACTH
	Non-functioning	Nil
	Associated tumours	
	Adrenal cortical	Hypercortisolaemia or primary hyperaldosteronism
	Carcinoid	↑ 5-HIAA
	Lipoma	Nil
MEN2a	Medullary thyroid carcinoma	Hypercalcitonaemia
	Phaeochromocytoma	↑ Catecholamines
	Parathyroid	Hypercalcaemia and ↑ PTH
MEN2b	Medullary thyroid carcinoma	Hypercalcitonaemia
	Phaeochromocytoma	↑ Catecholamines
	Associated abnormalities:	
	Mucosal neuromas	
	Marfinoid habitus	
	Medullated corneal nerve fibres	
	Megacolon	

Autosomal dominant inheritance of the MEN syndromes has been established.

of some endocrine tumours, for example, parathyroid tumours, gastrinomas and phaeochromocytomas, is different from that in non-MEN patients. In addition, the occurrence of a MEN syndrome in a patient is an indication for biochemical screening of the patient's family in order to achieve early detection of tumour development. In this chapter, the main clinical manifestations, biochemical features and management of MEN syndromes, together with their molecular genetic pathology, will be discussed. The diagnosis of sporadic pancreatic islet cell tumours is also discussed.

8.2 MULTIPLE ENDOCRINE NEOPLASIA TYPE 1 (MEN1)

8.2.1 CLINICAL FINDINGS

The clinical manifestations of MEN1 are related to the sites of the tumours and to their products of secretion (see Table 8.1). In addition to the triad of parathyroid, pancreatic and pituitary tumours, which constitute the major components of MEN1, adrenal cortical adenomas, thyroid adenomas, and carcinoid and lipomatous tumours have also been described.

8.2.2 PARATHYROID TUMOURS

Primary hyperparathyroidism is the most common feature of MEN1 and occurs in more than 95% of all MEN1 patients [2]. The clinical findings, diagnosis and localization of parathyroid tumours in patients with MEN1 is similar to that in non-MEN1 patients, and is discussed in Chapter 7. These are, in brief raised serum calcium, low serum phosphate, a raised urinary calcium excretion and a raised parathyroid hormone (PTH) level. Radionuclide imaging with MIBI/technetium substraction may show overactivity in all four glands.

The definitive treatment for primary hyperparathyroidism is parathyroidectomy, but in patients with MEN1, who have four-gland hyperplasia, total parathyroidectomy has been proposed as the definitive treatment to avoid the otherwise unavoidable recurrence of hypercalcaemia. It is recommended that such total parathyroidectomy should be reserved for the symptomatic hypercalcaemic patient with MEN1. The asymptomatic MEN1 patient who has mild hypercalcaemia should not have parathyroid surgery, but should have regular assessments for the onset of symptoms and complications, when total parathyroidectomy should be undertaken [3–6].

8.2.3 PANCREATIC TUMOURS

The incidence of pancreatic islet cell tumours in MEN1 patients varies from 30% to 80% in different series [1]. The majority of these tumours are functional, producing excessive amounts of hormone, such as gastrin, insulin, glucagon, vasoactive intestinal polypeptide (VIP), growth hormone releasing hormone (GHRH) and somatostatin, and are associated with distinct clinical syndromes.

Gastrinomas

These gastrin-secreting tumours represent over 50% of all pancreatic islet cell tumours in MEN1, and are the major cause of morbidity and mortality in MEN1 patients. This is due to the recurrent severe multiple peptic ulcers, which may perforate. This association of recurrent peptic ulceration, marked gastric acid production and non-β-islet cell tumours of the pancreas is referred to as Zollinger–Ellison syndrome. Additional prominent clinical features of this syndrome include diarrhoea and steatorrhoea.

Diagnosis

The diagnosis may be established by demonstration of a raised fasting serum gastrin concentration in association with an increased basal gastric acid secretion [7]. However, in patients with MEN1, the Zollinger–Ellison syndrome does not appear to occur in the absence of primary hyperparathyroidism [8,9], and hypergastrinaemia has been reported to be associated with hypercalcaemia [10]. Thus, the diagnosis of Zollinger–Ellison syndrome may be difficult in some MEN1 patients.

Table 8.2 Causes of elevated gastrin levels

Zollinger–Ellison syndrome
Gastrectomy
Vagotomy
Renal failure
Hypercalcaemia
Achlorhydria
H_2 receptor antagonists
G-cell hyperplasia

A number of conditions causing hypergastrinaemia are listed in Table 8.2.

Sporadic gastrinoma

Calcium challenge test

It has been shown that gastrin secretion can be stimulated by a calcium infusion. This test relies on the principle that a prolonged calcium infusion will cause a marked increase in both serum gastrin and gastric acid output.

Procedure

Following an overnight fast, a nasogastric tube is passed and residual gastric acid is aspirated and discarded. An intravenous normal saline infusion is then started at $24\,ml\,h^{-1}$. During the first hour, two venous samples are taken at 30-minute intervals for serum gastrin assays, and four separate 15-minute collections for gastric acid are made. In the second to fourth hours, calcium is added to the infusion in a dose of 15 mg calcium gluconate per kilogram and blood taken at 30-minute intervals for gastrin estimation, and gastric acid aspirated in 15-minute aliquots.

Interpretation

Calcium will stimulate a marked increase (>300%) in both gastrin and acid output whereas in patients with gastric hypersecretion, only a modest rise occurs.

Secretin stimulation test

Secretin decreases gastric acid output following pentagastrin stimulation, whereas given alone, it stimulates gastrin production. In gastrinomas, i.v. secretin produces an increase in both gastric acid secretion and serum gastrin concentration. This phenomenon forms the basis of a test that distinguishes between gastrinoma and other causes of raised gastrins.

Procedure

Secretin is given as an i.v. bolus in a dose of $2\,u\,kg^{-1}$ following an overnight fast, and blood taken for gastrin levels at 0, 2, 5 and 30 minutes.

Interpretation

In normal subjects, trivial rises in gastrin are seen, whereas in Zollinger–Ellison syndrome, the rise in gastrin is seldom less than 50% and usually well above 100%.

Gastric acid secretion

In Zollinger–Ellison patients, basal acid production is usually above 15 meq per hour in the intact stomach.

Imaging of pancreatic islet cell tumours

Computerized tomography (CT) scanning, arteriography, and intraoperative ultrasound are all helpful in delineating the larger tumours, although the smaller tumours may pose problems [11,12]. The use of transhepatic selective venous gastrin sampling to localize preoperatively the gastrinomas in MEN1 patients has been reported to improve the surgical outcome in one study [13]. Venous sampling in this study revealed that the MEN1 patients with Zollinger–Ellison syndrome had either diffuse gastrin secretion from multiple pancreatic sites or localized gastrin secretion from a single region. The patients in whom gastrin secretion was localized benefited from resection of the gastrinoma by a partial pancreatectomy, and required no postoperative drug therapy. Tumour localization studies using ultrasonography, CT or venous sampling have demonstrated that these techniques do not on the whole improve the surgical success rate [14].

Insulinoma

These β-islet cell tumours secreting insulin represent one-third of all pancreatic tumours in MEN1 patients [1]. Insulinomas also occur in association with gastrinomas in 10% of MEN1 patients, and the two tumours may arise at different times. The clinical manifestations, biochemical investigations and management of insulinomas in MEN1 patients are similar to that in non-MEN1 patients, and are discussed in Chapter 10.

Glucagonoma

These α-islet cell, glucagon-secreting pancreatic tumours have been reported in only five MEN1 patients [1]. The characteristic clinical manifestations of skin rash (necrolytic migratory erythema), weight loss, anaemia, stomatitis may be absent, and the presence of the tumour may be indicated only by glucose intolerance and hyperglucagonaemia. Psychiatric disturbance, venous thrombosis, hypoproteinaemia, zinc deficiency and hypoaminoacidaemia are associated features. Serum glucagon is usually markedly elevated.

Vipoma

Patients with vipomas, which are VIP secreting pancreatic tumours, develop watery diarrhoea (occasionally up to 20 l per day), hypokalaemic alkalosis and achlorhydria (WDHA; Verner–Morrisson syndrome). These features are secondary to the secretion of large quantities of bicarbonate-rich and potassium-rich fluid into the bowel. Vipomas have been reported in only a few MEN1 patients, and the diagnosis is established by documenting a markedly raised plasma VIP concentration. Raised VIP levels have been reported after extensive tissue ischaemia.

PPoma

These tumours, which secrete pancreatic polypeptide (PP), are found in a large number of patients with MEN1. No pathological sequelae of excessive PP secretion are apparent, and the clinical significance of PP is unknown, although the use of serum PP measurements has been suggested for the detection of pancreatic tumours in MEN1 patients, since elevated PP usually accompanies other pancreatic hormone production. Raised PP may also occur in the elderly, after bowel resection, in alcohol abuse and in some cases of pancreatitis. The release of PP from normal cells is under cholinergic control, and is suppressed by atropine. The atropine suppression test may be used to distinguish autonomous PP production from autonomous secretion.

Atropine suppression test

Procedure

Following an overnight fast of at least 10 hours, blood samples are taken for measurement of pancreatic polypeptide 30 minutes and 15 minutes before giving an intramuscular injection of atropine 1 mg. Further samples are taken at 15, 30, 45 and 60 minutes after injection.

In non-tumour cases, the PP level can be suppressed to <50% of the starting value, whereas in tumorous cases, there is no change in PP levels.

Somatostatinoma

In about half the cases of sporadic somatostatinoma, patients suffer from the syndrome of diabetes mellitus, gallstones, low acid output and weight loss. They are the slowest growing tumours of all. The diagnosis is made by measuring serum somatostatin levels. The somatostatinoma syndrome has not, to date, been reported to occur in a patient with MEN1.

8.2.4 PITUITARY TUMOURS

The incidence of pituitary tumours in MEN1 patients varies from 15% to 90% in different series [1]. Approximately 60% of MEN1 associated pituitary tumours secrete prolactin, 25% secrete growth hormone (GH), 3% secrete adrenocorticotropin (ACTH) and the remainder appear to be non-functioning.

The clinical manifestations depend upon the size of the pituitary tumour and its product of secretion. The diagnosis and management of pituitary tumours in MEN1 patients is similar to that in non-MEN1 patients, and is discussed in Chapters 2 and 4.

8.2.5 ASSOCIATED TUMOURS

Patients with MEN1 may have tumours involving glands other than the parathyroids, pancreas and pituitary. Thus, carcinoid, adrenal cortical, thyroid and lipomatous tumours have been described in association with MEN1.

Carcinoid tumours

Carcinoid tumours may be inherited as an autosomal dominant trait and occur more frequently in patients with MEN1. The carcinoid tumour may be located in the bronchi, the gastrointestinal tract, the pancreas or the thymus. Most patients are asymptomatic and do not suffer from the flushing attacks and dyspnoea associated with the carcinoid syndrome, which usually develops after the tumour has metastasized to the liver.

Diagnosis

The diagnosis relies on the demonstration of excessive 24-hour urinary excretion of 5-hydroxyindoleacetic acid (5-HIAA). Urine must be collected into glacial acetic acid. However, it is important to note that phenothiazines interfere with the biochemical assay and that the estimation of urinary 5-HIAA

Table 8.3 Factors interfering with 5-HIAA estimation

False positive
Foods
    Avocados
    Bananas
    Eggplants
    Pineapples
    Plums
    Walnuts
Drugs
    Paracetamol
    Caffeine
    Fluorouracil
    Lugol's solution
    Melphalan
    Reserpine

False negative
p-chlorphenylalanine
Heparin
Imipramine
Isoniazid
Methyldopa
Phenothiazine
Promethazine

may be falsely increased by the ingestion of foods containing serotonin, for example bananas, pineapple, plums and walnuts. A list of factors interfering with the determination of 5-HIAA is shown in Table 8.3.

Usually urinary levels exceed 30 mg per day in carcinoid tumours. Occasionally intestinal disorders such as non-tropical sprue will lead to sufficient 5-HT release to cause a modest elevation of urinary 5-HIAA.

Carcinoid tumours may occur more frequently in some MEN1 families, and a history of this condition in a relative is an indication for biochemical and radiological investigations to be undertaken.

Adrenal cortical tumours

The incidence of asymptomatic adrenal cortical tumours in MEN1 patients has been reported to be as high as 40%. The majority of these tumours are non-functioning. However, functioning adrenal cortical tumours in MEN1 patients have been documented to cause hypercortisolaemia and Cushing's syndrome, and hyperaldosteronism (Conn's syndrome) [15]. The diagnosis and management of these disorders in patients with MEN1 is similar to that in non-MEN1 patients and is discussed in Chapters 4 and 9.

Thyroid tumours

Thyroid adenomas, colloid goitres and carcinomas have been reported to occur in over 25% of MEN1 patients. However, the prevalence of thyroid disorders in the general population is high. It has been suggested that the association of thyroid abnormalities in MEN1 patients may be incidental and not significant.

8.2.6 FAMILY SCREENING

Attempts to screen for the development of MEN1 tumours in the asymptomatic relatives of an affected individual have depended largely on measuring the serum concentrations of calcium, gastrointestinal hormones and prolactin [16]. Parathyroid overactivity causing hypercalcaemia is invariably the first manifestation of the disorder, and this has become a useful and easy screening investigation [9].

Pancreatic involvement in asymptomatic individuals has previously been detected by estimating the fasting plasma concentrations of gastrin and PP. However, one recent study has reported that a stimulatory meal test is a better method for detecting pancreatic disease in individuals who show no demonstrable pancreatic tumours by CT [17]. An exaggerated increase in serum gastrin and/or PP proved to be a reliable early indicator for the development of pancreatic tumours in these individuals. Some asymptomatic pitui-

tary tumours may be detected by demonstration of hyperprolactinaemia.

Screening in MEN1 is difficult because the age-related penetrance (i.e. the proportion of gene carriers who have manifested symptoms or signs of the disease by a given age) has not been established. The proportion of affected individuals who have been detected at a certain age by clinical symptoms or biochemical screening in different series [1] has ranged from 11% to 47% at 20 years of age, 52% to 94% at 35 years and 83% to 100% at 50 years; biochemical screening, which detects asymptomatic patients, increased the proportion of affected individuals at all ages.

Thus, the likelihood of wrongly attributing an 'unaffected' status to an individual who has no manifestations of the disease at the age of 35 years may be as high as 1 in 2, or approaching 1 in 20, and depends on whether clinical symptoms alone or biochemical screening methods are used to detect the disease. In order to improve this situation, further biochemical screening and systematic family studies are required to clarify the age-related penetrances for MEN1, and a register for MEN1 patients has been established in Britain.

Preliminary results from two studies [18,19], in which 87 patients with familial MEN1 were investigated, are shown in Fig. 8.1.

This reveals that the age-related penetrances for MEN1 detected by clinical manifestations (symptomatic group) at 20, 35 and 50 years of age are 9%, 43% and 75%, respectively. The respective age-related penetrances for MEN1 detected by biochemical screening were markedly improved to 44%, 74% and 91%. At present it is suggested that relatives, especially first and second degree relatives, of an affected patient with MEN1 should be screened once a year.

Screening should commence in early childhood, as the disease has developed in some individuals by the age of 5 years, and should

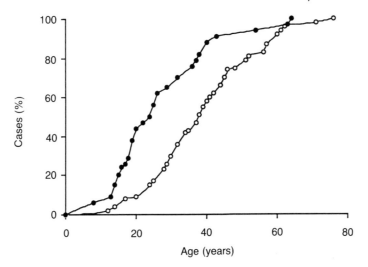

Fig. 8.1 Age-related penetrances of familial MEN1. The ages for diagnosis in 87 patients with familial MEN1 were found to range from 8 to 76 years. The patients were subdivided, depending on the method used to detect MEN1, into two groups. The symptomatic group (○) consisted of 53 patients and the age-related penetrances for MEN1 in these members at 20, 35 and 50 years of age were 9%, 43% and 75%, respectively. In another 34 asymptomatic patients MEN1 had been detected by biochemical screening (●) and the respective age-related penetrances in these members were increased to 44%, 74% and 91%. Thus, biochemical screening detected an earlier onset of MEN1 in all age groups. (Adapted from Vansen *et al.* [18] and Thakker *et al.* [19]).

continue for life, as some individuals have not developed the disease until the eighth decade. Screening history and physical examination should be directed towards eliciting the symptoms and signs of hypercalcaemia, nephrolithiasis, peptic ulcer disease, neuroglycopaenia, hypopituitarism, galactorrhoea and amenorrhoea in women, acromegaly, Cushing's syndrome, visual field loss and the presence of subcutaneous lipomata.

Biochemical screening should include serum calcium and prolactin estimations in all individuals, and measurements of gastrointestinal hormones, and more specific endocrine function tests should be reserved for individuals who have symptoms or signs suggestive of a clinical syndrome.

Recent molecular genetic studies which enable the detection of MEN1 gene carriers will further help to identify within these families those individuals who are at risk of devel-

oping MEN1. The recognition of MEN1 in a patient with an endocrine disorder is important as appropriate management decisions, for example in the treatment of parathyroid disease and gastrinoma, can be made and the prognosis improved.

8.2.7 MOLECULAR GENETICS OF MEN1

The development of tumours [20] has been shown to be associated with mutations and abnormal expression of normal cellular genes, which are called oncogenes. Two major types of oncogenes, described as dominantly or recessively acting, have been defined. Dominantly acting oncogenes have been shown to be associated with some diseases, for example chronic myeloid leukaemia and Burkitt's lymphoma, and in these conditions only one copy of the mutated gene is required within a cell for tumour formation.

149

In some inherited neoplasms, which may also arise sporadically, such as retinoblastoma, tumour development is associated with two recessive mutations in oncogenes, and these are referred to as recessive oncogenes. In the inherited tumours, the first of the two recessive mutations is inherited via the germ cell line and is present in all the cells. This recessive mutation is not expressed until a second mutation, within a somatic cell, causes loss of the normal dominant allele.

The mutations causing the inherited and sporadic tumours are similar, but the cell types in which they occur are different. In the inherited tumours, the first mutation occurs in the germ cell, whereas in the sporadic

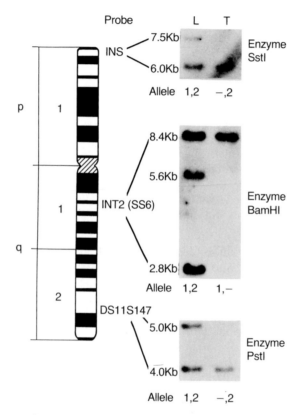

Fig. 8.2 Loss of alleles on chromosome 11 in a parathyroid tumour from a patient with familial MEN1. The RFLPs obtained from the patient's leukocyte (L) and parathyroid tumour (T) DNA using the probes insulin (INS), INT2(SS6) and D11S147 are shown. These probes are cloned human DNA sequences from chromosome 11, and are shown juxtaposed to their region of origin on the short (p) and long (q) arms of chromosome 11. The RFLPs are assigned alleles. For example, three BamHI-derived RFLPs were revealed by INT2(SS6): the 8.4 Kb fragment is assigned allele (1) and the 5.6 Kb and 2.8 Kb fragments are assigned allele (2). The leukocytes are heterozygous (allele 1, 2), but the tumour cells have lost the 5.6 Kb and 2.8 Kb fragments (allele 2) and are hemizygous (allele 1, –). An extensive loss of alleles involving the whole of chromosome 11 is observed in the parathyroid tumour of this patient with MEN1. In addition, the complete absence of bands suggests that this abnormality has occurred within all the tumour cells studied and indicates a monoclonal origin for this MEN1 parathyroid tumour. (From Thakker *et al.* [19]).

150

tumours both mutations occur in the somatic cell. This model [21], involving two or more mutations in the development of tumours, is known as the 'two hit' hypothesis. The normal function of these recessive oncogenes appears to be in regulating cell growth and differentiation, and these genes have also been referred to as anti-oncogenes or tumour suppressor genes.

The investigation of the mutations involved in tumour development and the search for the inherited cancer genes has become possible as a result of advances in molecular biology, which have provided cloned human DNA sequences to detect these mutations [20]. These cloned DNA probes identify restriction fragment length polymorphisms (RFLPs) that are the result of variations in the primary DNA sequence of individuals and may be due to either single base changes, deletions, additions or translocations.

Two complementary approaches have been used to identify the mutations involved in the development of tumours in MEN1 [22–24]. In one approach, RFLPs obtained from a patient's leucocyte DNA were compared to those obtained from tumour DNA and differences were sought. In the second approach, RFLPs were used as genetic markers in linkage studies of affected families in order to localize the gene responsible for MEN1.

Tumour studies

A comparison of leukocyte-derived and tumour-derived RFLPs has demonstrated allelic deletions involving chromosome 11 in parathyroid tumours and insulinomas from patients with MEN1 (Fig. 8.2).

Combined pedigree and tumour studies demonstrated that these tumour-related allelic deletions of chromosome 11 occurred on the chromosome inherited from the normal parent and not the one from the affected parent, and are in keeping with the 'two hit' hypothesis [24].

In addition, these molecular studies have revealed that some MEN1 parathyroid tumours have a monoclonal origin. The allelic deletions that occur in MEN1 parathyroid, pituitary and pancreatic tumours are also observed to occur, though less frequently, in sporadic non-MEN1 parathyroid and anterior pituitary tumours [25].

Further deletion mapping studies using parathyroid and anterior pituitary tumours from MEN1 and non-MEN1 patients have indicated that the mutant gene causing MEN1 is located in the pericentromeric region on the long arm of chromosome 11. Thus, the tumour suppressor gene involved in the development of MEN1 has been localized to 11q13.

Family linkage studies

RFLPs are inherited in a Mendelian manner and their inheritance can be followed together with a disease in an affected family [26]. The consistent inheritance of an RFLP allele with the disease indicates that the two genetic loci are close together, i.e. linked. Genes that are far apart do not consistently co-segregate but show recombination because of crossing over during meiosis. By studying recombination events in family studies, the distance between two genes and the probability that they are linked can be ascertained.

The distance between two genes is expressed as recombination fraction (θ), which is equal to the number of recombinants divided by the number of offspring resulting from informative meioses within a family. The value of θ can range from 0 to 0.5. A value of 0 indicates that the genes are very closely linked, while a value of 0.5 indicates that the genes are far apart.

The genetic distance, expressed as θ, does approximately correlate to the physical distance: for example, a recombination fraction of 10% ($\theta = 0.1$), which is also referred to as 10 centiMorgans, is equivalent to a physical

Family R/87

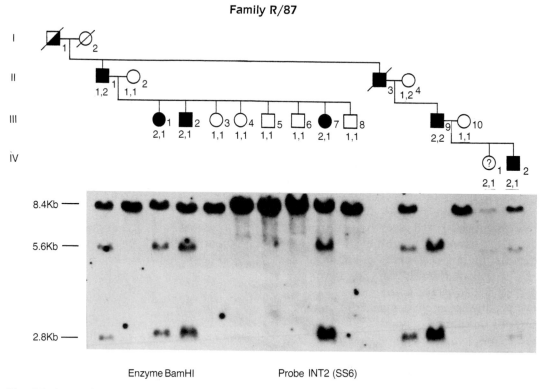

Fig. 8.3 Autoradiography obtained with probe INT2(SS6) hybridized to 5 μg genomic DNA digested with enzyme BamHI. The family, which suffers from MEN1, is drawn so that each member appears above his or her RFLP pattern. Alleles (1 and 2) have been assigned to each RFLP as indicated in Fig. 8.2. Individual II.1 is an affected male who is heterozygous (allele 1, 2) and is the father of eight children (three affected, five unaffected), in whom the paternal allele is shown on the left and the maternal allele on the right. All of the unaffected children have inherited allele 1, whereas the affected children have inherited allele 2. Thus, in this family the inheritance of MEN1 is associated with inheritance of allele 2 at the INT2(SS6) locus. The MEN1 phenotypes in this family were determined by biochemical screening and the age-related penetrance values derived from Fig. 8.1 were used in linkage analysis, as described in the text. (□), Normal male, (○); normal female; (■), affected male; (●), affected female. Individuals below the age of 20 years are shown as unknown (?) phenotype. (From Thakker *et al.* [19]).

distance of 10 million dinucleotide base pairs. The probability that the two loci are linked at these distances is expressed as an 'LOD score', which is log₁₀ of the odds ratio favouring linkage. The odds ratio favouring linkage is defined as the likelihood that two loci are linked at a specified recombination fraction (θ) versus the likelihood that the two loci are not linked.

An LOD score of +3, which indicates a probability in favour of linkage of 1000 to 1, establishes linkage between two loci. An

LOD score of −2, indicating a probability against linkage of 100 to 1, is taken to exclude linkage between two loci. LOD scores are usually evaluated over a range of θ, thereby enabling the genetic distance and the maximum (or peak) probability favouring linkage between two loci to be ascertained. This is illustrated for the family in Fig. 8.3.

In the family shown in Fig. 8.3, the disease and INT2 (SS6) loci are segregating together without recombination, and the likelihood of linkage at θ = 0 is therefore 1. If the disease and the INT2 (SS6) loci were not linked, then the disease would be associated with allele 1 in one half of the children and with allele 2 in the remaining half.

This is not observed in the eight children from the family of individual II.1, in which all three affected children have inherited allele 2 and all five unaffected children have inherited allele 1. The likelihood that the two loci are not linked is $(1/2)^8$. The odds ratio in favour of linkage between the disease and INT2 (SS6) loci at θ = 0, in this family, is therefore $1/(1/2)^8$, i.e. 256 to 1, and the LOD score = 2.4 (i.e. $\log_{10} 256$).

Additional studies from other families have also demonstrated positive LOD scores between MEN1 and the INT2 (SS6) locus. LOD scores from individual families have been summed, and the peak LOD score between MEN1 and INT2 (SS6) locus has exceeded +3, thereby establishing linkage between MEN1 and INT2 (SS6) loci [20].

Linkage between MEN1 and two other DNA probes, PYGM (glycogen phosphorylase in muscle, McArdle's syndrome) and the DNA segment D11S146 and INT2 (SS6), have all been localized to 11q13, and the results of these studies map the gene causing MEN1 to the pericentromeric region of the long arm of chromosome 11 (Fig. 8.4) [22,27].

This localization of the MEN1 gene will help in identifying individuals from affected families who are mutant gene carriers and therefore at a higher risk of developing the

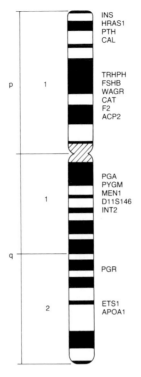

Fig. 8.4 Map of human chromosome 11 showing the locations of some genes encoding hormones, clinically useful DNA probes, oncogenes and disease loci. Chromosome 11 with Giemsa bands is schematically represented, and the probe and disease loci are shown juxtaposed to their regional localization, which has been ascertained by *in situ* hybridization, somatic cell hybrid or multipoint linkage studies. (INS), insulin; (HRAS1), harvey ras sarcoma 1 viral oncogene homologue; (PTH), parathyroid hormone; (CAL), calcitonin; (TRHPH), tryptophan hydroxylase; (FSHβ), follicle stimulating hormone, β polypeptide; (WAGR), Wilms' tumour, aniridia, genitourinary abnormalities and mental retardation complex; (CAT), catalase; (F2), coagulation factor II, prothrombin; (ACP2), acid phosphatase 2, lysosomal; (PGA), pepsinogen; (PYGM), phosphorylase glycogen muscle (McArdle's syndrome), glycogen storage disease type V; (MEN1), multiple endocrine neoplasia type 1; (D11S146), DNA segment; (INT2), murine mammary tumour virus integration site oncogene homologue; (PGR), progesterone receptor; (ETS1), avian erythroblastosis virus E26 oncogene homologue 1; and (APOA1), apolipoprotein A1.

disease. These individuals would then be advised to undergo regular screening, so that early effective therapy could be undertaken.

In addition, individuals from affected families who are not mutant gene carriers could be reassured and advised not to attend for regular screening. Further analysis to characterize the gene causing MEN1 is under way to elucidate the molecular basis for MEN1.

8.2.8 CIRCULATING GROWTH FACTORS IN MEN1

A factor with high parathyroid mitogenic activity has been identified in the plasma of MEN1 patients by *in vitro* studies, which used bovine parathyroid cells maintained in a long-term culture system [28]. Plasma from MEN1 patients stimulated these bovine parathyroid cells to rapidly incorporate [^{3}H] thymidine and to proliferate. This plasma mitogenic activity was markedly reduced by heat, acid and dithiothreitol treatment, indicating that the stimulatory properties may be due to a protein containing disulphide bonds.

This mitogenic factor was demonstrated to be a distinct factor from other growth factors such as epidermal growth factor (EGF), platelet derived growth factor (PDGF), nerve growth factor (NGF), fibroblast growth factor (FGF), insulin-like growth factor I (IGF-I) and tumour growth factor β (TGFβ), and was shown not to be an autocrine product from the parathyroid glands themselves.

This plasma mitogenic factor appeared to be specific for parathyroid cells and did not stimulate activity in anterior pituitary or pancreatic islet cells. More recent studies [29] have revealed that a basic fibroblast growth factor (bFGF) or a closely related factor is present in the plasma of patients with MEN1. The estimation of this parathyroid mitogenic factor is not generally available as a screening test, but the role of this mitogenic factor in MEN1 patients needs to be elucidated further.

8.3 MULTIPLE ENDOCRINE NEOPLASIA TYPE 2 (MEN2)

The clinical manifestations of MEN2 are related to the sites of the tumours and their products of secretion (Table 8.1). Genetic and molecular biological studies have helped to identify carriers of the mutant gene and to define the age-related penetrance of this autosomal dominant disease.

8.3.1 MULTIPLE ENDOCRINE NEOPLASIA TYPE 2A (MEN2a)

The triad of MTC, phaeochromocytoma and parathyroid tumours constitute the major components of MEN2a.

Medullary thyroid carcinoma (MTC)

MTC is the most common feature of MEN2a and occurs in almost all affected individuals. MTC represents 10% of all thyroid gland carcinomas, and 20% of MTC patients have a family history of the disorder [30]. Patients may be asymptomatic and the presence of MTC may have been detected by the demonstration of hypercalcitoninaemia at family screening.

However, MTC may also present as a palpable mass in the neck which causes symptoms of pressure or dysphagia in 16% of patients [30]. Diarrhoea may occur in 30% of patients [31] and is associated either with elevated circulating concentrations of calcitonin or tumour-related secretion of serotonin and prostaglandins. In addition, ectopic ACTH production by MTC may cause Cushing's syndrome [32].

Metastases of MTC, in the early stages, usually occur to the cervical lymph nodes, and in later stages to the mediastinal nodes, lung, liver, trachea, adrenal, oesophagus and bone. Radiography may reveal dense, irregular calcification within the involved portions of the thyroid gland and the lymph nodes involved with metastases. Radioiodine thyroid scans reveal the MTC tumours as cold nodules.

Diagnosis

The diagnosis of MTC relies on the demonstration of hypercalcitoninaemia either in the basal state ($>90 \, pg \, ml^{-1}$) or following stimulation with intravenous pentagastrin (0.5 $mg \, kg^{-1}$) and/or calcium infusion (2 $mg \, kg^{-1}$).

Procedure

Following an overnight fast, two basal blood samples for calcitonin are taken, following which pentagastrin (0.5 $mg \, kg^{-1}$) and calcium gluconate (2 $mg \, kg^{-1}$) are given as a bolus. Blood samples are taken at 1-minute intervals for 5 minutes for calcitonin levels.

Interpretation

Diagnostic criteria for MCT in MEN2 on the basis of the calcitonin testing are as follows: (i) a normal basal level of calcitonin (less than 200 $pg \, ml^{-1}$) that increases following the short pentagastrin/calcium infusion to greater than 300 $pg \, ml^{-1}$, or (ii) an elevated basal calcitonin level ($>300 \, pg \, ml^{-1}$) which if in the range 300–600 $pg \, ml^{-1}$ must rise at least fivefold following the provocative stimulus.

The previously used 'whisky test', in which elevations in circulating calcitonin were measured after drinking 50 ml of whisky or vodka, is not entirely reliable and has been replaced by the pentagastrin and calcium infusion tests. MTC in patients with a family history of MEN2a may be associated with phaeochromocytoma, therefore patients must be assessed and treated for these catecholamine secreting tumours prior to thyroidectomy, which is the definitive treatment for MTC.

Phaeochromocytoma

These noradrenaline and adrenaline secreting tumours occur in 50% of patients with MEN2a, and are a major cause of morbidity and mortality. Patients may have the symptoms and signs of excess catecholamine secretion or they may be asymptomatic and have been detected through biochemical screening, because of a history of either familial MEN2a or MTC.

The biochemical and radiological investigation of phaeochromocytoma in MEN2a patients is similar to that in non-MEN2 patients and is reviewed in Chapter 9. However, phaeochromocytomas in patients with MEN2a differ significantly in distribution when compared to those in non-MEN2 patients, and tend to be adrenal.

Bilateral adrenomedullary hyperplasia is the precursor to phaeochromocytoma in patients with MEN2. This is associated with the expansion of medullary tissue into the body and tail of the gland, with a decrease in corticomedullary ratio and nodular hyperplasia. Nodules exceeding 1 mm diameter are designated phaeochromocytomas.

The incidence of bilateral adrenal medullary tumours in MEN2a patients is 70%, in contrast to the 10% incidence observed in non-MEN2 patients [33,34]. In addition, extra-adrenal phaeochromocytomas, which occur in 10% of non-MEN2 patients, are rarely observed in MEN2a patients, and similarly malignancy in MEN2a phaeochromocytoma is much less common. Thus, a recommended treatment for phaeochromocytoma in patients with MEN2a is bilateral adrenalectomy, even in those MEN2a patients in whom only a unilateral tumour has been demonstrated by radiology [35].

Diagnosis

An early biochemical abnormality in MEN2 patients with phaeochromocytoma and medullary hyperplasia is an increase in the adrenalin/noradrenalin ratio to less than 0.15.

Parathyroid tumours

The incidence of parathyroid tumours in MEN2a patients varies from 40% to 80% in different series [36]. However, more than 50% of these patients do not have hypercalcaemia, and the presence of abnormally enlarged parathyroids, which are usually hyperplastic, is revealed in the normocalcaemic patient undergoing thyroidectomy for MTC. The biochemical investigation and management of the hypercalcaemic MEN2a patient is similar to that of the MEN1 patient.

8.3.2 MULTIPLE ENDOCRINE NEOPLASIA TYPE 2B (MEN2b)

In MEN2b, which has also been referred to as MEN type 3 (MEN3), the occurrence of MTC and phaeochromocytoma is associated with characteristic somatic features (see Table 8.1). Patients with MEN2b very rarely have parathyroid tumours but frequently suffer from a more aggressive form of MTC.

The diagnosis and management of each of these tumours are similar to those for the MEN2a tumours. However, the survival rates following thyroidectomy MTC in patients with MEN2b are significantly decreased [37], with the five-year survival rate being 80% and the ten-year survival rate being 50%.

The management of phaeochromocytoma in MEN2b patients is similar to that in MEN2a patients, and a conservative management is usually adopted for the mucosal neuromas.

8.3.3 MOLECULAR GENETICS OF MEN2

Molecular genetic studies in families suffering from MEN2a, MEN2b and MTC-only have localized these loci to the pericentromeric region of chromosome 10. All of these MEN2 variants show linkage to the same chromo-

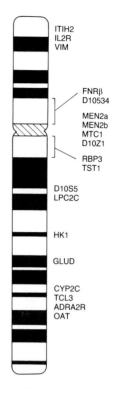

Fig. 8.5 Map of human chromosome 10 showing the locations of some genes encoding receptors, growth factors, enzymes, disease loci and some clinically useful DNA probes. Chromosome 10 with Giemsa bands is schematically represented, and the probe and disease loci are shown juxtaposed to their regional localization, which has been ascertained by *in situ* hybridization, somatic cell hybrid or multipoint linkage studies. (ITIH2), inter-alpha-trypsin inhibitor (protein HC) H2 polypeptide; (IL2R), interleukin 2 receptor; (VIM), vimentin; (FNRβ), fibronectin receptor, β polypeptide; (D10S34), DNA segment; (RBP3), interstitial retinol-binding protein 3; (TST1), transforming sequence, thyroid 1; (D10S5), DNA segment; (LPC2C), lipoprotein IIc; (HK1), hexokinase; (GLUD), glutamate dehydrogenase; (CYP2C), cytochrome P450, subfamily IIc, mephenytoin-4-hydroxylase; (TCL3), T cell lymphoma 3 associated breakpoint; (ADRA2R), adrenergic, alpha-2 receptor; and (OAT), ornithine aminotransferase.

some 10 markers, thereby indicating that each variant may be due to different mutant alleles at the same locus or that the pericentromeric region of chromosome 10 contains a group of genes involved in the development of neuroendocrine tumours.

Family linkage studies mapping MEN2

Linkage has been established between MEN2a and the retinol-binding protein (RBP3) locus and the D10S5 locus [38,39], thereby mapping the MEN2a gene to the pericentromeric region of chromosome 10.

In order to define a precise location for MEN2a, these studies have been extended in additional pedigrees using more DNA markers. The MEN2a gene has been mapped [40] between the DNA marker D10S34, which is located in the short arm region 10p12-p11, and the RBP3 locus which is located in the long arm region 10q11.2 (Fig. 8.5).

Genetic linkage studies in families affected with either MEN2b or MTC-only using DNA markers from the pericentromeric region of chromosome 10 have demonstrated that these loci are also located in the same region as MEN2a (see Fig. 8.5). Linkage was established between MEN2b and the D10Z1 locus, and between MTC-only and the D10Z1 locus [41].

These results, which demonstrate that the three clinically distinct variants of MEN2 (i.e., MEN2a, MEN2b and MTC-only) are located in the same chromosome region, suggest that either these MEN2 variants are allelic mutations at the same locus, or that this pericentromeric region of chromosome 10 contains a cluster of genes that are involved in the regulation of neuroendocrine tissue development.

Tumour studies

The molecular genetics of tumour development in MEN2 appears to be more complex than that described for MEN1 (see above).

Allele loss in MEN2a tumours is not observed to involve chromosome 10, and a detailed study of 42 MEN2a tumours using DNA markers from the short and long arms of chromosome 10 demonstrated allele loss in only one tumour [42].

However, allele loss in MEN2a tumours is frequently observed to involve the short arm of chromosome 1 (1p) [43]. Thus, there appear to be important differences in the genetic mechanisms involved in the development of MEN1 and MEN2 tumours. One possibility is that the genetic mechanism involved in MEN2 tumours may indeed be similar to that in MEN1 tumours, but that the allelic deletion in MEN2 tumours is confined to the MEN2 gene and that the current methods are not capable of detecting this small specific deletion.

MEN2 tumours with this small specific deletion of the MEN2 gene may be the only ones to develop if there were another gene close to the MEN2, hemizygous loss of which caused reduced viability to the cell. Thus, tumours with large deletions may be selected against, whereas tumours with small specific deletions involving the MEN2 gene may proliferate.

This possibility seems unlikely as one MEN2 tumour with allele loss involving a complete chromosome 10 loss has been observed [42]. However, the frequent occurrence of chromosome 10 loss in gliomas [44], which are also of neuroectodermal origin, argues against this possibility.

Tumour development in MEN2 may be more complex than in MEN1, and the situation may be analogous to that in colorectal carcinoma, where a progressive series of mutations is required for tumorigenesis [45]. The isolation of very closely linked probes and the cloning of the MEN2 gene will help to elucidate the factors regulating the growth and development of these neuroendocrine tumours.

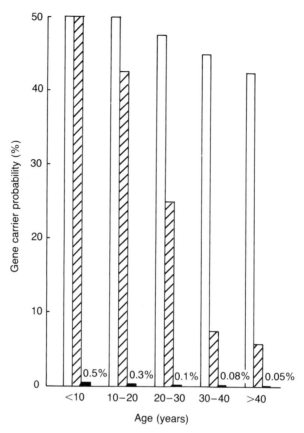

Fig. 8.6 Age-related penetrances and the probabilities for gene carriers of MEN2a. The probabilities (%) for a child of an affected MEN2a parent being a gene carrier following negative screening results using clinical history, pentagastrin-stimulated calcitonin and/or DNA marker studies (see Fig. 8:7) are shown for five age groups. The risk, assessed clinically at birth, of having inherited this autosomal dominant disorder is 50%, and a pentagastrin stimulated calcitonin is not useful in reducing this risk further. In contrast, DNA marker studies using flanking DNA probes can markedly reduce this risk of being a carrier to 0.5% (Fig. 8.7). With increasing age the clinically assessed risk for the unaffected child of an affected parent declines gradually from 50% to only 42.5% at the age of 40 years. However, the risk as assessed by the pentagastrin-stimulated calcitonin test declines more rapidly from 50% at birth to 25% by age 20 years and to 6% by age 40 years. These risks can be further decreased by the combined use of flanking DNA markers and the significantly lower 0.5% risk of being a gene carrier at birth is reduced to 0.05% at the age of 40 years. These risks are calculated for an individual whose mother was affected. For individuals whose father was affected, the above risk estimations after DNA marker tests will be lower because of the reduced probability of recombination in males. Thus, the use of DNA markers can help considerably in reassuring those individuals who are not gene carriers for MEN2a and in identifying those who are MEN2a gene carriers and who therefore require regular screening. (□), Clinical history; (□), pentagastrin-stimulated calcitonin; (■), DNA markers plus pentagastrin-stimulated calcitonin. (Adapted from Mathew *et al.* [40]).

8.3.4 FAMILY SCREENING

The detection by biochemical screening of the development of MEN2 tumours in asymptomatic members of families with MEN2 is of great importance, as earlier diagnosis and treatment of MTC and phaeochromocytoma reduces morbidity and mortality. Individuals within an affected family are at 50% risk of having inherited this autosomal dominant condition.

The disorder affects all age groups, with a reported age range of 2–60 years and a mean age of 25 years [46,47]. However, the clinical penetrance is incomplete and 40% of gene carriers remain asymptomatic at the age of 70 years [48].

The biochemical screening for MTC, which is invariably the earliest manifestation of MEN2, relies on the measurement of plasma calcitonin in both the basal state and following intravenous pentagastrin or calcium stimulation (see above). The estimation of plasma and urinary catecholamines is preferred for the detection of phaeochromocytomas [49,50], and the presence of hypercalcaemia and raised serum PTH concentrations indicates the development of parathyroid tumours.

Biochemical screening for MEN2 does involve a commitment to repeated tests from the age of 5 to at least 30 years. The pentagastrin test has become the most useful primary screening investigation for MTC, which is usually the first tumour to develop in MEN2. However, this test is mildly unpleasant and false positives do occur.

In addition, there are age-related penetrances for MEN2, and earlier detection of the disorder can be achieved more readily by a pentagastrin stimulation test rather than by clinical manifestations alone (Fig. 8.6).

For example, by the ages of 20 years and 30 years the disorder can be detected by clinical manifestations in only 3% and 15% of patients, respectively, whereas the pentagastrin stimulation test can detect 70% and 95% of patients at these respective ages [51].

Thus, identification of individuals at risk in an affected family can be difficult, and the recent availability of DNA markers for MEN2 has helped to reduce these problems. These DNA markers enable MEN2 gene carries to be detected within a family and thereby identify those individuals who need to undergo repeated screening tests for the development of tumours. This is illustrated in Fig. 8.7 for a family suffering from MEN2a.

The application of DNA markers to predictive testing has helped to determine the carrier risk status of many individuals, and this has substantially altered the screening strategy and clinical management of these patients [40]. It is recommended that DNA analysis should now be introduced in the screening programme of MEN2 families.

The advantages of DNA analysis are that it requires a single blood sample and does not need to be repeated, unlike the biochemical screening tests. This is because the analysis is independent of the age of the individual and provides an objective result. The limitations are that blood samples for DNA analysis must be available from two or more affected family members to conclude which allele of the marker is inherited with the MEN2a gene.

In addition, DNA analysis may be subject to a small but significant error rate because of recombination between the marker and the gene. This error rate can be minimized by the use of flanking DNA markers. The ultimate cloning of the gene itself will help to identify mutations directly and thereby remove this limited uncertainty. At present, an integrated programme of both DNA screening, to identify gene carries, and biochemical screening, to detect the development of tumours, is recommended.

Thus, a positive DNA test in an individual is likely to lead not to immediate surgery but to earlier and more frequent calcitonin

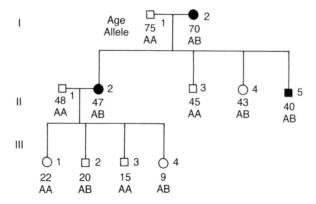

Fig. 8.7 Identification of gene carriers using DNA markers in family A, which suffers from MEN2a. The ages of each individual and the BglII derived RFLPs at the RBP3 locus, which reveals a <3% recombination rate with MEN2, are shown. The paternal alleles are shown on the left and the maternal alleles on the right. Individual I.2 is an affected female who is heterozygous (alleles AB) and is the mother of four children; her affected children II.2 and II.5 indicate segregation of allele B and the disease. Her unaffected daughter (II.4), who is 43 years old, has inherited allele B, and this indicates that she is highly likely (probability >97%) to be a MEN2a gene carrier. This individual (II.4) should undergo regular biochemical screening as she is at risk of developing the disease. However, it is important to note that not all gene carriers develop the disease, as the clinical presentation of MEN2 is incomplete and 40% of gene carriers do not present with symptoms by the age of 70 years. The unaffected son (II.3), who is 45 years old, has inherited allele A from his mother (I.2) and has a low probability (<3%) of being a gene carrier. The risk, for this age group, can be further reduced to 0.05% by the combined use of a flanking DNA marker and the pentagastrin-stimulated test (see Fig. 8.6). The four children (III.1 to III.4) of the affected female II.2 who is heterozygous (alleles AB), are in younger age groups and have not developed the disease. However, individuals III.2 and III.4 have inherited allele B from their affected mother, and are at risk of developing the disease as the probability of being gene carriers exceeds 97%. They should undergo regular biochemical screening. In contrast, individuals III.1 and III.3 have inherited allele A from their affected mother II.2, and this indicates a low probability (<3%) of their being gene carriers. The combined use of flanking DNA markers and the pentagastrin stimulation test in individual III.1, who is 22 years old, reduces this risk to 0.1% and in individual III.3, who is 15 years old, the risk is reduced to 0.3% (see Fig. 8.6). Thus, the use of DNA markers facilitates the identification of gene carriers and those individuals who need regular screening. (□), Normal male; (○), normal female; (■), affected male; (●), affected female. (Adapted from Mathew *et al.* [40]).

screening, whereas a negative DNA result that leaves an individual with a residual carrier risk of less than 1% will probably lead to a decision for either infrequent or no screening. Therefore, the recent advances in molecular biology, which have enabled the localization of the gene(s) causing MEN2a, MEN2b and MTC-only, have helped in the clinical management of patients and their families with these disorders.

8.4 CONCLUSION

Recent advances in the measurements of hormones and in molecular genetics have improved our understanding of the clinical varieties of the MEN syndromes, their presentation, age at onset, diagnosis and patterns of occurrences within families. These advances have facilitated the earlier detection and diagnosis of the disorders. Localization of the genes causing MEN1 and MEN2 to chromosome 11 and 10, respectively, is an important step towards the cloning of these genes. This will further help in family screening programmes and will also assist in elucidating the pathogenesis of these endocrine tumour syndromes.

REFERENCES

1. Thakker, R.V. and Ponder, B.A.J. (1988) Multiple endocrine neoplasia. In *Molecular Biology of Endocrinology. Bailliere's Clinical Endocrinology and Metabolism*, vol. 2, no. 4 (ed. M.C. Sheppard), Bailliere Tindall, London, pp. 1031–68.

2. Marx, S.J., Spiegel, A.M., Levine, M.A., Rizzoli, R.E., Lasker, R.D., Santora, A.C., Downs, Jr, R.V. and Aurbach, G.D. (1982) Familial hypocalciuric hypercalcaemia: the relation to primary parathyroid hyperplasia. *New Engl. J. Med.*, **307**, 416–26.

3. Rizzoli, R., Green, J. and Marx, S.J. (1985) Primary hyperparathyroidism in familial multiple endocrine neoplasis type 1. Long term follow-up of serum calcium levels after parathyroidectomy. *Am. J. Med.*, **78**, 467–74.

4. Wells, Jr, S.A., Fardon, J.R., Dale, J.K., Leight, G.S. and Dilley, W.G. (1980) Long-term evaluation of patients with primary parathyroid hyperplasia managed by total parathyroidectomy and heterotopic autotransplantation. *Ann. Surg.*, **192**, 451–8.

5. Saxe, A.W. and Brennan, M.F. (1982) Re operative parathyroid surgery for primary hyperparathyroidism caused by multiple-gland disease: total parathyroidectomy and autotransplantation with cryopreserved tissue. *Surgery*, **91**, 616–21.

6. Mallette, L.E., Blevins, T., Jordan, P.H. and Noon, G.P. (1987) Autogenous parathyroid grafts for generalised primary hyperplasia: contrasting outcome in sporadic versus multiple endocrine neoplasia type I. *Surgery*, **101**, 738–45.

7. Wolfe, M.M. and Jensen, R.T. (1987) Zollinger–Ellison syndrome. Current concepts in diagnosis and management. *New Engl. J. Med.*, **317**, 1200–9.

8. Betts, J.B., O'Malley, B.P. and Rosenthal, F.D. (1980) Hyperparathyroidism: a prerequisite for Zollinger–Ellison syndrome in multiple endocrine adenomatosis type 1 – report of a further family and a review of the literature. *Q. J. Med.*, **193**, 69–76.

9. Benson, L., Ljunghall, S., Akerstrom, G. and Oberg, K. (1987) Hyperparathyroidism presenting as the first lesion in multiple endocrine neoplasia type 1. *Am. J. Med.*, **82**, 731–7.

10. Thompson, M.H., Sanders, D.J. and Grund, E.R. (1976) The relationship of the serum gastrin and calcium concentrations in patients with multiple endocrine neoplasia type 1. *Br. J. Surg.*, **63**, 779–83.

11. Delcore, R., Hermreck, A.S. and Friesen, S.R. (1989) Selective surgical management of correctable hypergastrinemia. *Surgery*, **106**, 1094–102.

12. Sheppard, B.C., Norton, J.A., Dopmann, J.L., Maton, P.N., Gardner, J.D. and Jensen, R.T. (1989) Management of islet cell tumours in patients with multiple endocrine neoplasia: a prospective study. *Surgery*, **106**, 1108–18.

13. Thompson, N.W., Bondeson, A.G., Bondeson, L. and Vinik, A. (1989) The surgical treatment of gastrinoma in MEN1 syndrome patients. *Surgery*, **106**, 1081–6.

14. Wise, S.R., Johnson, J., Sparks, J., Carey, L.C. and Ellison, E.C. (1989) Gastrinoma: the predictive value of preoperative localisation. *Surgery*, **106**, 1087–93.

15. Fertig, A., Webley, M. and Lynn, J.A. (1980) Primary hyperparathyroidism in a patient with Conn's syndrome. *Postgrad. Med. J.*, **56**, 45–7.

16. Marx, S.J., Vinik, A.I., Santen, R.J., Floyd, J.C., Mills, J.L. and Green, J. (1986) Multiple endocrine neoplasia type 1: assessment of laboratory tests to screen for the gene in a large kindred. *Medicine*, **65**, 226–41.

17. Skogseld, B., Oberg, K., Benson, L., Lindgren, P.S., Lörelius, L.E., Lundquist, G., Wide, L. and Wilander, E. (1987) A standardized meal stimulation test of the endocrine pancreas for early detection of pancreatic endocrine tumours in multiple endocrine neoplasia type 1 syndrome: five years experience. *J. Clin. Endocrinol. Metab.*, **64**, 1233–40.

18. Vansen, H.F.A., Lamers, C.B.H.W. and Lips, C.J.M. (1989) Screening for multiple endo-

crine neoplasia syndrome type 1. A study of 11 kindreds in the Netherlands. *Archs Intern. Med.*, **149**, 2717–22.

19. Thakker, R.V., Bouloux, P., Wooding, C., Chotai, K., Broad, P.M., Spurr, N.K., Besser, G.M. and O'Riordan, J.L.H. (1990) The molecular basis of parathyroid tumours in multiple endocrine neoplasia type 1. In *Calcium Regulation and Bone Metabolism*, vol. 10 (eds D.V. Cohn, T.J. Martin and P.J. Meunier), Elsevier, Amsterdam.

20. Thakker, R.V., Davies, K.E. and O'Riordan, J.L.H. (1989) Gene mapping of mineral metabolic disorders. *J. Inherited Metab. Dis.*, **12** (suppl. 1), 231–46.

21. Knudson, A.G., Strong, L.C. and Anderson, D.E. (1973) Hereditary and cancer in man. *Progr. Med. Genet.*, **9**, 113–58.

22. Larsson, C., Skogseld, B., Oberg, K., Nakamura, Y. and Nordenskjöld, M. (1988) Multiple endocrine neoplasia type 1 gene maps to chromosome 11 and is lost in insulinoma. *Nature*, **332**, 85–7.

23. Friedman, E., Sakaguchi, K., Bale, A.E., Falchelti, A., Streeten, E., Zimering, M.B., Weinstein, L.S., McBride, W.O., Nakamura, Y., Brandi, M.L., Norton, J.A., Aurbach, G.D., Spiegel, A.M. and Marx, S.J. (1989) Clonality of parathyroid tumours in familial multiple endocrine neoplasia type 1. *New Engl. J. Med.*, **321**, 213–18.

24. Thakker, R.V., Bouloux, P., Wooding, C., Chotai, K., Broad, P.M., Spurr, N.K., Besser, G.M. and O'Riordan, J.L.H. (1989) Association of parathyroid tumours in multiple endocrine neoplasia type 1 with loss of alleles on chromosome 11. *New Engl. J. Med.*, **321**, 218–24.

25. Byström, C., Larsson, C., Blomberg, C., Sandelin, F., Falkmer, U., Skogseld, B., Oberg, K., Werner, S. and Nordenskjöld, M. (1990) Localisation of the MEN1 gene to a small region within chromosome 11q13 by deletion mapping in tumours. *Proc. Natl. Acad. Sci.*, **87**, 1968–72.

26. Thakker, R.V. and O'Riordan, J.L.H. (1988) Inherited forms of rickets and osteomalacia. In *Metabolic Bone Disease. Bailliere's Clinical Endocrinology and Metabolism*, vol. 2, no. 1 (ed. T.J. Martin), Bailliere Tindall, London, pp. 157–91.

27. Nakamura, Y., Larsson, C., Julier, C., Byström, C., Skogseld, B., Wells, S., Oberg, F., Carlson, M., Taggart, T., O'Connell, P., Leppert, M., Lalouel, J.M., Nordenskjöld, M. and White, R. (1989) Localisation of the genetic defect in multiple endocrine neoplasia type 1 within a small region of chromosome 11. *Am. J. Hum. Genet.*, **44**, 751–5.

28. Brandi, M.L., Aurbach, G.D., Fitzpatrick, L.A., Quarto, R., Spiegel, A.M., Bliziotes, M.M., Norton, J.A., Doppman, J.L. and Marx, S.J. (1986) Parathyroid mitogenic activity in plasma from patients with familial multiple endocrine neoplasia type 1. *New Engl. J. Med.*, **314**, 1287–93.

29. Zimering, M.B., Brandi, M.L., de Grange, D.A., Marx, S.J., Streeten, E., Katsumata, N., Murphy, P.R., Sato, Y., Friesen, H.G. and Aurbach, G.D. (1990) Circulating fibroblast growth factor like substance in familial multiple endocrine neoplasia type 1. *J. Clin. Endocrinol. Metab.*, **70**, 149–54.

30. Hill, Jr, C.S., Ibanez, M.L., Samaan, N.A. *et al.* (1973) Medullary (solid) carcinoma of the thyroid glands: an analysis of the M.D. Anderson Hospital experience with patients with the tumour, its special features and its histogenesis. *Medicine*, **52**, 141–71.

31. Cox, T.M., Fagan, E.A., Hillyard, C.J. *et al.* (1979) Role of calcitonin in diarrhoea associated with medullary carcinoma of the thyroid. *Gut*, **20**, 629–33.

32. Melvin, K.E.W., Tashjian, Jr, A.J., Cassidy, C.E. *et al.* (1970) Cushing's syndrome caused by ACTH and calcitonin-secreting medullary carcinoma of the thyroid. *Metabolism*, **19**, 831–8.

33. Lips, C.J.M., van der Sluys Veer, J., Struyvenberg, A. *et al.* (1981) Bilateral occurrence of phaeochromocytoma in multiple endocrine neoplasia type 2a (Sipple's syndrome). *Am. J. Med.*, **70**, 1051–60.

34. Webb, T.A., Sheps, S.G. and Carney, J.A. (1980) Differences between sporadic phaeochromocytoma and phaeochromocytoma in multiple endocrine neoplasia type 2. *Am. J. Surg. Path.*, **4**, 121–6.

35. Freier, D.T., Thompson, N.W., Sisson, J.C. *et al.* (1977) Dilemmas in the early diagnosis and treatment of multiple endocrine adenomatosis, type II. *Surgery*, **82**, 407–13.

36. Keiser, H.R., Beaven, M.A., Doppman, J. *et al.* (1977) Sipple's syndrome: medullary thyroid carcinoma, phaeochromocytoma, and parathyroid disease: studies in a large family. *Ann. Intern. Med.*, **78**, 561–79.

37. Carney, J.A., Sizemore, G.W. and Hayles, A.B. (1979) C-cell disease of the thyroid gland in multiple endocrine neoplasia, type 2b. *Cancer*, **44**, 2173–83.

38. Mathew, C.G.P., Chink, S., Easton, D.G. *et al.* (1987) A linked genetic marker for multiple endocrine neoplasia type 2a on chromosome 10. *Nature*, **328**, 527–8.

39. Simpson, N.E., Kidd, K.K., Goodfellow, P.J. *et al.* (1987) Assignment of multiple endocrine neoplasia type 2a on chromosome 10 by linkage. *Nature*, **328**, 528–30.

40. Mathew, C.G.P., Easton, D.F., Nakamura, Y. and Ponder, B.A.J. (1991) Presymptomatic screening for multiple endocrine neoplasia type 2a with linked DNA markers. *Lancet*, **337**, 7–11.

41. Lairmore, T.C., Howe, J.R., Korte, J.A., Dilley, W.G., Aine, L., Aine, E., Wells, Jr, S.A. and Donis-Keller, H. (1991) Familial medullary thyroid carcinoma and multiple endocrine neoplasia type 2b map to the same region of chromosome 10 as multiple endocrine neoplasia type 2a. *Genomics*, **9**, 181–92.

42. Ponder, B.A.J., Smith, B.A., Marcus, E.M., Nakamura, Y., Landsvater, R.M., Buys, C.H.C.M. and Mathew, C.G.P. (1989) Genetic events in tumorigenesis in multiple endocrine neoplasia type 2. *Cancer Cells*, **7**, 219–21.

43. Mathew, C.G.P., Smith, B.A., Thorpe, K., Wong, Z., Royle, N.J., Jeffreys, A.J. and Ponder, B.A.J. (1989) Deletion of genes on chromosome 1 in endocrine neoplasia. *Nature*, **328**, 524–6.

44. Bigner, S.H., Mark, J., Burger, P.C. *et al.* (1988) Specific chromosome abnormalities in malignant human gliomas. *Cancer Res.*, **88**, 405–11.

45. Fearon, E.R. and Vogelstein, B. (1990) A genetic model for colorectal tumorigenesis. *Cell*, **61**, 759–67.

46. Lips, C.J.M., Vaseu, H.F.A. and Lamers, C.B.H.W. (1984) Multiple endocrine neoplasia syndromes. *CRC Crit. Rev. Oncol./Haematol.*, **2**, 117–84.

47. Gagel, R.F., Jackson, C.E., Block, M.A., Feldman, Z.T., Reichlin, G., Hamilton, B.P. and Tashjian, Jr, A.H. (1982) Age-related probability of development of hereditary medullary thyroid carcinoma. *J. Pediat.*, **101**, 941–6.

48. Easton, D.F., Ponder, M.A., Cummings, T. and the CRC Medullary Thyroid Group (1989) The clinical and screening age-at-onset distribution for the MEN2 syndrome. *Am. J. Hum. Genet.*, **44**, 208–15.

49. Sheps, S.G., Jiang, N.S. and Kless, G.G. (1988) Diagnostic evaluation of phaeochromocytoma. *Endocrinol. Metab. Clin. North Am.*, **17**, 397–414.

50. Vistele, R., Grulet, H., Gibold, C., Chafour-Higel, B., Delemer, B., Fay, R., Delisle, M.J. and Caron, J. (1991) High permanent plasma adrenaline levels: a marker of adrenal medullary disease in medullary thyroid carcinoma. *Clin. Endocrinol.*, **34**, 133–8.

51. Ponder, B.A.J., Ponder, M.A., Coffey, R., Pembrey, M.E., Gagel, R.F., Telenius-Berg, M., Semple, P. and Easton, D.F. (1988) Risk estimation and screening in families of patients with medullary thyroid carcinoma. *Lancet*, **i**, 397–401.

163

9

Endocrine hypertension

P.L. PADFIELD and C.R.W. EDWARDS

9.1 INTRODUCTION

There can be no doubt that hypertension is common. Estimates of prevalence vary with diagnostic criteria, numbers of measurements and the populations studied, but a conservative estimate for the western world is that some 10% of the adult population have raised blood pressure.

There is even more uncertainty regarding the true prevalence of secondary or endocrine hypertension, given that most studies have been performed in selected patients. Even within the 95% or more of patients with raised blood pressure in whom no demonstrable cause can be found, it is conceivable that endocrine disorders may play a part [1].

Hypertension may be commoner among diabetic patients [2] and is probably present more often than chance would dictate in both hypothyroidism [3] and acromegaly [4]. In addition, up to 40% of patients with hyperparathyroidism have been found to be hypertensive, although blood pressure may not always be affected by parathyroidectomy [5].

It is not, however, the purpose of this chapter to consider these specific conditions, but more those which may be considered in patients presenting with raised blood pressure in whom there is reason to believe that a secondary cause may be involved.

The value of the various diagnostic tests in both primary and secondary mineralocorticoid excess, together with those in renal artery stenosis, will be reviewed. In addition, a brief comment will be made upon hypertension in glucocorticoid excess.

9.2 ADRENOCORTICAL DISORDERS

9.2.1 MINERALOCORTICOID HYPERTENSION

Physiology of the renin–angiotensin system and the control of aldosterone production

Aldosterone is regulated primarily via the renin–angiotensin system [6] (see Fig. 9.1).

Angiotensin II is an octapeptide generated within the circulation by the action of two enzymes on a precursor α_2-globulin (angiotensinogen) from the liver. The first enzyme, renin, is secreted by the renal juxta-glomerular cells in response to a variety of stimuli but mainly a fall in effective circulating blood volume or pressure. Renin cleaves the largely inactive decapeptide angiotensin I from angiotensinogen and the so-called converting enzyme, a dipeptidase, removes a further two amino acids to produce angiotensin II, the main effector of the system.

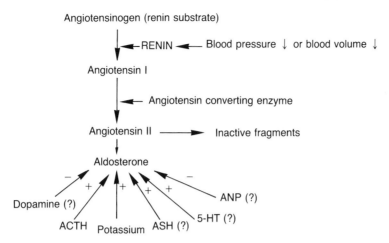

Fig. 9.1 The control of aldosterone production. Only angiotensis II is of clear physiological significance. ACTH, adrenocorticotropic hormone; ASH, aldosterone stimulating hormone; 5-HT, serotonin; ANP, atrial natriuretic peptide.

Circulating angiotensin II stimulates the conversion of cholesterol to pregnenolone (the rate limiting step in the formation of all steroid hormones) and also probably acts later in the pathway, converting corticosterone to aldosterone [7].

In supine humans, plasma aldosterone levels parallel those of adrenocorticotropic hormone (ACTH) and cortisol, although this circadian effect is not present in ambulatory subjects where the postural increase in renin/angiotensin II secretion more than overcomes any decrease in ACTH effect as the day progresses [8]. ACTH is at least as potent as angiotensin II as an aldosterone secretagogue *in vitro* [9] but chronic administration *in vitro* or *in vivo* does not result in sustained stimulation [10], nor does the acute suppressive effect of dexamethasone on aldosterone production persist with continued use.

Potassium is also a potent secretagogue *in vitro* [9] and *in vivo* [11]. Effects on both the early and late steroid metabolic pathways have been described [12]. The potency of potassium seems to be very much dependent upon the presence of angiotensin II and is thus diminished in the presence of a high salt intake [13] or following administration of a converting enzyme inhibitor [14].

The role of a pituitary factor other than ACTH remains speculative but may be important in some forms of 'primary aldosterone excess' (see below). The physiological effects of serotonin and the inhibitors dopamine and atrial natriuretic hormone are speculative and will not be discussed further (Fig. 9.1). For a more detailed assessment the reader is referred to the review by Shenker [15].

9.2.2 ACTIONS OF ALDOSTERONE

Aldosterone is produced exclusively in the zona glomerulosa of the adrenal cortex. Its main site of action is the distal renal tubule where it acts to increase the reabsorption of sodium, promoting excretion of potassium and hydrogen ions (the latter mostly as ammonia). Aldosterone is metabolized predominantly by the liver but a proportion is excreted in the urine as the glucoronide form.

165

Table 9.1 Sub-types of low renin aldosteronism (primary aldosteronism)

Type	Approximate frequency (%)	Site	Responsiveness	
			ANG11	ACTH
1. Aldosterone-producing adenoma	64[a]	Unilateral	−	+
2. Idiopathic aldosteronism	32[a]	Bilateral	+	−
3. Glucocorticoid suppressible aldosteronism	1	Bilateral	−	+
4. Primary adrenal hyperplasia	<1	Unilateral	−	+
5. Aldosterone-producing AII responsive adenoma	<1	Unilateral	+	−
6. Aldosterone-producing carcinoma	<1	Unilateral	−	−

[a] More recent diagnostic criteria indicates an increase in frequency of IHA in comparison to APA [18].

9.3 PRIMARY ALDOSTERONISM (PRIMARY HYPERALDOSTERONISM)

The original description by Conn [16] of a golden yellow adrenal tumour producing aldosterone remains the archetype for this condition but there are now at least five other subtypes under the above broad heading. The term 'primary aldosteronism' does not always appear to fit (see Table 9.1), and as all are characterized by an increased production of aldosterone together with a decreased level of circulating renin a better term is 'low-renin aldosteronism' (LRA).

This allows a clear distinction from secondary or 'high-renin aldosteronism', and we will use the term LRA in this review.

The true prevalence of this condition is unknown but may lie between 0.5% and 2% of patients who are hypertensive. As will be discussed later, the prevalence may be critically related to diagnostic criteria used, and a possible blurring between the condition of low-renin hypertension and idiopathic aldosteronism [17] may be the explanation for an apparent increase in prevalence of idiopathic aldosteronism among patients who have LRA.

9.4 SUB-TYPES OF LRA

9.4.1 ALDOSTERONE-PRODUCING ADENOMA

Most aldosterone-producing adenomas (APAs) are about 1 cm in size (Fig. 9.2) and are rarely greater than 3 cm.

The condition appears commoner in women than men and is more often found on the left side [18]. Histologically, the tumour more closely resembles zona fasciculata than zona glomerulosa tissue [19]. The cause is unknown but aldosterone is at least partly autonomous in that it is unresponsive to angiotensin II [15] but retains normal circadian rhythm and responds acutely to changes in ACTH [20].

In general, biochemical abnormalities are

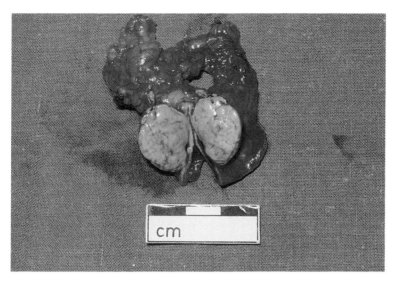

Fig. 9.2 A typical golden yellow aldosterone-producing adenoma.

more pronounced than in idiopathic aldosteronism and this has formed the basis of statistical tests for the separation of the two conditions [21,22].

9.4.2 IDIOPATHIC ALDOSTERONISM

The second commonest variety of LRA is characterized by bilateral abnormalities comprising nodular hyperplasia of the adrenal glands. The nodules are not capable of secreting aldosterone *in vitro*, however [17], and hypertension is rarely, if ever, cured by a sub-total or even bilateral adrenalectomy, suggesting that aldosterone excess may not be the cause of hypertension in this condition [17,23]. The intriguing observation that aldosterone was exquisitely sensitive to small changes in circulating angiotensin II [24] and that aldosterone levels increased with the assumption of the erect posture [25] led to the inevitable assumption that this was not true primary aldosteronism but related in some way to an enhanced adrenal sensitivity to angiotensin II. Indeed, whereas the relationship between circulating levels of angiotensin

II and aldosterone is a negative one in patients with APA, it is positive in idiopathic aldosteronism (IHA) [26].

Although most texts would indicate that two-thirds of LRA is caused by APA and about one-third by IHA (Table 9.1), it has been suggested recently that IHA may be much commoner [18,27]. Between 1970 and 1978 at the Mayo Clinic the prevalence of IHA was 26% of all patients with LRA but between 1978 and 1987 it had increased to 45% [18]. It is likely that this apparent increase in the prevalence of IHA reflects changing diagnostic criteria. Among patients with essential hypertension, a significant proportion have low renin hypertension [17,28] and this condition is also characterized by an enhanced adrenal sensitivity to angiotensin II [29] and by a relative failure to suppress aldosterone in the salt-loaded state [30]. It seems likely that more patients with low renin hypertension are now being classified as IHA (see below).

The reason for the enhanced adrenal sensitivity to angiotensin II in IHA may lie within the pituitary gland. It is possible that

167

the putative aldosterone stimulating hormone may be elevated in this condition, and there is good evidence that the serotonin antagonist cyproheptadine acts centrally to suppress aldosterone production [31].

9.4.3 GLUCOCORTICOID SUPPRESSIBLE ALDOSTERONISM

Glucocorticoid suppressible aldosteronism (GSA) was first described by Sutherland and colleagues [32]. It is inherited as an autosomal dominant condition and is characterized by a similar parallelism between cortisol and ACTH as is seen in APA. Aldosterone secretion is bilateral, however, and is suppressed both acutely and chronically by the exogenous administration of a glucocorticoid [33]. Chronic glucocorticoid suppression restores aldosterone responsiveness to normal [32,34]. Until recently it was believed that patients with GSA had transitional adrenocortical cells [35,36] with the characteristics of both the zona glomerulosa and the zona fasciculata [33,37]. But there is now good evidence that the genetic defect for this condition involves a mutation whereby the 5' regulatory region of 11β-hydroxylase is fused to decoding sequences of aldosterone synthase on chromosome 8 [37a]. This unequal crossing over allows the expression of aldosterone synthase in the zona fasciculata so that aldosterone can then be produced under continuing ACTH control [37a].

9.4.4 PRIMARY ADRENAL HYPERPLASIA AND ALDOSTERONE PRODUCING RESPONSIVE ADENOMA

These represent two recent additions to the list of LRA [38–40]. Patients with aldosterone producing responsive adenoma (AP-RA) maintain the normal physiological responses to the assumption of the erect posture and thus behave in a similar way to IHA. Hypertension is corrected by unilateral adrenalec-tomy [39]. Patients with primary adrenal hyperplasia (PAH) have physiological responses similar to patients with APA but have no demonstrable tumour [41]. Again, unilateral adrenalectomy is successful in controlling blood pressure [39].

9.4.5 FAMILIAL ALDOSTERONE-PRODUCING ADRENAL ADENOMA

Until recently the only hereditable form of LRA was thought to be glucocorticoid-suppressible (see above). A number of Australian families have now been described with angiotensin II unresponsive adrenal adenomata, with several members of the family affected. It is not clear what form of inheritance pattern is present, nor, indeed, how important this condition is likely to be in the future [41].

9.4.6 ALDOSTERONE-PRODUCING CARCINOMA

This is a particularly rare condition and is characterized by the presence of a large adrenal tumour (usually >3 cm). Tumours often produce multiple hormones [15].

9.4.7 CLINICAL AND BIOCHEMICAL PRESENTATION

Most patients with LRA have no symptoms and are discovered incidentally by the presence of hypokalaemia in a hypertensive patient. Although hypokalaemia can induce a mild nephrogenic diabetes insipidus and a proximal myopathy, such symptoms are uncommon.

The clinical suspicion is first raised in a hypertensive patient who has an unprovoked hypokalaemic alkalosis (<3.5 mmol l^{-1}) or whose serum potassium drops below 3 mmol l^{-1} during therapy with a thiazide diuretic. Measurement of serum sodium at this stage may not be diagnostic although a normal-to-high sodium is supportive of LRA (secondary aldosterone excess is generally associated with a low serum sodium). If possible hypokalaemia should be confirmed off all therapy for at least one month while on a normal (>150 mmol day^{-1}) sodium intake. The high/normal sodium intake is important as normokalaemic LRA has been described [42]. The frequency of this lies between 7% and 38% in various series [18]. A relatively low sodium intake will mask hypokalaemia and in most patients a higher sodium intake will lower the potassium.

If it is not considered possible to remove antihypertensive therapy, drugs which do not have chronic effects on the renin–angiotensin system should be used (e.g. bethanidine or prazosin) [43]. Hypokalaemia is associated with inappropriate kaliuresis (>30 mmol day^{-1}) and the same urine specimen can be used to ensure the adequacy of sodium intake. For the assessment of the renin–angiotensin–aldosterone axis at this stage it is not necessary to control sodium intake, only to ensure that it is not reduced, and for simplicity basal measurements of renin and aldosterone (supine after overnight fast and recumbency) are combined with a study of the effect of posture (see below). Such measurements should be done on two occasions (see Fig. 9.3).

Measurement of plasma renin (usually as

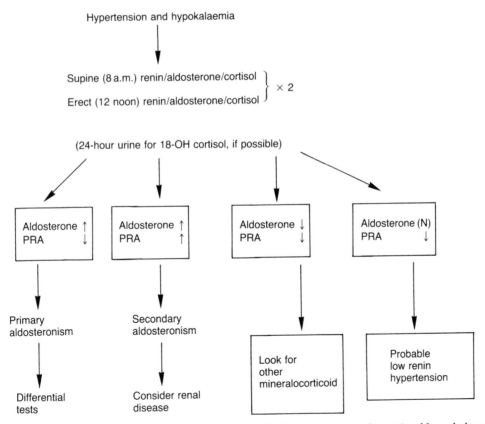

Fig. 9.3 Suggested series of investigations in patients with hypertension and sustained hypokalaemia or hypokalaemia unmasked by high sodium intake. PRA, plasma renin activity; N, normal.

169

plasma renin activity) is critical in differentiating primary from secondary aldosterone excess states.

The combination of a low renin and high aldosterone confirms the diagnosis, and investigation to determine the cause should proceed (Fig. 9.3). If both renin and aldosterone levels are suppressed then an endogenous or exogenous mineralocorticoid other than aldosterone is likely to be present. A proportion of patients with mild or borderline serum potassium will have suppressed renin but normal aldosterone levels. The majority of these will have so called 'low renin hypertension' [17] although some may have mild primary aldosterone excess which may be unmasked by a repeat study following oral or intravenous saline loading [44]. Such patients with mildly abnormal biochemistry are most likely to have PAH and it is the authors' contention that this is likely to differ quantitatively rather than qualitatively from low renin hypertension [17].

9.4.8 DIFFERENTIAL DIAGNOSIS OF LRA

For most practical purposes differential diagnosis lies between APA and IHA, the other conditions being extremely uncommon. Surgical removal of an APA is likely to be successful in curing hypertension in at least 50% of cases [45], whereas surgical intervention for IHA has proved unsuccessful [44]. GSA, although uncommon, is effectively treated with glucocorticoids and is thus worth diagnosing.

Hormone studies

Posture

Between 8 a.m. and 12 noon plasma levels of ACTH and hence cortisol decline, as does aldosterone, providing the supine posture is maintained. If a normal subject stands

between these times the effect of a rise in angiotensin II overcomes the fall in ACTH and aldosterone levels increase. In a patient with APA or GSA, or even the more unusual PAH, a fall in aldosterone levels will be observed, whereas in IHA and AP-RA aldosterone will increase [39,40]. In normal subjects aldosterone increases between two- and fourfold on assumption of the erect posture, and in patients with IHA the increase is at least 33% over baseline. In most patients there will be no detectable change in renin levels although it is assumed that small changes are occurring below the limits of sensitivity to the assay. A concurrent measurement of cortisol is critical to ensure that the patient is not stressed at the time of the second measurement. If stress occurs and ACTH levels (measured as cortisol) rise, then the test is invalid and needs to be repeated [46]. In their review of the literature Young and Klee [18] found that this test had a diagnostic accuracy in patients with surgically proven APA of 85% (data from 47 reports).

18-Hydroxycorticosterone (18-OHB)

18-OHB is either the immediate precursor of aldosterone or a separate compound formed from 18-hydroxylation of corticosterone [47–49]. Plasma levels in the supine position are generally at least five times normal in APA but nearer normal in patients with IHA [50]. However, this assay is unlikely to be readily available.

The captopril suppression test

The heightened sensitivity of the adrenal cortex to angiotensin II in IHA has been used in the reverse sense. The use of the short-acting ACE inhibitor captopril to reduce circulating angiotensin II has helped differentiate between IHA and APA. Although there may be little blood pressure effect following the acute administration of the ACE

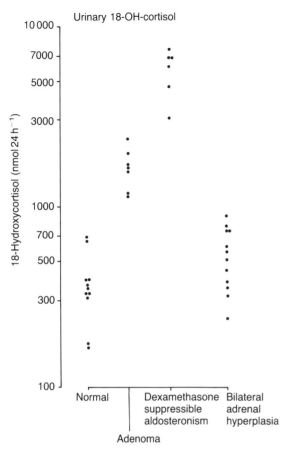

Fig. 9.4 24-hour urinary excretion of 18-hydroxycortisol in normal subjects and patients with APA, GSA and IHA. (From *Handbook of Hypertension*, vol. 13 [46]).

inhibitor, patients with IHA will reduce plasma aldosterone levels whereas there will be no effect in patients with APA [51]. Although positive results are quite helpful, this test has been thought to have been unhelpful by some (R.D. Gordon, personal communication).

18-Hydroxycortisol

Ulick and Chu were the first to show that 18-hydroxycortisol (18-OH F) might be a useful diagnostic marker for some types of mineralocorticoid hypertension [52]. Subsequently, a specific radioimmunoassay for this steroid was developed in this department [53] and this has been found to be a useful marker for APA with a clear distinction from IHA (see Fig. 9.4).

Levels are extremely high in GSA and APA [53] and may occasionally be high in secondary aldosterone excess, hence the importance of establishing LRA prior to acting on the information provided by this assay. The most recently discovered form of LRA, AP-RA, has consistently shown normal levels of 18-OH F [37,39]. Given the limited experience with this assay, its promise cannot yet be translated into accurate figures of specificity or sensitivity.

Adrenal imaging

Current adrenal ultrasound techniques lack sufficient sensitivity to detect small adenomata and the common modalities of imaging are adrenal computerized tomography (CT) and scintigraphy. Most recently magnetic resonance imaging (MRI) has been used and may be of equivalent accuracy to modern CT scanners [54].

It is difficult to be dogmatic regarding the relative merits of scintigraphy and CT scanning as review of the literature spans some 10 years, during which time CT scanners have improved and the techniques of adrenal scintigraphy have altered, probably increasing sensitivity. It is likely that the two imaging techniques are broadly comparable in patients with unequivocal biochemical diagnoses and neither test should be performed without this prerequisite [55]. The CT scan can never reflect function and given that the frequency of non-functioning adrenal nodules lies somewhere between 0.6% and 1.3% of the general population [56] there is perhaps more scope for error with CT, although it is much simpler to use and delivers less radiation to the patient. Review of the literature by Young and Klee revealed a 73% accuracy with CT scanning and 72% with iodocholesterol scintigraphy. Such figures necessarily cover the very good and the very bad [18].

The adrenocortical imaging agents are [131]I-6β-iodomethylnorcholesterol (NP59) and [75]Se-6β-selenomethylnorcholesterol. Uptake by the adrenal gland is mediated via the LDL receptor and is inversely proportional to circulating cholesterol levels [57]. Most experience in the United States has been with NP59 and selenocholesterol is the only isotope available in the United Kingdom [58]. The Ann Arbor group, who have the largest published experience, have been able to enhance the accuracy of adrenal scintigraphy by prior treatment with dexamethasone to remove glucocorticoid function. A somewhat empirical dosage regime used is 1 mg four times daily for 3 days prior to the administration of the isotope and for a week thereafter. It is clearly important if an iodinated label is used to give exogenous iodine to prevent thyroid uptake. This is not necessary with selenocholesterol.

The entero-hepatic circulation of both agents can obscure imaging of the adrenal glands and laxative therapy can be helpful to clear the bowels. An advantage of selenium is its increased half-life, which allows imaging after a much longer period of time (2 weeks or more) when all liver uptake will have disappeared, enhancing particularly the right adrenal gland [58] (Fig. 9.5).

Normal adrenals are not visualized before the fifth day using the dexamethasone pretreatment protocol [55], whereas adrenal adenomas are usually visualized prior to this. Bilateral uptake earlier than the fifth day is suggestive of adrenal hyperplasia but has also been seen in patients with low renin hypertension [59], adding further support to the view that this represents a similar condition to IHA.

It must be emphasized that the diagnosis of LRA should be clear prior to scintigraphy as all forms of secondary aldosteronism will result in bilateral uptake of the isotope. For a

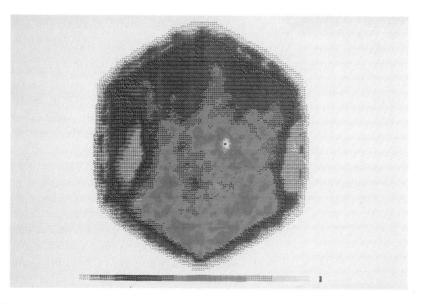

Fig. 9.5 Unilateral uptake of selenocholesterol in a patient with a right-sided APA, two weeks after administration of the isotope.

detailed assessment of the accuracy of both scintigraphy and adrenal scanning the reader is referred to recent reviews [18,55].

Adrenal venous catheterization

This is often regarded as the gold standard for the assessment of unilateral or bilateral secretion of aldosterone but suffers from the obvious problems of difficulties of catheterization of the adrenal veins, particularly the right. The procedure fails in approximately 25% of cases and is operator-dependent [18]. Simultaneous measurement of cortisol is helpful in assessing the degree of dilution of adrenal venous blood and some authors have advised continuous infusion of ACTH during the procedure to remove the possibility of surges of ACTH, due to stress, affecting aldosterone levels [42].

Most patients suspected of LRA are investigated in a specialized unit but Fig. 9.6 outlines an algorithm for the suggested investigation of patients in whom LRA has been proven.

The authors recommend both CT scanning and isotopic imaging. These tests are complementary, given that CT does not provide information on function. Venous catheterization should be reserved for equivocal cases.

9.4.9 OTHER MINERALOCORTICOID EXCESS SYNDROMES

When both PRA and aldosterone are low in patients with clinical and biochemical features of mineralocorticoid excess there are several possibilities.

Excess production of either deoxycorticosterone (DOC) or corticosterone

Two forms of congenital adrenal hyperplasia are associated with hypertension. These are the 17α-hydroxylase and 11β-hydroxylase deficiency states, both well reviewed by White *et al.* [60]. In 17α-hydroxylase deficiency, excess ACTH production stimulates both DOC and corticosterone, resulting in suppression of the renin–angiotensin system, hypo-

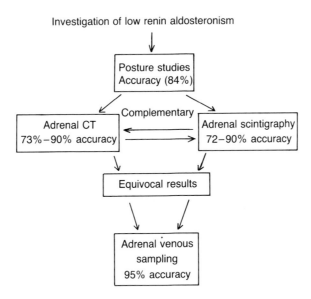

Fig. 9.6 Investigation of patients with proven low renin aldosteronism. It is suggested that both adrenal CT and scintigraphy be combined in all patients.

kalaemia and low aldosterone production. Females present with primary amenorrhoea because of a similar defect in the gonads and males have pseudohermaphroditism.

In 11β-hydroxylase deficiency, DOC accumulates and there is increased androgen production. Clinical features in the female are clitoromegaly and hirsutism as well as mineralocorticoid hypertension [61].

In both conditions glucocorticoid replacement therapy is effective although occasionally in the 11β-hydroxylase deficiency state a salt-losing crisis can occur following therapy, suggesting the possibility of defective aldosterone production. This might be because the defect occurs within the zona glomerulosa as well as the fasciculata [48].

In some patients with adrenal tumours there will be an isolated production of DOC or corticosterone [56] and this may be more common in adrenocortical carcinomas.

The apparent mineralocorticoid excess syndrome

This extremely rare condition, first described by Werder *et al.* [62], usually presents in childhood but has been described in an adult [63] and is now known to occur as a result of a deficiency of the enzyme 11β-hydroxysteroid dehydrogenase (11β-OHSD) [64]. 11β-OHSD regulates the conversion of cortisol to cortisone [63]. The kidney is responsible for much of this conversion and in the absence of 11β-OHSD cortisol has direct access to the type 1 (mineralocorticoid) receptor, giving rise to a mineralocorticoid excess syndrome. Such patients will have normal levels of ACTH and plasma cortisol but urinary free cortisol is increased [63]. The diagnosis is made on the basis of a marked elevation of cortisol metabolites (tetrahydrocortisol and allotetrahydrocortisol) in comparison to those of cortisone (tetrahydrocortisone). It has been shown that the urinary tetrahydrocortisol (THF) + allotetrahydrocortisol/tetrahydro-

cortisone ratio is markedly abnormal in these subjects and is a clue to diagnosis. Dexamethasone represents rationale therapy.

Exogenous mineralocorticoid excess

The most well known of these syndromes is that due to ingestion of liquorice or carbenoxolone. It is now know that both of these drugs inhibit the 11β-hydroxysteroid dehydrogenase enzyme, producing the syndrome of apparent mineralocorticoid excess [65].

Liddle's syndrome

This unusual condition is thought to relate to a primary renal abnormality in which there is enhanced sodium potassium exchange in the distal tubule [66]. The patient therefore has sodium dependent hypertension with kaliuresis but it is not truly mineralocorticoid in origin. Both renin and aldosterone levels are low and blood pressure responds to amiloride or triamterine but not to spironolactone.

9.5 SECONDARY ALDOSTERONISM (HIGH RENIN ALDOSTERONISM)

The association of a high circulating renin and aldosterone occurs in many disorders which do not present with hypertension (e.g. diuretic abuse, Bartter's syndrome, the nephrotic syndrome and cirrhosis) and some (e.g. congestive cardiac failure) which may or may not be associated with raised blood pressure. Conventional antihypertensive doses of thiazide diuretics do not result in chronic activation of the circulating renin–angiotensin–aldosterone system although excessive dosing may cause this [67].

Hypertension and secondary aldosteronism is most commonly seen in patients with accelerated phase hypertension (formerly known as malignant phase hypertension) or renovascular disease. It may, however, occur in any patient with chronic renal failure and has been described in most forms of renal disease, whether unilateral or bilateral [68]. The purest form of the condition arises as a result of the rare renin secreting tumour [68,69]. In this condition a benign haemangiopericytoma of juxta-glomerular cells overproduces renin with resultant angiotensin II and aldosterone excess. Patients are usually children or young adults and present with severe hypertension and marked hypokalaemia. This condition is clear evidence that sustained angiotensin II production can cause persistent hypertension.

In the absence of diuretic excess the hypertensive patient presenting with secondary aldosteronism is usually one who has accelerated phase hypertension. This condition occurs most commonly in males who are smokers and unless occurring as part of a systemic disorder (systemic lupus erythematosus or polyarteritis nodosa) blood pressure is likely to be extremely high, with diastolics in excess of 120 or 130 mmHg. Pulmonary oedema and proteinuria are commonly associated features. Intra-renal fibrinoid necrosis is a likely cause of overproduction of renin, together with a concomitant tendency to salt depletion [70]. The simple biochemical clue is the presence of a hypokalaemic alkalosis with hyponatraemia and mild to moderate renal impairment. Hyponatraemia occurs not only because of salt depletion but is also related to overproduction of vasopressin [71], resulting in a dilutional state. The incidence of renovascular hypertension is particularly common in patients presenting in the accelerated phase and may be as high as 50% [72].

9.6 RENOVASCULAR HYPERTENSION

9.6.1 PATHOPHYSIOLOGY OF RENOVASCULAR HYPERTENSION

It is now more than half a century since the classic Goldblatt experiments demonstrated that blood pressure could be elevated by inducing renal ischaemia with a renal artery clip in an animal [73]. The role of the renin–angiotensin system in the initiation and maintenance of hypertension has, however, remained controversial to this day [68,74,75]. Most information on pathophysiology has been extrapolated from experimental animals and it seems clear from a variety of studies [68] that the acute rise in blood pressure following the development of renal artery stenosis in dogs and rats is related to the rise in circulating angiotensin II. Both the increase in angiotensin II and the rise in blood pressure can be aborted by pretreatment with either a converting enzyme inhibitor or the angiotensin II receptor blocker, saralasin [68] and the role of angiotensin II in the initial onset of hypertension seems relatively clear. Such a situation is rarely observed in man, however, and most controversy is related to the role of the renin–angiotensin system in chronic renal artery stenosis associated with hypertension.

In the experimental animal it is clear that although blood pressure continues to rise following clipping of a renal artery, renin levels (and presumably angiotensin II) tend to fall towards baseline after several weeks [76]. In this situation renal artery stenosis is still the cause of hypertension, which can be reversed by removal of the clip. In the animal model a stage is reached when removal of the clip no longer reverses hypertension and this may be analogous to the situation often seen in man.

It is known that chronic infusion of doses of angiotensin II which are acutely subpressor can raise blood pressure [77] and it is thus possible that even 'normal' circulating angiotensin II may relate to the maintenance of high blood pressure in patients with renal artery stenosis. It is beyond the scope of this review to discuss in detail the potential mechanisms for maintaining blood pressure in renovascular hypertension and the reader is referred to more detailed reviews on this subject [68,75,78–80].

An important clinical problem relates to the observation that renal artery stenosis is a term not necessarily synonymous with renovascular hypertension. Arteriographic evidence of stenotic renal arteries may be present in as many as one-third of patients investigated for peripheral vascular disease who are normotensive [81–83]. Among a similar population of patients who are hypertensive the prevalence may be as high as 60%–70% [81]. In an autopsy series of almost 300 patients, moderate or severe renal artery stenosis was found in 50% of patients who were known to be normotensive during life [84]. Renal artery stenosis may therefore cause hypertension (renovascular hypertension), may be the consequence of hypertension (accelerated atheromatous production) or may occur coincidentally in a patient who has essential hypertension. The clinical dilemma is obvious.

Further problems arise in that the simple biochemical clue (hypokalaemia) so important in the diagnosis of primary aldosterone excess is not always present in renovascular hypertension. In a large co-operative study of renovascular hypertension [85], hypokalaemia ($<3.4\,\mathrm{mmol\,l^{-1}}$) was present in between 14% and 17% of patients with renovascular hypertension. It was also present in 7% of those labelled as having essential hypertension.

For the clinician it is worth considering renovascular hypertension, particularly in patients who are young (<25 years), who present in the accelerated phase, have evidence of arterial disease elsewhere or in whom hypertension appears to have been relatively sudden in onset [79]. Clinical clues are unhelpful other than the presence of vascular disease and, although approximately 50% of patients with renovascular hypertension will have an abdominal bruit [85] this may be heard in 7% of those with essen-

tial hypertension, so a hypertensive patient with an abdominal bruit is more than twice as likely to have essential hypertension as to have renovascular hypertension.

The advent of percutaneous transluminal renal angioplasty as a relatively simple way of correcting the angiographic abnormalities [86,87] has led to a wave of intervention procedures with little evidence of clinical benefit. A recent review of the available literature [88] has revealed that although the procedure is technically successful in up to 88% of patients with atherosclerotic renal artery stenosis, hypertension is cured in only 24%. Improvements are said to occur in up to 43% but this figure is variably defined and has not been compared against placebo intervention. The same review indicates that significant complications are reported in 9% of cases, with a mortality of 0.4%. If it were possible to predict those patients who might be cured by this procedure then even if it did not affect ultimate outcome, benefit would accrue by virtue of removal of antihypertensive drugs. Unfortunately we are not in a position to make such a prediction, although certain tests may increase the likelihood for success.

9.6.2 THE AETIOLOGY OF RENAL ARTERY STENOSIS

The majority of arteriographic lesions are atheromatous in nature and most commonly occur in the proximal third of the renal artery (often involving the ostia) [78]. Severe stenosis may progress to occlusion in a relatively short time-scale [89]. Approximately 25% of patients (mostly the young) have fibromuscular hyperplasia. This term includes both the commoner medial hyperplasia (70%) and intimal fibroplasia [78]. Progression to occlusion never occurs and the arteriographic appearance of beading is characteristic. Other rarer causes include external compression, Takayasau's disease and polyarteritis nodosa [78].

9.6.3 DIAGNOSIS OF RENOVASCULAR HYPERTENSION

In approaching this problem there are two schools of thought. There are those who utilize predictive tests (see Table 9.2) prior to the use of angiography and only perform intra-arterial studies at the time of planned angioplasty [79] and those in whom some form of arteriographic study is done first and only then are the full range of tests designed to predict the response to subsequent angioplasty performed [68].

The problem with this latter approach, of course, is that two arteriographic procedures are involved.

9.6.4 DIAGNOSTIC OR PREDICTIVE TESTS (Table 9.2)

Peripheral plasma renin activity

Remembering the experience from the animal model, it is not perhaps surprising to learn that not all patients with renovascular hypertension have a high circulating renin. In the co-operative study [85] an elevated renin was present in 80% of patients with renovascular hypertension but was also a feature in 15% of essential hypertensives. If one assumes, therefore, a rather generous prevalence rate

for renovascular hypertension of 5% of a hypertensive population [90] then of 1000 patients with raised blood pressure 40 (80%) of those with renovascular disease would have a high renin whereas 143 (15%) of those with essential hypertension would be similarly categorized. It is true that, as a group, patients with renovascular hypertension have higher levels of circulating renin than a comparable group of patients with essential hypertension, but the overlap is considerable and attempts to predict success of revascularization by virtue of the peripheral plasma renin have been unsuccessful [68]. Others have claimed, however, that if peripheral plasma renin activity is carefully related to sodium intake (as measured by urinary sodium excretion) the test is more accurate [91,92] but even here the specificity and sensitivity are only around 70%.

Captopril test

As a screening test this has a lot to recommend it in terms of simplicity and currently appears to be the most sensitive test available. Case and Laragh [93] were the first to demonstrate that patients with renovascular hypertension had a greater renin response to the administration of an oral dose of captopril than did patients with essential hypertension. This was accompanied by a greater blood pressure fall although the magnitude of this difference was not sufficient to clearly separate the two groups. The same workers went on to develop pro-

Table 9.2 Diagnosis of renovascular disease

1. Peripheral plasma renin activity
2. Captopril test
3. Differential renal vein renin determinations
4. Intravenous urogram
5. Digital subtraction angiography
6. Isotope renography
7. Captopril renography
8. Arteriography
9. Angioplasty

Table 9.3 Original criteria for a positive captopril test in the diagnosis of renovascular hypertension

1. Stimulated PRA of $12\,\mathrm{ng^{-1}\,ml^{-1}\,h^{-1}}$ or more
2. Absolute increase of PRA of $10\,\mathrm{ng^{-1}\,ml^{-1}\,h^{-1}}$ or more
3. Per cent increase of PRA of 150% or more or 400% or more if baseline PRA $<3\,\mathrm{ng^{-1}\,ml^{-1}\,h^{-1}}$

spective criteria for defining a positive test (see Table 9.3) and in their hands a specificity and sensitivity of 95% was seen [94].

In their studies it seemed clear that patients with renal insufficiency gave responses which were less accurate but an important observation was that the concomitant use of antihypertensive drugs, including betablockers, did not reduce the accuracy of the test. More recently, Frederickson and colleagues [95] further refined the test but demonstrated a 90% sensitivity with an 80% specificity. Postma and colleagues [96] found the test to be highly specific at 96% but poorly sensitive at only 39%. The reason for this difference is not immediately clear. It would appear necessary that each institution develops its own experience with this test.

Differential renal vein renin determinations

The theoretical argument behind this test is that the ischaemic kidney will produce more renin, most of which will pass into the renal vein. The concomitant increased production of angiotensin II and the raised blood pressure will suppress renin secretion in the contralateral kidney, and thus the amount of renin in the contralateral renal vein should approximate to that which enters the kidney via the renal artery. As arterial renin levels are similar to those measured in the vena cava the test has been performed with simultaneous measurements of renin, in both renal veins, together with a measurement from the inferior vena cava. Various criteria for positivity have been advanced, the simplest being a ratio of >1.5:1 from abnormal to normal side. This ratio was derived on theoretical grounds and confirmed by observations in patients with essential hypertension [97]. Limitations of this simple assessment were first highlighted by Marks and Maxwell [98] and may have occurred because hypertensive damage to the contralateral kidney can result in increased renin secretion. A

more accurate predictive test can be derived if it is also shown that the contralateral kidney produces no renin. This test has been claimed to have a specificity as high as 100% but the sensitivity can be as low as 75% [79]. Laragh and colleagues have shown that concomitant use of captopril enhances the accuracy of renal vein renin estimations by increasing secretion from the ischaemic kidney [99]. The authors claim that this increases the sensitivity of the test, although figures are not quoted. It is important to emphasize the need for accurate collection of blood from renal veins and for theoretical reasons [79] it is important to show that the increment of renin from renal veins to peripheral blood is at least 50% or the test has been technically compromised. Abnormal renal vein renin ratios have tended to return to normal following successful angioplasty [100].

Not all have found this test so successful, however, and Marks and Maxwell [98], reviewing 21 published series, pointed out that the degree of confidence with which surgical success could be predicted depended upon the ratio used (e.g. 81% confidence with a ratio of 1.5:1 and 95% confidence with a ratio of 1.6:1 or greater). In the same analysis, 51% of patients who had a ratio of <1.5:1 showed improvement of blood pressure following surgical correction of the renal artery stenosis. Others suggest, however, that these tests were probably flawed technically [79]. One further problem with this test is that it is likely to be inaccurate in patients with bilateral renal artery lesions.

Imaging techniques

Several imagining procedures have been used to diagnose renovascular disease, some of which have fallen into disfavour [101]. Although classic features on the intravenous urogram have been described, false negatives occur in between 7% and 28% of patients and false positives in as many as 11% of those with essential hypertension [102]. Digital subtraction angiography with intravenous injection of contrast has replaced conventional arteriography in some centres. The need for much larger boluses of contrast material together with poor visualization of anything other than mainstem renal artery lesions has cast some doubt on the suitability of this as a screening test, however [101].

The captopril renogram

In 1984 Wenting and colleagues [103] demonstrated that some patients with arteriographically proven renal artery stenosis had a fall in GFR (measured isotopically) in the affected kidney following the administration of an ACE inhibitor. In patients with bilateral renal artery stenosis acute renal failure may occur, although this is generally reversible [104]. The pathophysiology is thought to relate to the role of angiotensin II in maintaining efferent arteriolar tone in kidneys that are ischaemic. If renal blood flow falls then angiotensin II becomes important in maintaining the tone of the efferent arteriole, hence maintaining the pressure in the glomerulus [105]. Thus if a renal artery stenosis is functionally significant, removal of angiotensin II with an ACE inhibitor would result in dilatation of the efferent arteriole and a drop in glomerular pressure, hence a fall in GFR. This has been used as the basis of a test to demonstrate functionality of an arteriographically demonstrated stenosis and, indeed, to predict subsequent intervention. Earlier reports suggested a sensitivity of 80% and a specificity of 100% [106]. Some have suggested an improved predictive effect with prior administration of frusemide [107]. More recently, using ^{99m}Tc, diethylene triaminepenta-acetic acid (DTPA), a sensitivity of 91% with a specificity of 93% has been reported [108]. Most studies have shown the test to be more specific than sensitive [109] and others have reported 92% sensitivity and 97% specificity [110]. It is difficult, therefore, from reviewing the literature to be absolutely certain how good this test is, and different authors have made different measurements, ranging from an absolute measurement of the GFR to the shape of the renogram curve. Another confounding variable is that different doses of captopril have been used and it is unclear whether 25 mg or 50 mg would produce different results. This test cannot be described as being simple and takes the best part of two days, having to be done with and without captopril (an exception to this is the modified test by Chen and colleagues [108], where the whole study is performed at a single sitting). The need for each institution to define its own characteristics probably means that the test is unlikely to be widely applied.

Angioplasty

The use of angioplasty as a diagnostic test for renovascular hypertension is acceptable only if the procedure is without risk and this cannot be said to be true (see above). In young patients renal artery stenosis is more likely to be caused by the condition of fibromuscular hyperplasia [101] and the success rates of angioplasty are greater than 50% in this group [88]. There is thus an argument for performing angioplasty in such patients without recourse to predictive tests.

9.6.5 CONCLUSIONS

It is difficult to be dogmatic about the approach to renal artery stenosis and renovascular hypertension but it is the authors' experience that most investigators in the United Kingdom will perform arteriography or digital vascular imaging in patients as defined above or in those with resistant hypertension rather than perform any other predictive test first. A demonstration of an angiographic abnormality should thereafter be followed by some attempt to predict the success or otherwise of intervention. As all tests have their problems, a combination is likely to enhance diagnostic accuracy and the best test would appear to be the captopril stimulation test and renal vein renins. The authors have used the captopril renogram increasingly in recent years but have encountered both false positive and false negative tests. It is probably not appropriate to proceed directly to angioplasty in patients with atherosclerotic disease.

Some authors have suggested that the blood pressure response to the chronic administration of an ACE inhibitor [111] predicts ultimate success of surgical or angioplasty intervention but there remains a need for carefully controlled trials of intervention against more conventional forms of antihypertensive therapy. There is a justifiable concern that chronic ACE inhibition may produce irreversible renal damage in the kidney distal to the stenosis.

9.7 GLUCOCORTICOID-INDUCED HYPERTENSION (CUSHING'S SYNDROME)

Cortisol is the major glucocorticoid in man, being the ultimate product of the zona fasciculata function in the adrenal cortex. Its control is regulated ultimately by a complex stimulation of the pituitary corticotrophs by corticotropin-releasing hormone (CRH) or hormones [112]. A circadian rhythm of both ACTH and cortisol exists, with peak levels in the early hours of the morning, and cortisol itself modulates secretion of ACTH by the classic negative feedback of cortisol on both pituitary and hypothalamus. It is clear that stress can play an overriding part in the central secretion of cortisol [113].

9.7.1 PATHOPHYSIOLOGY

Endogenous Cushing's syndrome, with its characteristic clinical features [114,115] is a rare condition. The various causes of this syndrome can be broadly classified according to whether or not the glucocorticoid excess is ACTH-dependent or independent. The true prevalence of the various types depends upon the series cited, on referral patterns, but best estimates are obtained from data published by the Mayo Clinic. In the 15-year period to 1988, 312 patients with Cushing's syndrome were seen (108 male). Of these, 72% had true ACTH-dependent Cushing's disease, 11% had the ectopic ACTH syndrome, 7% had adrenal adenoma and 6% had adrenal carcinoma. The remaining small group comprised 11 patients with nodular adrenal hyperplasia which was ACTH-independent [116]. More recently, cases of ectopic production of CRH have been described [117].

Most textbook descriptions include hypertension as an integral part of the syndrome, being described in approximately 85% of cases [118]. Exogenously administered glucocorticoid also raises blood pressure [119] but less consistently than in the endogenous condition. We make the point to remind readers that it remains uncertain as to whether the hypertensive effects of a pure glucocorticoid are the same as those caused by ACTH induced changes in adrenal steroid output [120,121].

Glucocorticoids act on both type 1 (mineralocorticoid) and type 2 (glucocorticoid) receptors [122] and thus hypertension may result from activation at either or both sites in man; the acute administration of ACTH or cortisol results in similar short-term effects on blood pressure [123] which parallel a rise in cardiac output and an increase in plasma volume. In the long term, as for most other forms of raised blood pressure, plasma volume is nearer normal and peripheral resistance is elevated [120]. It seems likely that there are species differences in ACTH mediated effects on blood pressure which are beyond the scope of this review [121]. For a fuller review of the several postulated mechanisms for raised blood pressure in Cushing's syndrome the reader is referred to recent reviews [48,120].

9.7.2 DIAGNOSIS AND DIFFERENTIAL DIAGNOSIS

The diagnosis of Cushing's syndrome depends upon the demonstration of relatively non-suppressible cortisol secretion and correct management thereafter depends upon adequate differential diagnoses. The reader is referred to two recent reviews detailing the relative merits of the available diagnostic tests [122,123], and the discussion in Chapter 4.

9.7.3 CONCLUSIONS

There can be little doubt that the investigation of patients with secondary hypertension presents an exciting challenge to the clinician. Although rare, such disorders may yet allow us valuable insights into the pathophysiology of the much commoner and as yet unexplained condition of essential hypertension [1].

REFERENCES

1. Edwards, C.R.W. and Carey, R.M. (ed.) *Essential Hypertension as an Endocrine Disease*, Butterworths, London.
2. McLellan, A.R. and Connell, J.M.C. (1988) Diabetes and hypertension. *Curr. Opin. Cardiol.*, **3**, 666–74.
3. Streeten, D.H., Anderson, G.H., Howland, T., Chiang, R. and Smulyan, H. (1988) Effects of thyroid function on blood pressure. Recognition of hypothyroid hypertension. *Hypertension*, **11**, 78–83.
4. Nabarro, J.D.N. (1987) Acromegaly. *Clin. Endocrinol.*, **26**, 481–512.
5. Sangal, A.K. and Beevers, D.G. (1983) Parathyroid hypertension. *Brit. Med. J.*, **286**, 498–9.
6. Brown, J.J., Fraser, R., Lever, A.F. *et al.* (1977) Renin–angiotensin system in the regulation of aldosterone in humans. In *Hypertension: Physiopathology and Treatment* (ed. J.J. Genest, E. Koiw and O. Kuchel), McGraw-Hill, New York, p. 874.
7. Fraser, R. and Padfield, P.L. (1985) Role of mineralocorticoids in essential hypertension. In *Essential Hypertension as an Endocrine Disease* (ed. C.R.W. Edwards and R.M. Carey), Butterworths, London, p. 158.
8. Katz, F.H., Romfh, P. and Smith, J.A. (1975) Diurnal variation of plasma aldosterone, cortisol and renin activity in supine man. *J. Clin. Endocrinol. Metab.*, **40**, 125.
9. Haning, R., Tait, S.A.S. and Tait, J.F. (1970) *In vitro* effects of ACTH, angiotensins, serotonin, and potassium on steroid output and conversion of corticosterone to aldosterone by isolated adrenal cells. *Endocrinology*, **87**, 1147.
10. Gaillard, R.C., Riondel, A.M., Faroud-Coune, C.A., Valloton, M.B. and Muller, A.F. (1983) Aldosterone escape to chronic ACTH administration in man. *Acta Endocrinol., Copenhagen*, **103**, 116–24.
11. Campbell, W.B. and Schmitz, J.M. (1978) Effect of alterations in dietary potassium on the pressor and steroidogenic effects of angiotensin II and III. *Endocrinology*, **103**, 2098.
12. McKenna, T.J., Island, D.P., Nicholson, W.E. *et al.* (1978) The effects of potassium on early and late steps in aldosterone biosynthesis in cells of the zona glomerulosa. *Endocrinology*, **103**, 1411.
13. Fraser, R., Mason, P.A. and Buckingham, J.C. (1979) The interaction of sodium and potassium status, of ACTH and of angiotensin II in the control of corticosteroid secretion. *J. Steroid Biochem.*, **11**, 1039.
14. Parkinson, C.A., Belton, S.J. and Pratt, J.H. (1984) The effects of captopril on potassium-induced stimulation of aldosterone production in vitro. *Endocrinology*, **114**, 1567.
15. Shenker, Y. (1989) Medical treatment of low-renin aldosteronism. *Endocrinol. Metab. Clin. North Am.*, **18**, 415–42.
16. Conn, J.W. (1955) Presidential address: part I. Painting background. Part II. Primary aldosteronism, a new clinical syndrome. *J. Lab. Clin. Med.*, **45**, 3.
17. Padfield, P.L., Brown, J.J., Davies, D. *et al.* (1981) The myth of idiopathic hyperaldo-

steronism. *Lancet*, ii, 83–4.

18. Young, Jr, W.F. and Klee, G. (1988) Primary aldosteronism. *Endocrinol. Metab. Clin. North Am.*, **17**, 367–95.

19. Carbailleira, A., Fishman, L.M., Brown, J.W. and Trujillo, D. (1989) Content and biosynthesis of cortisol in aldosterone-producing mass. *J. Lab. Clin. Med.*, **114**, 120–8.

20. Ganguly, A., Dowdy, A.J., Leutscher, J.A. *et al.* (1973) Anomalous postural response of plasma aldosterone concentration in patients with aldosterone-producing adrenal adenoma. *J. Clin. Endocrinol. Metab.*, **36**, 401.

21. Ferris, J.B., Beevers, D.G., Brown, J.J. *et al.* (1978) Low-renin ('primary') hyperaldosteronism. *Am. Heart J.*, **95**, 641–58.

22. Leutscher, J.A., Ganguly, A., Melada, G.A. *et al.* (1974) Preoperative differentiation of adrenal adenoma from idiopathic adrenal hyperplasia in primary aldosteronism. *Circulation Res.*, **34/35** (suppl. 1), 175.

23. Baer, L., Brunner, H.R., Buhler, F. and Laragh, J.H. (1972) Pseudo-primary aldosteronism, a variant of low renin essential hypertension. In *Hypertension '72* (ed. J. Genest and E. Koiw), Springer-Verlag, Berlin, pp. 459–72.

24. Wisgerhof, M., Carpenter, P.C. and Brown, R.D. (1978) Increased adrenal sensitivity to angiotensin II in idiopathic hyperaldosteronism. *J. Clin. Endocrinol. Metab.*, **47**, 938.

25. Schambelan, M., Brust, N.L., Chang, B., Slater, K.L. and Biglieri, E.G. (1976) Circadian rhythm and effect of posture on plasma aldosterone concentration in primary aldosteronism. *J. Clin. Endocrinol. Metab.*, **43**, 115–31.

26. Davies, D.L., Beevers, D.G., Brown, J.J. *et al.* Aldosterone and its stimuli in normal and hypertensive man: are essential hypertension and primary hyperaldosteronism without tumour the same condition? *J. Endocrinol.*, **81**, 79–91.

27. Streeten, D.H., Tomycz, N. and Anderson, G.H. (1979) Reliability of screening methods for the diagnosis of primary aldosteronism. *Am. J. Med.*, **67**, 403.

28. Padfield, P.L., Beevers, D.G. and Brown, J.J. (1974) Is low-renin hypertension a stage in the development of essential hypertension or a diagnostic entity? *Lancet*, i, 548–50.

29. Wisgerhof, M. and Brown, R.D. (1979) Increased adrenal sensitivity to angiotensin II in low renin hypertension. *J. Clin. Invest.*, **64**, 1456–62.

30. Khokhar, A.M., Slater, J.D.H., Jowett, T.P. and Payne, N.N. (1976) Suppression of the renin aldosterone system in mild essential hypertension. *Clin. Sci. Molec. Med.*, **50**, 269–76.

31. Gross, M.D., Grekin, R.J., Gniadek, T.C. and Villareal, J.Z. (1981) Suppression of aldosterone by cyproheptadine in idiopathic aldosteronism. *New Engl. J. Med.*, **305**, 181.

32. Sutherland, J.D.A., Ruse, J.L. and Laidlaw, J.C. (1966) Hypertension, increased aldosterone secretion and low plasma renin activity relieved by dexamethasone. *Can. Med. Ass. J.*, **95**, 1109.

33. Connell, J.M., Kenyon, C.J., Corrie, J.E.T. *et al.* (1986) Dexamethasone-suppressible hyperaldosteronism: adrenal transition cell hyperplasia? *Hypertension*, **8**, 669.

34. Woodland, E., Tunny, T.J., Hamlet, S.M. *et al.* (1985) Hypertension corrected and aldosterone responsiveness to renin–angiotensin restored by long term dexamethasone in glucocorticoid-suppressible hyperaldosteronism. *Clin. Exp. Pharmacol. Physiol.*, **12**, 245.

35. Gomez-Sanchez, C.E., Clore, J.N., Estep, H.L. and Watlington, C.O. (1988) Effect of chronic adrenocorticotropin stimulation on the excretion of 18-hydroxycortisol and 18-oxocortisol. *J. Clin. Endocrinol. Metab.*, **67**, 322–6.

36. Ganguly, A. (1991) Glucocorticoid-suppressible hyperaldosteronism: a paradigm of arrested adrenal zonation? *Clin. Sci.*, **80**(10), 1–7.

37. Hamlet, S.M., Godon, R.D., Gomez-Sanchez, C.E., Tunny, T.J. and Klemm, S.A. (1988) Adrenal transitional zone steroids, 18-oxo and 18-hydroxycortisol, useful in the diagnosis of primary aldosteronism, are ACTH-dependent. *Clin. Exp. Pharmacol. Physiol.*, **15**, 317–22.

37a. Lifton, R.P., Dhluy, G., Powers, M. *et al.* (1992) A chimaeric 11β-hydroxylase/aldosterone synthase gene causes glucocorticoid-remedial aldosteronism and human hypertension. *Nature*, **355**, 262–5.

38. Gordon, R.D., Hamlet, S.M., Tunny, T.J. and Klemm, S.A. (1987) Aldosterone-producing adenomas responsive to angiotensin pose problems in diagnosis. *Clin. Exp. Pharmacol. Physiol.*, **14**, 27–31.

39. Biglieri, E.G., Irony, I. and Kater, C.E. (1989) Identification and implications of new types of mineralocorticoid hypertension. *J. Steroid Biochem.*, **32**, 199–204.

40. Irony, I., Kater, C.E., Biglieri, E.G. and Shackleton, C.H. (1990) Correctable subsets of primary aldosteronism. Primary adrenal hyperplasia and renin responsive adenoma. *Am. J. Hypertension*, **3**, 576–82.

41. Banks, W.A., Kastin, A.J., Biglieri, E.G. and Ruiz, A.G. (1984) Primary adrenal hyperplasia: a new subset of primary hyperaldosteronism. *J. Clin. Endocrinol. Metab.*, **58**, 783–5.

42. Melby, J.C. (1984) Primary aldosteronism. *Kidney Int.*, **26**, 769.

43. Young, Jr, W.F. and Hogan, M.J. (1990) Primary aldosteronism: diagnosis and treatment. *Mayo Clin. Proc.*, **65**, 96–110.

44. Bravo, E.L. (1989) Primary aldosteronism. *Urol. Clin. North Am.*, **16**, 481–6.

45. Ferris, J.B., Brown, J.J., Fraser, R. *et al.* (1975) Results of adrenal surgery in patients with hypertension, aldosterone excess, and low plasma renin concentration. *Brit. Med. J.*, **1**, 35.

46. Lardinois, C.K., Mazzaferri, E.L. and McGregor, D.B. (1984) Plasma cortisol and primary aldosteronism (letter). *Ann. Intern. Med.*, **100**, 917.

47. Fraser, R. and Lantos, C.P. (1978) 18-Hydroxy-corticosterone: a review. *J. Steroid Biochem.*, **9**, 273.

48. Edwards, C.R.W. (1990) Hypertension and the adrenal cortex. In *The Management of Hypertension: Handbook of Hypertension*, vol. 13 (ed. F.R. Buhler and J.H. Laragh), Elsevier, Amsterdam.

49. Biglieri, E.G. and Schambelan, M. (1979) The significance of elevated levels of plasma 18-hydroxycorticosterone in patients with primary aldosteronism. *J. Clin. Endocrinol. Metab.*, **49**, 87.

50. Kem, D.C., Tang, K., Hanson, C.S. *et al.* (1985) The prediction of anatomical morphology of primary aldosteronism using serum 18-hydroxycorticosterone levels. *J. Clin. Endocrinol. Metab.*, **60**, 67.

51. Muratani, H., Abe, I., Tomita, Y. *et al.* (1986) Is single oral administration of captopril beneficial in screening for primary aldosteronism? *Am. Heart J.*, **112**, 361.

52. Ulick, S. and Chu, M.D. (1982) Significance of the secretion of 18-hydroxycortisol by the human adrenal cortex. In *Endocrinology of Hypertension* (ed. F. Mantero, E.G. Biglieri and C.R.W. Edwards), Academic Press, London, p. 23.

53. Corrie, J.E.T., Edwards, C.R.W. and Budd, P.S. (1985) A radioimmunoassay for 18-hydroxycortisol in plasma and urine. *Clin. Chem.*, **31**, 849.

54. Ikeda, D.M., Francis, I.R., Glazer, G.M. *et al.* (1989) The detection of adrenal tumours and hyperplasia in patients with primary aldosteronism: comparison of scintigraphy, CT, and MR imaging. *Am. J. Radiol.*, **153**, 301–6.

55. Gross, M.D. and Shapiro, B. (1989) Scintigraphic studies in adrenal hypertension. *Sem. Nucl. Med.*, **XIX**, 122–43.

56. Ross, N.S. and Aron, D.C. (1990) Hormonal evaluation of the patient with an incidentally discovered adrenal mass. *New Engl. J. Med.*, **323**, 1401–5.

57. Valk, T.W., Gross, M.D., Swanson, D.P. *et al.* (1980) The relationship of serum lipids to adrenal gland uptake of 6B-131-I-iodomethyl-19-norcholesterol in Cushing's syndrome. *J. Nucl. Med.*, **21**, 1069–72.

58. Shapiro, B., Britton, K.E., Hawkins, L.A. and Edwards, C.R.W. (1981) Clinical experience with ^{75}Se selenomethylcholesterol adrenal imaging. *Clin. Endocrinol.* **15**, 19–27.

59. Rifai, A., Beierwaites, W.H., Freitas, J.E. *et al.* (1978) Adrenal scintigraphy in low renin essential hypertension. *Clin. Nucl. Med.*, **3**, 282–6.

60. White, P.C., New, M.I. and Dupont, B. (1987) Congenital adrenal hyperplasia. *New Engl. J. Med.*, **316**, 1580–6.

61. Fraser, R. (1983) Inborn errors of corticosteroid biosynthesis: their effects on electrolyte metabolism and blood pressure. In *Handbook of Hypertension*, vol. 2 (ed. J.I.S. Robertson), Elsevier, Amsterdam, pp. 162–88.

62. Werder, E., Zachmann, M., Vollmin, J.A. *et al.* (1974) Unusual steroid excretion in a child with low renin hyperplasia. *Res. Steroids.*, **6**, 385.

63. Stewart, P.M., Corrie, J.E.T., Shackleton, C.H.L. and Edwards, C.R.W. (1988) Syndrome of apparent mineralocorticoid excess: a defect in the cortisol–cortisone shuttle. *J. Clin. Invest.*, **82**, 340.

64. Ulick, S., Levine, L.S., Gunczler, P. *et al.* (1979) A syndrome of apparent mineralocorticoid excess associated with defects in the peripheral metabolism of cortisol. *J. Clin. Endocrinol. Metab.*, **49**, 757.

65. Stewart, P.M., Wallace, A.M., Valentino, R. *et al.* (1987) Mineralocorticoid activity of liquorice: 11β-hydroxysteroid dehydrogenase deficiency comes of age. *Lancet*, **ii**, 821.

66. Liddle, G.W., Bledsoe, T., Coppage, Jr, W.S. (1963) A familial renal disorder stimulating primary aldosteronism but with negligible aldosterone secretion. *Trans. Ass. Am. Physns*, **76**, 199.

67. Carlsen, J.E., Kober, L., Torp-Pedersen, C. and Johansen, P. (1990) Relation between dose of bendrofluazide, antihypertensive effect and adverse biochemical effects. *Br. Med. J.*, **300**, 975–8.

68. MacKay, A., Brown, J.J., Lever, A.F., Morton, J.J. and Robertson, J.I.S. (1983) Unilateral renal disease in hypertension. In *Handbook of hypertension*, vol. 2 (ed. J.I.S. Robertson), Elsevier, Amsterdam, pp. 33–79.

69. Robertson, P.W., Klidjian, A., Harding, L.K. *et al.* (1967) Hypertension due to a renin-secreting renal tumour. *Am. J. Med.*, **43**, 963.

70. Barraclough, M.A. (1966) Sodium and water depletion with acute malignant hypertension. *Am. J. Med.*, **40**, 265–72.

71. Padfield, P.L., Brown, J.J., Lever, A.F. *et al.* (1981) Blood pressure in acute and chronic vasopressin excess. *New Engl. J. Med.*, **304**, 1067–70.

72. Davis, B.A., Crook, J.E., Vestal, R.E. *et al.* (1979) Prevalence of renovascular hypertension in patients with grade II or IV hypertensive retinopathy. *New Engl. J. Med.*, **30**, 273.

73. Goldblatt, H., Lynch, J., Hanzal, R.F. *et al.* (1934) Studies on experimental hypertension. I. The production of persistent elevation of systolic blood pressure by means of renal ischemia. *J. Exp. Med.* **59**, 347–78.

74. Davies, D.L., McElroy, K., Atkinson, A.B. *et al.* (1979) Relationships between exchangeable sodium and blood pressure in different forms of hypertension in man. *Clin. Sci.*, **57** (suppl. 5), 69.

75. Luscher, T.F., Jager, K., Muller, F.B. and Buhler, F.R. (1990) Renovascular hypertension: update on diagnosis and treatment. In *The Management of Hypertension. Handbook of Hypertension*, vol. 13 (ed. F.R. Buhler and J.H. Laragh), Elsevier, Amsterdam.

76. Brown, J.J., Cuesta, V., Davies, D.L. *et al.* (1976) Mechanism of renal hypertension. *Lancet*, 5 June, 1219–21.

77. Dickinson, C.J. and Yu, R. (1967) Mechanisms involved in the progressive pressor response to very small amounts of angiotensin in conscious rabbits. *Circulation Res.*, **21** (suppl. 2), 157.

78. Pickering, T.G. (1989) Renovascular hypertension: etiology and pathophysiology. *Sem. Nucl. Med.* **XIX**, 79–88.

79. Pickering, T.G. (1990) Renovascular hypertension. Medical evaluation and non-surgical treatment. In *Hypertension: Pathophysiology, Diagnosis and Management*, vol. 2 (ed. J.H. Laragh. and B.M. Brenner), Raven Press, New York, pp. 1539–59.

80. Grim, C.E. (1983) Renovascular hypertension: the medical point of view. In *Clinical Aspects of Renovascular Hypertension* (ed. R. van Schilfgaarde, J.C. Stanley, P. van Brummelen and E.H. Oberbosch), Martinus Nijhoff, The Hague, pp. 243–58.

81. Eyler, W.R., Clark, M.E., Garman, J.E. *et al.* (1962) Angiography of the renal areas including a comparative study of renal arterial stenoses with and without hypertension. *Radiology*, **78**, 879–91.

82. Choudhri, A.H., Cleland, J.G.F., Rowlands, P.C. *et al.* (1990) Unsuspected renal artery stenosis in peripheral vascular disease. *Br. Med. J.*, **301**, 1197–8.

83. Main, J., Ward, M., Loose, H. and Wilkinson, R. (1991) Renal artery stenosis. *Br. Med. J.* **302**, 115.

84. Holley, K.E., Hunt, J.C., Brown, A.L., Kin-

caid, O.W. and Sheps, S.G. (1964) Renal artery stenosis. A clinical–pathologic study in normotensive and hypertensive patients. *Am. J. Med.*, **37**, 14–22.

85. Maxwell, M.H., Bleifer, K.H., Franklin, S.S. and Varady, P.D. (1972) Co-operative study of renovascular hypertension: demographic analysis of the study. *J. Am. Med. Ass.*, **220**, 1195.

86. Millan, V.G. and Madias, N.E. (1979) Percutaneous transluminal angioplasty for severe renovascular hypertension due to renal artery medial fibroplasia. *Lancet*, **i**, 993–5.

87. Sos, T.A., Pickering, T.G., Sniderman, K. *et al.* (1983) Percutaneous transluminal renal angioplasty in renovascular hypertension due to atheroma or fibromuscular dysplasia. *New Engl. J. Med.*, **309**, 274–9.

88. Ramsay, L.E. and Waller, P.C. (1990) Blood pressure response to percutaneous transluminal angioplasty for renovascular hypertension: an overview of published series. *Br. Med. J.*, **300**, 569–72.

89. Schreiber, M.J., Pohl, M.A. and Novick, A.C. (1984) The natural history of atherosclerotic and fibrous renal artery disease. *Urol. Clin. North Am.*, **11**, 383–92.

90. Gifford, R. (1969) Evaluation of the hypertensive patient with emphasis on detecting curable causes. *Millbank Mem. Fund Q.*, **47**, 170–86.

91. Vaughan, Jr, E.D., Buhler, F.R., Laragh, J.H. *et al.* (1973) Renovascular hypertension: renin measurements to indicate hypersecretion and contralateral suppression, estimate renal plasma flow, and score for surgical curability. *Am. J. Med.*, **55**, 402–14.

92. Vaughan, Jr, E.D., Carey, R.M., Ayers, C.R. *et al.* (1979) A physiological definition of blood pressure response to renal revascularization in patients with renovascular hypertension. *Kidney Int.*, **15**, 83–92.

93. Case, D.B. and Laragh, J.H. (1979) Reactive hyper-reninemia in renovascular hypertension after angiotensin blockade with saralasin or converting enzyme inhibitor. *Ann. Intern. Med.*, **91**, 153–60.

94. Muller, F.B., Sealey, J.E., Case, D.B. *et al.* (1986) The captopril test for identifying reno-

vascular disease in hypertensive patients. *Am. J. Med.*, **80**, 633–44.

95. Frederickson, E.D., Wilcox, C.S., Bucci, M. *et al.* (1990) A prospective evaluation of a simplified captopril test for the detection of renovascular hypertension. *Archs Intern. Med.*, **150**, 569–72.

96. Postma, C.T., van der Steen, P.H.M., Hoefnagels, W.H.L., de Boo, T, and Thien, T. (1990) The captopril test in the detection of renovascular disease in hypertensive patients. *Archs Intern. Med.*, **150**, 625–8.

97. Sealey, J.E., Buhler, F.R., Laragh, J.H. and Vaughan, Jr, E.D. (1973) The physiology of renin secretion in essential hypertension: estimation of renin secretion rate and renal blood flow from peripheral and renal vein renin levels. *Am. J. Med.*, **55**, 391–401.

98. Marks, L.S. and Maxwell, M.H. (1975) Renal vein renin value and limitations in the prediction of operative results. *Urol. Clin. North Am.*, **2**, 311–25.

99. Vaughan, Jr, E.D., Pickering, T.G. and Laragh, J.H. (1987) Identifying patients with renovascular hypertension. In *The Kidney in Hypertension: Clinical Aspects*, vol. 1 (ed. N. Kaplan, B.M. Brenner and J.H. Laragh), Raven Press, New York, pp. 91–108.

100. Pickering, T.G., Sos, T.A., Vaughan, Jr, E.D. *et al.* (1985) Predictive value and changes of renin secretion in hypertensive patients with unilateral renovascular disease undergoing successful renal angioplasty. *Am. J. Med.*, **76**, 398–404.

101. Luscher, T.F., Lie, J.T., Stanson, A.W. *et al.* (1987) Arterial fibromuscular dysplasia. *Mayo Clin. Proc.*, **62**, 931.

102. Bookstein, J.J., Abrams, H.L., Buenger, R.E. *et al.* (1972) Radiologic aspects of renovascular hypertension. 2. The role of urography in unilateral renovascular disease. *J. Am. Med. Ass.*, **220**, 1225.

103. Wenting, G.J., Tan-Tjiong, H.L., Derkx, F.H.M. *et al.* (1984) Split renal function after captopril in unilateral renal artery stenosis. *Br. Med. J.*, **288**, 886–90.

104. Hricik, D.D., Browning, P.J. and Kopelman, R. (1983) Captopril-induced functional renal insufficiency in patients with bilateral renal artery stenosis or renal artery stenosis in a

185

solitary kidney. *New Engl. J. Med.*, **308**, 373.

105. Ichikawa, I., Ferrone, R.A., Duchin, K.L. *et al.* (1983) Relative contribution to vasopressin and angiotensin II to the altered renal micro-circulatory dynamics in two-kidney Goldblatt hypertension. *Circulation Res.*, **53**, 592–602.

106. Geyskes, G.G., Oei, H.Y., Puylaert, C.B.A.J. and Dorhout Mees, E.J. (1987) Renovascular hypertension identified by captopril-induced changes in the renogram. *Hypertension*, **9**, 451–8.

107. Kopecky, R.T., Thomas, F.D. and McAfee, J.G. (1987) Furosemide augments the effects of captopril on nuclear studies in renovascular stenosis. *Hypertension*, **10**, 181–8.

108. Chen, C.C., Hoffer, P.B., Vahjen, G. *et al.* (1990) Patients at high risk for renal artery stenosis: a simple method of renal scintigraphic analysis with Tc-99m DTPA and Captopril[1]. *Radiology*, **176**, 365–70.

109. Fine, E.J. and Sarkar, S. (1989) Differential diagnosis and management of renovascular hypertension through nuclear medicine techniques. *Sem. Nucl. Med.*, **19**, 101–5.

110. Dondi, M., Franchi, R., Levorato, M. *et al.* (1989) Evaluation of hypertensive patients by means of a captopril enhanced renal scintigraphy with technetium-99m DTPA. *J. Nucl. Med.*, **30**, 615–21.

111. Atkinson, A.B., Brown, J.J., Cumming, A.M.M. *et al.* (1982) Captopril in renovascular hypertension: long-term use in predicting surgical outcome. *Br. Med. J.*, **284**, 689.

112. Gilles, G. and Grossman, A. (1985) The CRFs and their control: chemistry, physiology and clinical implications. *J. Clin. Endocrinol. Metab.*, **14**, 821–41.

113. Udelsman, R., Norton, J.A., Jelenick, S.A. *et al.* (1987) Responses on the hypothalamic-pituitary-adrenal and renin-angiotensin axes and the sympathetic system during controlled surgical and anesthetic stress. *J. Clin. Endocrinol. Metab.*, **64**, 986–94.

114. Cushing, H. (1932) The basophil adenomas of the pituitary body and their clinical mani-festations (pituitary basophilism). *Bull. Johns Hopkins Hosp.*, **50**, 127.

115. Findling, J.W., Aron, D.C. and Tyrell, J.V. (1985) Cushing's disease. In *The Pituitary Gland* (ed. H. Imura), Raven Press, New York, pp. 441–54.

116. Carpenter, P.C. (1988) Diagnostic evaluation of Cushing's syndrome. *Endocrinol. Metab. Clin. North Am.*, **17**, 445–72.

117. Schteingart, D.E., Lloyd, R.V., Akil, H. *et al.* (1986) Cushing's syndrome secondary to ectopic corticotropin-releasing hormone – adrenocorticotropin secretion. *J. Clin. Endocrinol. Metab.*, **63**, 770–5.

118. Greminger, P., Tenschert, W. and Vetter, W. (1982) Hypertension in Cushing's syndrome. In *Endocrinology of Hypertension* (ed. F. Mantero and E.G. Biglieri), Academic Press, London, pp. 103–110.

119. Plotz, C., Knowlten, A. and Ragan, C. (1962) Growth hormone in cardiac hypertrophy induced by nephrogenous hypertension. In *Recent Advances in Studies on Cardiac Structure and Metabolism*, vol. 8 (ed. P.E. Roy and P. Harris), University Park Press, Baltimore, pp. 413–25.

120. Fraser, R., Davies, D.L. and Connell, J.M.C. (1989) Hormones and hypertension. *Clin. Endocrinol.*, **31**, 701–46.

121. Scoggins, B.A., Denton, D.A., Whitworth, J.A. and Coghlan, J.P. (1984) ACTH-dependent hypertension. *Clin. Exp. Hypertension*, **A6**, 599–646.

122. Edwards, C.R.W., Stewart, P.M., Burt, D. *et al.* (1988) Tissue localisation of 11β-hydroxysteroid dehydrogenase-tissue specific protector of the mineralocorticoid receptor. *Lancet*, **ii**, 986.

123. Connell, J.M.C., Whitworth, J.A., Davies, D.L. *et al.* (1987) Effects of ACTH and cortisol administration on blood pressure, electrolyte metabolism, atrial natriuretic peptide and renal function in normal man. *J. Hypertension*, **5**, 425–33.

10

Diagnostic tests in diabetes mellitus and hypoglycaemia

S.A. AMIEL and E.A.M. GALE

10.1 DIABETES MELLITUS

10.1.1 CLASSIFICATION

Diabetes mellitus is a heterogeneous group of disorders characterized by chronic hyperglycaemia associated with inadequate insulin action. Although diabetes mellitus is defined in terms of high blood glucose levels, inadequate insulin action results in multiple metabolic, endocrine and haematological derangements which may be equally important in the pathogenesis of the disease and its complications, but usually improve as glucose levels are brought under control (Table 10.1).

Primary diabetes mellitus (Table 10.2) is conveniently divided into two main syndromes, although each syndrome almost certainly includes a range of diseases and may indeed merge into the other.

The currently agreed version of the classification divides primary diabetes mellitus into insulin dependent (IDDM or Type I) and non-insulin dependent (NIDDM or Type 2) diabetes mellitus. A third category, malnutrition related diabetes mellitus (MRDM), is common in the Third World [1]. Two variants of this are recognized: fibrocalcific disease of the pancreas and protein deficient pancreatic diabetes.

IDDM is primarily a disease of young people, resulting from autoimmune destruction of the beta cells of the islets of Langerhans. Because it is due to failure of insulin production it may lead to overproduction of ketones, and diabetic ketoacidosis is the hallmark of this type of diabetes.

NIDDM, in contrast, is commonly (though not exclusively) a disease of older people and is frequently associated with obesity. There is a strong element of insulin resistance in its aetiology, although some degree of beta cell failure is implied, since a healthy beta cell mass could otherwise maintain normoglycaemia, at the cost of hyperinsulinaemia.

MRDM typically presents in adolescence or early adult life in individuals with a history of malnutrition; ketosis does not develop.

Diabetes mellitus can almost always be diagnosed on clinical grounds on the basis of symptoms and acute or chronic complications, in association with clearly elevated random blood glucose levels. The oral glucose tolerance test (Table 10.3) is useful in defining borderline diabetes, impaired glucose tolerance and a low renal threshold.

The impaired glucose tolerance syndrome, which can be diagnosed only by the glucose tolerance test, has uncertain clinical significance. The rate of progression to frank

Table 10.1 Circulating derangements of uncontrolled diabetes mellitus

Metabolic

Carbohydrate metabolism
Increased:
    glycogenolysis   hyperglycaemia
    gluconeogenesis   glycosuria   polyuria
                         osmotic diuresis polydipsia
                                          dehydration

Decreased:
    glucose oxidation
    glucose storage

Protein metabolism
Increased:
    protein breakdown   circulating   muscle wasting
                        amino acids

Decreased:
    protein synthesis

Lipid metabolism
Increased:
    lipolysis   NEFA   may contribute to
                        hyperlipidaemia atherogenesis
    ketogenesis   ketosis   nausea
                        acidosis   hyperventilation
                        aciduria   dehydration

Decreased:
    fat synthesis

Endocrine
Increased:
    stress hormones   increased effects
                        of insulin lack
    growth hormone
Decreased:
    IGF-1   decreased linear growth

Haematological
Increased:
    fibrinogen and other   may contribute to
    clotting factors   acceleration of vessel
                                    wall damage

Decreased:
    neutrophil phagocytosis   risk of infection

Table 10.2 Typical features of the main diabetes mellitus syndromes

	IDDM	NIDDM	MRDM
Age at onset (years)	<30 (peak incidences at 5 years and puberty)	>40	<30
Prodrome	Clinical symptoms for weeks or days	Clinical symptoms may be for years	Clinical symptoms may be for years
Genetics:			
HLA association	DR3 & DR4	None	None
Family history	+ve in 10%	+ve in 30%	
Concordance in twins	50%	100%	
Ketosis-prone	Yes	No	Not usually
Need for insulin	Yes	Not usually	Yes
Obesity related	No	Yes	No
Autoimmune			
Islet cell antibodies	Yes	No	No
Other autoimmune disease	Yes (1b)	No	No
Exocrine pancreatic disease	No	No	Yes (fibrocalculous, not protein deficient)
Microvasular disease at presentation	Rare	Common	
Risk for microvascular disease	High	High	
Risk for macrovascular disease	High	High	

diabetes is approximately 4% per year, while the remainder either revert to normal glucose tolerance or remain unchanged. Individuals with impaired glucose tolerance have an increased risk of macrovascular disease but are unlikely to develop microvascular lesions. Concerns that hyperinsulinaemia secondary to impaired glucose tolerance might increase susceptibility to ischaemic heart disease or cerebrovascular disease remain speculative but there is increasing evidence to suggest an underlying mechanism for such a causal relationship. Individuals in this category should be advised to keep lean, to exercise and to reduce other cardiovascular risk factors.

Gestational diabetes is diabetes developing in pregnancy. This, unless carefully controlled, is associated with neonatal hypoglycaemia and macrosomia. Diagnosis is important, although still controversial. About 70% of the women who develop diabetes in pregnancy will revert to normal glucose tolerance postpartum, but the remainder will remain diabetic or will develop diabetes shortly afterwards. The overall majority – about three-quarters within 24 years [2] – will develop NIDDM as they age, although this risk can be greatly reduced by the avoidance of obesity [3].

Secondary diabetes mellitus results from either pancreatic destruction (e.g. pancreatitis, trauma, surgery or haemochromatosis) or from insulin resistance. States of insulin resistance are most commonly seen secondary to either drug therapy (notoriously

Table 10.3 Oral glucose tolerance test: WHO criteria (75 g oral glucose, 395 ml chilled Lucozade, given after basal blood sample obtained)

		Whole blood		Plasma	
		Venous	*Capillary*	*Venous*	*Capillary*
		(glucose mmol l⁻¹)		*(glucose mmol l⁻¹)*	
Diabetes	Basal	>6.7	>6.7	>7.8	>7.8
mellitus	after 2 hrs	>10.0	>11.1	>11.1	>12.2
IGT	Basal	>6.7	>6.7	>7.8	>7.8
	after 2 hrs	6.7–10.0	7.8–11.1	7.8–11.1	8.9–12.2
Normal	Basal	<6.7	<6.7	<7.8	<7.8
	after 2 hrs	<6.7	<6.7	<7.8	<7.8

thiazide diuretics and anti-inflammatory doses of corticosteroids) or excessive production of hyperglycaemic hormones as in Cushing's syndrome and disease, acromegaly, phaeochromocytoma or glucagonoma. Abnormalities of the insulin receptor may also produce insulin resistance which, if not fully compensated by increased insulin secretion, will lead to clinical diabetes mellitus. Receptor concentration falls in obesity, acromegaly, uraemia and Type A insulin receptor defect syndrome [4], a rare condition of insulin resistance, ovarian dysfunction and usually hypertriglyceridaemia. In contrast, reduced receptor affinity, probably secondary to anti-receptor antibody formation, may be the principal cause of the insulin resistance of the Type B syndrome, where severe insulin resistance is seen in association with pseudoacanthosis nigricans [5].

10.1.2 ORAL GLUCOSE TOLERANCE TEST

Diabetes is defined according to the effects of a standardized glucose challenge on blood or plasma glucose profiles. A 75 g oral dose of glucose, often given as 395 ml chilled Lucozade (the chilling is useful in reducing nausea), is taken by an overnight fasted individual at rest, after at least 3 days on a diet containing a minimum of 200 g of carbohydrate. The numerical values for glucose (Table 10.3) depend on the nature of the sample taken: capillary blood gives higher values than venous, and plasma gives readings about 10% higher than whole blood.

Strip tests, even used in association with reflectance meters, should not be used to establish a diagnosis [6,7], despite recent claims that a false negative rate of 20% in one study still did not miss any important cases [8].

The oral glucose tolerance test is not ideal. It lacks reproducibility, with a coefficient of variation of around 25% at the 2-hour mark [9]. Nevertheless, and despite its faults, it remains the gold standard for diagnosis, although it should not be forgotten that diabetes can usually be diagnosed by a single fasting or post-prandial venous plasma glucose over 11.1 mmol l⁻¹ in the presence of symptoms without recourse to a formal test. According to WHO criteria, only a fasting and 2-hour post-glucose load glucoses are needed, although intermediate readings with paired urine samples are useful in diagnosing a low renal threshold for glucose. Despite an extensive literature, high intermediate glucose values ('lag curve' or 'steeple') and flat glucose tolerance curves have no prognostic significance.

10.1.3 DIAGNOSIS OF DIABETES MELLITUS IN PREGNANCY

Glycosuria is common in pregnant women because of a lowered renal threshold for glucose. Diagnosis is complicated by the effect of normal pregnancy on glucose tolerance – fasting glucoses are lower than in the non-pregnant state while stimulated glucose levels may be higher. A large study of normal pregnant women recently suggested that plasma glucose levels of 7.5 and 9.6 mmol l^{-1} two hours after a 75 g oral glucose load should be accepted as normal for women in the second and third trimesters of pregnancy, respectively, although pregnancy outcome was not examined [10].

What are the risks of glucose intolerance in pregnancy? In 1964, O'Sullivan and Mahan [11] defined abnormal glucose tolerance in pregnancy on the basis of a 3-hour 100 g oral glucose tolerance test. Their data were later adjusted for changes in the method of glucose measurement and conversion to the use of plasma rather than blood glucose, and gestational diabetes was diagnosed if any two of the pre-load or hourly post-load values were more than two standard deviations from the norm (5.3, 10, 8.6 and 7.8 mmol l^{-1} before and at 1, 2 and 3 hours post-load, respectively) [12]. Because these criteria identified a population of pregnancies with a fourfold increase in perinatal mortality, and a 60% prevalence of abnormal glucose tolerance 16 years later, they have been the basis for much subsequent work. More recently, it has been reported that glucose levels below 10 mmol l^{-1} two hours after 100 g oral glucose or 8.9 mmol l^{-1} one hour after 50 g of glucose do not appear to be associated with increased neonatal risk [13]. Despite this, debate continues concerning diagnostic criteria for gestational diabetes. O'Sullivan and Mahan's criteria gained much favour in America, and the American National Diabetes Data Group still recom-

mends a 100 g oral glucose tolerance test for the diagnosis of diabetes in pregnancy. The WHO, however, recommends the 75 g glucose tolerance test and the same diagnostic criteria as in the non-pregnant state, and this is our usual practice.

When, who and how to screen

Most authorities agree that screening should be performed on all pregnant women between the 24th and 28th weeks of pregnancy. The reasons for screening are more compelling for women over 24 years of age, in whom the prevalence of gestational diabetes is perhaps tenfold higher, although not all would agree that younger women should be excluded [14].

10.1.4 PREDICTIVE TESTS FOR DIABETES MELLITUS

There have been hopes that it will be possible to diagnose diabetes mellitus before the onset of the disease. This is especially true for IDDM, which has an autoimmune aetiology and is potentially open to preventive therapy. IDDM is associated with the histocompatibility antigens DR3 and DR4, which may even play a role in the pathogenesis of the disease. Most recently, the high prevalence of a particular amino acid at position 57 on the DQ-beta chain of the HLA antigen in people with IDDM has given rise to suggestions that its effect on the tertiary structure of the molecule may be important in its recognition by the immune system and subsequent activation of the immune system [15]. Refinement of the identification of the genetic features associated with IDDM continues, but as yet genetic grounds alone are only weakly predictive of diabetes.

The concept that Type 1 diabetes is a disease of autoimmunity has built up steadily over the past 20 years. Evidence for this included the description of lymphocytic infiltration of the islets, followed by the discovery of a variety of circulating autoantibodies in patients with established Type 1 diabetes. The most important of these have been islet cell antibodies (ICA), insulin autoantibodies (IAA), and glutamic acid decarboxylase (GAD) [16]. ICA are directed against an unknown antigen (probably a glycolipid) present on all islet endocrine cells. Antibodies against insulin itself (IAA) were next reported; and insulin is at present the only antigen that is clearly beta cell specific. More recently, a 64 K antigen present in the islet cells of humans and the BB rat has been identified as GAD, an enzyme also found in nerve cell endings and involved in the synthesis of the inhibitory neurotransmitter GABA. GAD peptides are expressed at the surface of beta cells and presented by class I receptors there. These peptides are recognized by cytotoxic T cells, and could thus have the potential to initiate a process leading to beta cell destruction [17].

ICAs are the most useful marker of future diabetes, and may precede impairment of islet function by many years. Recently, international consensus has been reached about the quantification of these antibodies in 'JDF units', and high titres of these antibodies are closely correlated with risk for development of IDDM. Methods for detecting islet cell antibodies usually depend on immunochemical or immunofluorescent identification of their binding to fixed or unfixed human or animal pancreatic tissue. The methods are very variable indeed and have equally variable detection limits. A standard serum containing 80 JDF units of activity is now used to standardize the various assays, which should now be more readily compared [18]. The risk of developing diabetes has been shown to rise in parallel with titres of islet cell antibodies.

IAAs are also strongly predictive in the presence (but not in the absence) of ICA.

Combination of ICA, IAA and a reduced first phase insulin response to intravenous glucose can offer highly specific prediction in family members, but different screening strategies are needed for prediction in families and in the general population [19].

10.1.5 MONITORING DIABETES AND ITS COMPLICATIONS

(a) Monitoring glycaemic control

Clinical assessment

The clinical history is an important guide to management of a patient with diabetes, but should be supported by reliable tests reflecting glycaemic control.

Measurement of blood glucose

Older methods of blood glucose measurement using *o*-toluidine or depending upon detection of reducing substances in the blood have largely been replaced by more specific enzymatic methods using, for example, glucose oxidase immobilized on electrodes. A current is generated when oxygen is released from the glucose molecule. Hexokinase and glucose dehydrogenase are also used in assay systems. Immobilization of the enzyme plus either an electronic or colorimetric assay system on a small pad on a plastic strip provides the basis for strip tests for home blood glucose monitoring. It should be remembered that whole· blood preserved with fluoride (to inhibit cellular metabolism of glucose) shows an initial rapid fall in glucose content of up to 10% at room temperature but is more stable thereafter. Whole blood glucose reads 10%–15% lower than plasma if the haematocrit is normal, because red cells contain less glucose than plasma, and arterial glucose at normal concentrations is 7% higher than the corresponding venous reading, although this ratio depends upon the glucose concentration and alters after meals.

Urine versus blood tests

Urine testing has largely been superseded by home blood glucose monitoring, but it continues to have a use in older patients in whom strict blood glucose control is not indicated. Fehling's test detected the presence of reducing substances in the urine, of which glucose is but one, and Clinitest – still used by many patients – relies on reduction of a copper salt to produce a colour change. It is, however, cumbersome and is being replaced by the more acceptable strip methods. These consist of a filter paper impregnated with glucose oxidase, a peroxidase and a colour indicator. Held in the urine flow, glucose in the urine is oxidized to produce hydrogen peroxide, which alters the colour. Glucose appears in the urine only if the renal threshold for glucose has been exceeded at some point while the urine was formed. A low renal threshold for glucose will result in glycosuria in the presence of normal blood glucoses. This is typical of pregnancy and is of no pathological significance. Conversely, in a patient with a high renal threshold, significant hyperglycaemia can exist with negative urine tests. Urine testing for glucose is a useful indicator of control in elderly patients, even though many appear to have a high renal threshold for glucose, and can supplement home blood glucose testing results. It has major limitations if good (i.e. nearly normal) blood glucose control is required.

Home blood glucose monitoring

The principles are similar to those of strip tests for urine. The finger is pricked and a drop of blood allowed to flow over a reagent pad on a plastic strip. After a specified time interval the blood is wiped or blotted away, and a colour change develops which can be read by eye or with the aid of a reflectance meter.

Used correctly, the test strips can be very accurate, but results are very operator-dependent – more so with some strips than with others. Timing is critical and errors introduced by inadequate technique, e.g. smearing of the sample, are common. Inaccuracies of hypoglycaemic levels are also common [6]. The newest devices for home glucose monitoring rely on the generation of an electrical potential by oxidation of the glucose in the blood sample.

Home blood glucose monitoring is essential for intensified insulin therapy. Since this therapy increases the risk of hypoglycaemia, it is only safe if the patient can measure blood glucose frequently and adjust insulin therapy accordingly. This involves regular glucose profiles, before and at least 90 minutes after meals and occasionally at night. Blood tests taken within 90 minutes of a meal and glucose profiles collected in hospital are hard to interpret and hence of limited value. Blood glucose monitoring techniques can and should be checked, in both patients and staff.

Ketones

Urine tests for ketones are cheap, simple and easy to perform. Again, tests for urinary ketones are available in the older tablet form (Acetest, containing sodium nitroprusside, glycine and disodium phosphate, specific for the detection of beta-hydroxybutyrate and acetoacetate) or in more easily quantified strip form (e.g. Ketostix). The role of urine testing for protein is considered later.

Medium term control: Glycation products

Glucose attaches to amines in proteins and polypeptide chains, first by a reversible condensation to form a Schiff base, and then by a slow structural rearrangement to create a more stable glycosylated protein, the Amadori product. Although the Amadori rearrangement is reversible, the rate constant for the forward reaction is much greater than that for the dissociation. The rate of glycosylation is determined by four factors – temperature, pH, protein concentration and type – which are effectively fixed *in vivo*, and two variables, ambient glucose and the length of exposure to the glucose. The proportion of any glycosylated product thus depends upon the rate of formation and the rate of removal.

Glycation of haemoglobin

Haemoglobin has a long half-life and is susceptible to glycation. Glycated haemoglobin (HbA1) is more negatively charged than the non-glycated form and can readily be separated from it by electrochemical means. HbA1c fraction is much more resistant to the influences of temperature and time in sampled blood than HbA1a and 1b, and is therefore more reliable as a clinical test. The percentage of haemoglobin that is glycated reflects the integrated glucose over the preceding eight to twelve weeks, and can be used as an objective measure of the mean blood glucose over that time.

HbA1 or HbA1c is most commonly measured by cation exchange chromatography, using either microcolumns or high performance liquid chromatography (HPLC). The latter is preferable if enough samples are generated to make it economical. In cation exchange chromatography, the more negatively charged particles elute first and can be measured spectroscopically. These systems can be used to separate HbA1, both from HbA0 and into its components HbA1a, 1b and 1c. The assay is affected by temperature, pH, ionic strength of the eluting fluids and column size, and all these factors must be controlled. Partly because of this, and

because no single standard is available, it should be noted that each laboratory will have its own normal range and no direct comparisons can be made. Since laboratory values often drift over time, small changes in HbA1 should be interpreted with caution. Glycation products will remain stable for about a week if kept at 4°C and for several months if frozen at −70°C.

Haemolysis, blood loss and pregnancy all increase red cell turnover and cause a corresponding reduction in HbA1 independent of glycaemic exposure. Triglycerides and bilirubin interfere with the assay, leading to overestimation of HbA1 and 1c levels in severe hypertriglyceridaemia or jaundice, and haemoglobinopathies may affect results by altering the charge of the molecule. HbC and HbS decrease, while HbF increases, the percentage glycation. Other substances which bind to haemoglobin can also lead to overestimation of glycation: this effect is seen in opiate addiction, uraemia, alcoholism and high dose aspirin therapy.

Other methods for estimating HbA1 include agar gel electrophoresis, which measures HbA1 as a single entity. It is quick but expensive, unless many samples are to be measured. HbF and pre-A1 interfere with results, but HbS and HbC do not. None of the haemoglobinopathies affects results generated by isoelectric focusing, in which electrophoresis is applied across a gel in which a pH gradient has been established, so that individual haemoglobins separate out according to their isoelectric points. This does distinguish HbA1c from other haemoglobin components but pre-HbA1 must be removed first. Other methods do not depend on the electrical charge of the molecules and measure additional glycated haemoglobin molecules, giving higher results. They include a colorimetric assay, in which glucose is released from the haemoglobin by heat and acid, to generate a colour with hydroxymethylfurfural thiobarbituric acid

194

(TBA); and affinity chromatography, in which the glucose moieties on the haemoglobin form complexes with boronic acid ligands supported on a cross-linked agarose gel matrix and are then washed off (after washing through the unbound, non-glycated haemoglobin) for quantization with a sorbitol buffer. Results with colorimetry are relatively unaffected by storage of samples, haemoglobinopathy or non-glucose adducts of haemoglobin, but assay units have not been standardized. Affinity chromatography likewise gives stable results not much affected by variations in sample collection and storage, and although very sensitive to differences in the gels themselves, the estimation of glycated haemoglobin is not affected by haemoglobinopathy or nonglucose adducts of haemoglobin.

Perhaps the biggest problem in estimations of glycated haemoglobin is the lack of standardization, and the National Institutes of Health are developing a standard to work with all systems. Within a single laboratory, the test can be of great clinical utility – a 1% change in glycated haemoglobin probably represents a change in mean plasma glucose of $1.7 \, \text{mmol} \, l^{-1}$. Since the principal use of the test is to monitor long-term glycaemic control and response to therapy, good quality control within the laboratory is essential.

Fructosamine

The fructosamine test measures the extent of glycation of serum proteins. The ketoamine in the glycated proteins will, in alkaline conditions, reduce and open the ring structure of the redox dye nitro blue tetrazolium chloride, altering the absorption spectrum of the dye to a degree proportional to the concentration of glycated protein in the original sample. The result shows linear correlation with the concentration of total protein in the sample, decreasing by about 1% for every gram of albumin in plasma samples. It is probably better expressed corrected for the total protein content of the sample [20] or as a ratio with albumin [21]. Alterations in protein concentration during pregnancy, for example, pose a theoretical problem, although fructosamine measurements have been clinically useful. Lipid abnormalities also affect the fructosamine assay, and removing lipid from samples may reduce the variability of the assay, provided that the treatment does not also remove protein [22]. Finally, it should be noted that the labile form of fructosamine does not appear to affect the estimation to a clinically relevant degree, except in cases of extreme hyperglycaemia.

Several studies have failed to show a correlation between HbA1 levels and fructosamine. Although this may be due to inherent problems in the fructosamine assay, it is more likely to reflect the different half-lives of plasma protein and haemoglobin. Thus, while fructosamine correlates well with other indices of glucose control over the preceding week or two [23], HbA1 shows its best correlation with glucose control over the previous three months. Despite the cheapness and ease of fructosamine measurement, most clinicians consider HbA1 to provide a more reliable index of glycaemic control.

In the attempt to find the perfect test to reflect short-term glycaemic control, other glycation products have been examined. The ease and inexpensive nature of the fructosamine assay does have great appeal, but other potential candidates include glycosylated serum albumin, for which a simple precise assay is now available [24].

In summary, despite its expense, glycated haemoglobin, especially in the stable form, is the most reliable measure of mid-term glycaemic control currently available. Its limitations are in circumstances where shorter periods of glucose control are important, especially in pregnancy.

(b) Screening for complications

Measurement of renal function

Diabetes affects the kidneys, with structural changes in the microcirculation (thickening of endothelial basement membrane, increased mesangial tissue, sclerosis of glomeruli) and functional changes, one of the earliest of which may be hyperfiltration (increased glomerular filtration rate). This may be followed by increased leakiness of the glomerular basement membrane, with leakage of albumin into the glomerular filtrate and hence into the urine. Thus, albuminuria is one of the earliest easily detectable signs of developing diabetic nephropathy, although other causes of proteinuria must first be excluded.

Tests for urine albumin

Standard clinic testing of spot urines using the commercially available strips detects albumin concentrations of $300–500\,\mathrm{mg\,l^{-1}}$. For practical purposes this represents irreversible renal disease. More sensitive tests are needed if abnormalities are to be detected at a time when intervention may yet be successful. Radioimmunoassay to detect low concentrations of albumin in urine [25] has been replaced with more rapid radioimmunoassays, radial immunodiffusion assays, immunoturbidimetric assays and enzyme-linked immunosorbent assays (ELISAs), facilitating laboratory measurement of small quantities of albuminuria. Non-diabetics have an albumin excretion rate of $12\,\mathrm{\mu g\,min^{-1}}$ or less, and there is a consensus that an albumin excretion rate of $30\,\mathrm{\mu g\,min^{-1}}$ or more is predictive of diabetic renal disease [26]. This has been termed microalbuminuria.

Albumin measurement is best performed on a timed urine collection, to estimate the *rate* of albumin secretion. Overnight collections, i.e. the first urine passed on rising, are especially useful because they eliminate effects of posture and exercise. Because of difficulties of sample collection, the albumin/creatinine ratio in the overnight urine is a useful alternative. Tests have also been designed to measure low rates of albumin excretion (as single concentrations) in spot urines in the diabetes clinic. Currently, available tests (Microalbutest, Ames Laboratories and Albusure, Cambridge Life Sciences) can detect urinary albumin concentrations in excess of $24\,\mathrm{mg\,l^{-1}}$. Most studies have used early morning urines to investigate the new tests [27]. The cut-off for these tests may still be too high for really effective screening, and they are at a further disadvantage because they measure concentration only [28]. They are not specific for albumin and are not quantitative. Overnight albumin/creatinine ratios therefore remain the best screening test, backed up by measurement of overnight excretion rate if positive. In NIDDM, microalbuminuria also indicates high risk of cardiovascular disease.

Measurements of renal function in established disease

Once clinical proteinuria has been detected, renal function can be assessed in a variety of ways. Probably the most useful parameter to follow is the glomerular filtration rate (GFR), quantified by the excretion rate of radiolabelled EDTA, a molecule which is filtered and not resorbed. For an individual, the decline in GFR is linear with time [29]. Creatinine clearance can be a useful parameter if access to GFR testing is limited. Plasma creatinine is also a useful parameter to follow in established nephropathy and its rise is related both to poor glycaemic control and to hypertension. The reciprocal of serial measurements of plasma creatinine reflects a decline in GFR [30]. Once creatinine levels have reached $200\,\mu\text{mol}\,l^{-1}$, end-stage renal failure can be expected in a mean of 26 months. Measures to interfere with the progression of renal failure should be instituted before impairment in these parameters occurs, but further measures such as treatment of hypertension [31] may delay deterioration even in established disease. Dietary protein restriction and referral for consideration of renal replacement therapy should be instituted as creatinine clearance falls below $30\,\text{ml}\,\text{min}^{-1}$.

Hyperfiltration may be an early marker of diabetic renal disease. This is detected by measuring glomerular filtration rate by EDTA. It is suggested that this early hyperfiltration (GFR in excess of $150\,\text{ml}\,\text{min}^{-1}$ $1.73\,\text{m}^{-2}$) is related to leakage of protein into the mesangium and later development of nephropathy. Later on, GFR falls as renal damage persists.

Non-diabetic causes of proteinuria must be excluded. Recurrent urinary tract infections should prompt intravenous urography and micturating cystograms to exclude reflux. Renal ultrasound is useful to exclude obstructive nephropathy, especially in hypertensive patients; renal scintigraphy can show a small kidney, characteristic of diffuse small blood vessel disease. Although the typical diabetic kidney is large, atheroma occurs early in diabetic patients and ischaemic nephropathy may lead to a shrinkage of kidney size. It should be borne in mind that while intravenous urography does not cause renal impairment in otherwise healthy diabetic patients, highly concentrated contrast media can cause further impairment in the presence of renal disease, and dehydration.

Renal biopsy, though usually definitive, should be reserved for those cases in which there is real reason to doubt that diabetes is the only pathology. It is traditionally considered if there is no detectable retinopathy, since these two microvascular complications almost invariably go together, but has a low yield even in this situation. Early diabetic nephropathy shows as a thickening of the basement membrane of the glomerular capillaries. Recent elegant electron microscope studies have shown a change in the structure of the fenestrae of the basement membrane as an early change in the disease. Basement membrane thickening is associated with increased polysaccharide content and loss of protein cross-linkages, which may enhance permeability. Fibrin and fibrin derivatives are deposited into basement membrane, and expand the mesangium with PAS positive material. Mesangial cell numbers also increase. Blood vessels are occluded and the final picture is one of diabetic glomerulosclerosis. This includes diffuse, generalized hyalinization of glomeruli, starting from the peripheral capillaries of the glomerulus; a rather less specific leakage of intensely acidophilic protein and fibrin derived material into the glomerular lumen and increasing numbers of glomeruli becoming hyalinized and then fibrosed and shrunken. The characteristic feature of diabetic nephropathy on light microscopy is the nodular deposit within the glomerulus. Nodular glomerulosclerosis, although pathognomic of diabetes, is not the typical lesion, and diffuse glomerulosclerosis is much more common. Functioning glomeruli initially enlarge to compensate for the loss of others, but more and more will become sclerotic as the disease progresses, leading to end-stage renal failure.

Assessment of retinopathy

Diabetes mellitus can affect all parts of the eye but it is its effect on the retina that rank diabetes as the commonest cause of blindness in young people in the Western world [32], and 1.2% per year develop sight threatening complications [33]. Because 70% of blindness due to diabetic retinopathy is preventable if therapy begins early enough [34], early diagnosis of retinopathy and regular screening are mandatory for all people with diabetes past puberty.

The early stages of retinal disease manifest microscopically as a thickening of capillary basement membrane, loss of pericytes and initial increase followed by loss of capillary endothelium, all of which predate clinically apparent disease. After some years of diabetes, the capillaries lose their endothelial lining and may close [35]. Capillary non-perfusion may in turn trigger proliferative changes in the retina.

The retina must be examined through dilated pupils to detect or exclude such retinopathy. Fundal photography is a useful way of augmenting direct clinical examination, and, when films are examined by an ophthalmologist, provides a useful way of expanding the number of diabetic patients who can have such expert assessment. However, the efficacy of fundal photography compared with ophthalmoscopy remains uncertain. Probably the best pick-up of retinopathy would be achieved by expert assessment through dilated pupils, but the expertise of many fundoscopists may be open to doubt. In such circumstances, the best pick-up rate is achieved by combining clinical examination with photography.

It is not clear how many fields in the eye should be photographed. Studies are under way to determine how much is missed by a single wide angle view centred on the disc. Certainly, dilatation of the pupil improves diagnosis even with so-called 'non-mydriatic' cameras. Early retinopathy is most common just lateral to the macula, which must be included in any assessment.

Small microaneurysms (saccular dilatations of capillaries) are the earliest signs of retinopathy and are found surrounding areas of non-perfusion. Fluorescein angiography detects not only clinically invisible areas of capillary non-perfusion (later seen as cotton wool spots on ophthalmoscopy) and leakage, but also smaller microaneurysms than are detectable by ophthalmoscopy or colour photography (12 μm and above, versus 35 μm and above). Similarly, fluorescein angiography will detect dilatation of capillaries not visible by other means until leakage from the dilated vessels has produced hard exudates (usually temporarily). Fluorescein angiography can detect retinopathy earlier than other means, but these early changes are unlikely in themselves to threaten vision, and angiography is generally used as a prelude to laser therapy rather than as a screening technique.

Vitreous fluorophotometry, in which fluorescein light-sensitive probes are used to detect leakage of fluorescein into the vitreous, was initially thought to identify a very early stage of incipient retinopathy [36]. With more sophisticated equipment, it has not proved possible reliably to distinguish diabetes with pathology from non-diabetics [37].

Detection of early 'background' retinopathy is useful, but about a third of patients with IDDM never progress beyond it [38]. Nevertheless, its detection is important and it is in those patients with early changes that preventive measures should be attempted. Furthermore, in long-standing diabetes, maculopathy may accompany background retinopathy without proliferative changes. Maculopathy is best detected by declining visual acuity – pupils should not be dilated for retinal inspection until this simple test has been performed. In NIDDM, retinopathy can progress rapidly, and may be present at diagnosis. However, in statistical terms, proliferative retinopathy is less common. Occurring in only 20%–40% of patients [39], it is none the less important because of the much greater number of patients who have NIDDM.

The appearances of pre-proliferative retinopathy include more than five cotton wool spots in a single eye; cluster and blot hae-morrhages; venous beading, looping and reduplication; intra-retinal microvascular abnormalities; blood vessel sheathing and occlusion; and loss of striation of the retina (atrophy). New vessel formation, the hall-mark of proliferative retinopathy, is best treated before bleeding and later traction have impaired visual function. It should be noted that there is considerable evidence to suggest that retinopathy is more likely to occur in long-term poorly controlled diabetes [40–42], and that although the institution of improved glycaemic control may produce initial deterioration in retinal appearances, the long-term benefit of improved control may be real [43,44]. Pre-proliferative and proliferative retinopathy should be stabilized with laser therapy before any major im-provement in control is attempted.

Assessment of diabetic neuropathy

Damage to the nervous system may com-plicate all forms of diabetes mellitus, regard-less of aetiology [45]. Classically, the term diabetic neuropathy is used to describe the syndromes due to damaged peripheral and autonomic nerves, although it seems un-likely that the brain alone is immune from the disease process. A spectrum of neuro-pathies is seen in diabetes mellitus, differ-entiated by clinical, electrophysiological or histopathological criteria, but often a mixed picture will be found in any individual patient.

Sensory neuropathy presents with dys-aesthesia of the hands and feet. It predisposes to foot ulceration, to which the anhydrosis of autonomic neuropathy may contribute. Motor neuropathies include focal lesions involving only isolated nerves. These may be transient (most commonly involving cranial nerves, especially the sixth) or multiple (mononeuritis multiplex) or may reflect the increased susceptibility of diabetic nerves to trauma, carpal tunnel syndrome and ulnar nerve and lateral popliteal nerve lesions all being more common in diabetes. Diabetic amyotrophy is a generalized painful pro-ximal myopathy, associated with systemic illness, wasting and fasciculation of the affected proximal muscles, and weight loss [46]. An often unrecognized variant is truncal neuropathy, which may clinically resemble herpetic neuralgia [47]. Autonomic neuro-pathy may present with postural hypoten-sion; persistent or intermittent diarrhoea (especially nocturnal), often alternating with constipation; bladder dysfunction; erectile impotence; and abnormalities of sweating (decreased sweating in lower limbs with compensatory increased sweating in the upper part of the body), akin to the effects of lumbar sympathectomy [48], night sweats or gustatory sweating probably due to dis-organized regeneration of damaged nerves [49].

Initial diagnosis is by physical examina-tion. Sensory neuropathy produces a loss of pinprick, touch, temperature and vibration perception initially at the feet and spreading progressively proximally. The hands will be involved as the level of damage in the legs is detectable at mid-thigh level, because the presentation depends upon the length of the nerves involved. Reduced or absent reflex jerks must be interpreted with caution in older patients – they are lost in 25% of healthy individuals over 60! Motor neuro-pathy presents as localized or proximal muscle weakness and autonomic neuropathy may be reflected by resting tachycardias, a drop in systolic blood pressure in excess of 15 mmHg, measured immediately or within 5 minutes of standing from the supine posi-tion. This postural drop in blood pressure will be markedly exacerbated by dehydration and may occur in response to insulin injec-tion, when it may be confused with hypo-glycaemia. Other causes of neuropathy –

vitamin B12 deficiency, syphilis, alcoholism, uraemia and porphyria – should be excluded.

Laboratory tests of nerve function

Electrophysiology: the electromyogram (EMG) may differentiate neuropathy from myopathy, although both may occur in diabetes [50]. Test electrodes in the muscles record spontaneous activity in resting muscle, motor unit activity during minimal activity and recruitment and interference patterns during increasing effort. Denervated muscle shows spontaneous fibrillation potentials with large motor unit potentials, reduced recruitment and interference due to the loss of functioning motor units.

Nerve conduction studies measure conduction velocity and amplitude, primarily features of large myelinated fibre activity, which may be normal in the small fibre damage associated with painful diabetic neuropathy [51]. However, nerve conduction is slowed in diabetes [52]. Abnormalities at diagnosis probably reflect the high ambient glucose at the time of testing [53]. There is rather poor correlation between abnormal conduction studies and the clinical severity of the disease. The most useful diagnostic test may be conduction in the lateral popliteal nerve [53], and the resistance of the diabetic nerve to ischaemia during testing [54] is useful, although this is also seen in uraemia. Conduction studies are useful to confirm a diagnosis of carpal tunnel syndrome or ulnar nerve damage.

Nerve biopsy shows demyelination and remyelination in asymptomatic patients while fibre loss and demyelination are seen in patients with symptoms [55]. The pathogenesis of the neuropathy is multiple, with ischaemic injury segmental demyelination and abnormalities of axonal transport, potential generation and nodal membranes. Diabetic peripheral nerves have a high sorbitol content, consequent upon excessive glucose entry into the glucose-6-phosphate pathway and synthesis of the sorbitol by aldose reductase. This is associated with low levels of inositol, which may be causally related. Inositol is an integral part of phospholipid metabolism, diacylglycerol formation and therefore activation of protein kinase c and of membrane sodium potassium ATPase.

Peripheral nerve function tests: patient cooperation and observer bias are major problems in reliable quantification of diabetic neuropathy [56]. Computer assisted devices for the assessment of sensory perception thresholds are described [57]. Biosthesiometry, to measure detection thresholds for vibration sensation, has long been used clinically, but its poor reproducibility is well documented [58]. Thermal perception thresholds test the integrity of small fibres and, although really a sensory test, therefore correlate well with autonomic damage [59].

Autonomic nerve function tests: the best documented tests of autonomic function centre around tests of cardiovascular innervation as described and validated by Ewing and Clarke [60]. Resting tachycardia, loss of sinus arrythmia and loss of the reflex tachycardia and rebound bradycardia during a Valsalva manoeuvre describe sympathetic function. Loss of sinus arrythmia is best seen as a variation of less than 10 beats per minute (between 10 and 15 is borderline) during regular deep breathing at a rate of 6 breaths per minute, best timed by an oscillator. The maximum and minimum heart rates from each respiratory cycle are calculated by the gap between R waves on the ECG, either manually or by computer. It is the response to the first breath that shows the greatest variation [60,61]. The Valsalva manoeuvre calculates the difference between maximum and minimum R to R interval during three forced expirations in which the subject attempts to blow an anaeroid manometer to 40 mmHg for 20 seconds. The ratio should be more than 1.21, with less than 1.1 as frankly abnormal. Diastolic blood pressure, measured at intervals of 1 minute before and during 5 minutes of sustained gripping of a dynamometer to 30% of the subject's own maximal effort, should rise by more than 16 mmHg, and a rise of less than 10 mmHg is frankly abnormal. Finally, the reflex tachycardia and overshoot bradycardia that occur on standing after a period of lying supine are measured as the ratio between the R–R interval at the 30th beat to the 15th beat on the ECG taken during the procedure. Less than 1 is frankly abnormal, less than 1.04 may be. A postural fall in blood pressure of more than 30 mmHg is grossly abnormal and suggests parasympathetic damage. Anything more than 10 mmHg is suspicious. This test should be conducted very carefully. The patient should be supine for 20 minutes before standing and blood pressure recorded, preferably by a random zero sphygmomanometer, at intervals of 1 minute, before and for at least 5 minutes after standing.

Other signs of cardiovascular denervation, not in general diagnostic use but reflective of potentially lethal pathology, include the number of changes in heart rate during 24-hour monitoring, standing to lying changes in heart rate and blood pressure, heart rate response to cough, cold pressor testing (immersion of one hand into iced water) and measurement of QT prolongation. Pupil size may be reduced and speed of response to changes in light intensity [62] or pharmacological stimulation occur in diabetes [63], and the size of the pupil in the dark has been suggested as an indicator of autonomic dysfunction. Polaroid photography [64] or infrared photography [65] can be used to measure the pupil responses. Infective, inflammatory and allergic causes of diarrhoea must be sought in diabetics presenting with diarrhoea. Measurement of gastric impedance [66] and gastric emptying time measured by following the disposal of a radiolabelled test meal may help diagnose gut involvement in autonomic neuropathy.

Tests of bladder dysfunction include cystometry, sphincter EMG, urethral flow patterns, urethral manometry and electrophysiology [67]. These invasive tests are for the specialist centres, and useful clinical clues are obtained from ultrasound measurement of residual volumes and conventional radiography [68]. A neuropathic basis for impotence is suggested by the finding of abnormal thermal detection thresholds in the feet, denoting small fibre damage. A good response to intracavernosal papaverine is useful in diagnosis, as well as being a form of treatment [69].

Old tests of sudomotor function measured responses to thermal, electrical or pharmacological stimuli, but chemical indicators of sweating (starch and iodine, for example) are not quantitative and are very messy [70]. Galvanic skin responses where a potential can only be conducted in the presence of moisture of the skin is cleaner and correlates well with small fibre dysfunction, but poorly with tests of cardiovascular denervation. Changes in humidity after stimulation of sweating induced by acetylcholine [71] and the sweat imprint in a silastic mould after pilocarpine [72] are claimed to give quantitative assessments. For clinical use, a rather neat method using starch powder on the feet has recently been described [73].

Some authorities suggest that the conditions under which autonomic neuropathy is tested are important [74]. Ewing, however, states that if the patients are comfortable, other features (fasting or not, for example) are not major determinants of the response to tests [75,76]. Age and sex may influence results. In non-diabetics, female sex and increasing age are related to slower nerve conduction, but in diabetics, duration of diabetes alone correlated with slowing of conduction velocity [77]. Nevertheless, tables of normal values adjusted for age and sex do show variation in results of the tests described above. Despite the wide range of tests available, in clinical practice, most use will be made of the simple cardiovascular tests, abnormalities of which correlate well with the symptoms of autonomic neuropathy and may highlight an increased risk of sudden death or progressive disability.

The diabetic foot

Foot ulceration in diabetes has many causes. Neuropathy can be sought as described above. Arterial disease may well underlie ulceration and it is an important distinction because (i) a foot with easily palpable pulses is almost certainly retrievable even in the presence of quite gross ulceration and infection, (ii) a local operation to relieve an obstructed arterial supply to an infected foot may allow the healing of the foot and avoid amputation, and (iii) compression bandaging may help to heal ulceration secondary to venous stasis and varicose oedema but will not benefit a foot ischaemic because of arterial pathology. Measurement of pedal blood pressure and the pedal to brachial pressure ratio (which should be over 1) using a sphygmomanometer and a Doppler probe, Doppler angiography and ultimately radiographic angiography are all useful diagnostic tests.

Ischaemic heart disease and early atheroma

Atheroma occurs prematurely in diabetic patients. Hyperinsulinism has been blamed but this remains contentious. Research into the underlying pathology continues but meanwhile clinical examination for carotid, femoral, abdominal and renal bruits with ultrasonic imaging should be used to identify problems in individual patients. Invasive angiography for investigation and treatment of poor perfusion can often help the healing of an ischaemic foot lesion and prevent amputation. Recently it has been suggested that asymptomatic ischaemic heart disease should be sought actively in patients with diabetes, with exercise ECG testing or ambulatory cardiac monitoring, especially if an active exercise programme is to be advised. In NIDDM microalbuminuria (q.v.) suggests especially high risk.

Bone changes in diabetes mellitus

In the early 1970s several reports were published suggesting that diabetes was found twice as commonly in patients with osteopaenic fractures as in the general population. This led to the impression that diabetes mellitus might be associated with osteoporosis, although later studies failed to demonstrate the reverse association – increased incidence of osteopaenic fractures in diabetic populations. Nevertheless, the evidence to date, neatly summarized by McNair [78], does suggest that there is an increased bone loss in insulin dependent diabetic patients. The phenomenon is associated with low ionized calcium, relatively high phosphate and low magnesium, parathyroid hormone and 1,25 vitamin D. Urine excretion of calcium and magnesium may be high. The explanation of the bone loss remains to be elucidated but probably relates to glycaemic control [79] rather than to microangiopathy, since it can be demonstrated early (McNair, indeed, suggests that bone mass stabilizes after 5 years [78]) and is not related to retinal changes or albuminuria.

Bone demineralization probably does occur to an exaggerated degree in insulin dependent diabetes and increased bone density in non-insulin dependent people probably relates to their obesity. New techniques of measuring bone mass may help to elucidate further the importance of these phenomena and perhaps to determine causal relationships, but at present there is no indication for routine measurement of bone mass in diabetic patients.

10.1.6 SCREENING PEOPLE WITH DIABETES MELLITUS

The aims of diabetes treatment are threefold. The first is to control blood glucose in the short term so as to remove symptoms and allow the patient to pursue an active lifestyle. High blood glucose levels are associated with disturbed nights, dehydration, weight loss, lethargy and impaired defences against infection, and, in IDDM, ketosis. The second aim of diabetes therapy is to prevent the development of diabetic complications. The evidence suggests that good glycaemic control will be beneficial in this respect, but the case is far from proved and the risks of intensified therapy still not fully appreciated. Prevention of diabetic complications, therefore, also entails the detection and removal of additional risk factors such as smoking, hypertension and hyperlipidaemia. And, finally, if complications cannot be avoided, early detection may allow treatment before they have caused significant morbidity. Thus, 70% of blindness from retinopathy is preventable by laser therapy, provided such therapy is instituted before the retinopathy itself has caused visual impairment. Neuropathic foot ulcers, developing unnoticed from minor injuries and infections in insensitive feet, can be cured with aggressive antibiotic therapy and prevented by measures such as protective footwear, professional chiropody, treatment of interdigital fungal infection with surgical spirit and antifungal creams, treatment of dry and cracking skin with emollient creams and removal of oedema fluid. Even arteriopathic ulcers can heal after angioplasty and varicose ulceration can be helped by suitable diuretic therapy and support hose. Such measure can avoid the tragedy of amputation. Current work suggests that renal disease may be reversed, or at least retarded, by dietic manipulation and the aggressive treatment of even mild hypertension, if detected early enough.

Annual screening of diabetic patients for risk factors and for early complications is thus a very worthwhile exercise. Although there is no agreement as to how frequent such screening should be (estimates range from annually to 5-yearly), current recommendations are that screening should be considered at least annually for all diabetics post puberty and/or with more than 5 years duration of disease. For NIDDM, where patients often present late, such screening should be instituted from diagnosis. Frequency of monitoring, if early complications are detected, depends upon the nature of the problem.

A screen for risk factors must include:

Estimate of glycaemic control (HbA1c)

Fasting lipids: cholesterol, HDL cholesterol, LDL cholesterol, triglyceride

Urinalysis for albuminuria

Erect and supine blood pressure

Assessment of peripheral nerve function

Assessment of peripheral circulation, including pedal pulses, blood pressures if indicated and carotid inspection

Assessment of state of skin of feet

Visual acuity

Inspection of optic lenses

Inspection for retinopathy through dilated pupils

Consider need for assessment of thyroid function.

10.1.7 SCREENING FOR DIABETES MELLITUS

Screening populations for diabetes mellitus may not be practicable, given a national incidence of approximately 1.2%. Certain high risk populations would, however, benefit from screening, and probably the most reliable screening test is the fasting 2-hour post-prandial glucose, although testing for glycosuria is simple and cheap. Pregnant women should certainly be screened with blood tests because of the risks to the foetus of undiagnosed diabetes even quite late in pregnancy. Women with gestational diabetes should be screened postpartum and dietary advice given to those with normal glucose tolerance but obesity, and all should be warned of the risk of obesity in later life.

10.2 HYPOGLYCAEMIA

10.2.1 INTRODUCTION

Under normal conditions of feeding, fasting and exercise arterial blood glucose levels are maintained within narrow limits. This is due mainly to the ability of the liver to absorb carbohydrate after meals, and to secrete glucose at other times at rates precisely matched to peripheral glucose uptake. This function is regulated by portal insulin delivery, modified in important respects by the hepatic and/or peripheral effects of other hormones such as glucagon, adrenalin and cortisol.

The central nervous system is, under normal circumstances, almost entirely dependent upon circulating glucose levels for its energy needs. These are high because of the need to generate ATP to maintain the electrical potential across nerve membranes, and it has been estimated that in a 70 kg man the brain normally consumes some 50% of the total glucose production by the liver, equivalent to 100–120 g per day [80].

Although the term is widely used in the clinical sense, it is helpful to reserve the term 'hypoglycaemia' for the biochemical abnormality – defined as a statistical deviation below the normal range – and to refer to the clinical syndrome that results as 'neuroglycopenia' [80]. Neuroglycopenia is among the most intensively studied of all physiologi-

cal responses, and as a result considerable effort has been expended in the attempt to equate symptoms and neuroendocrine responses with plasma glucose levels.

Physiology and pathophysiology

Introduction of the slow-fall hypoglycaemic clamp technique has confirmed that responses to hypoglycaemia are not unitary ('all or none') but sequential. It has also confirmed the clinical impression that non-diabetic individuals show remarkable uniformity of response, whereas responses in patients with recurrent neuroglycopenia are much more heterogeneous.

In healthy subjects neuropsychological performance deteriorates at plasma glucose levels of 3.0–3.6 mmol l^{-1} [81], and small increments in counter-regulatory hormones have been detected at slightly higher glucose levels. Subjective perception of hypoglycemia develops at around 2.7–2.9 mmol l^{-1}, and unequivocal EEG changes at about 2 mmol l^{-1} or below [82]. Patients exposed to recurrent hypoglycaemia (whether due to intensively treated diabetes or insulinoma) have a lowered threshold for symptom perception but, paradoxically, develop EEG changes earlier than non-diabetic controls [83]. Conversely, patients with poorly controlled diabetes experience symptoms at higher plasma glucose levels, extending well into the range of normoglycaemia [84].

10.2.2 CLINICAL PRESENTATION

In common usage symptoms are categorized as *adrenergic* (ignoring the fact that sweating is cholinergic) or *neuroglycopenic*, but we believe it is more comprehensible and correct to speak of *peripheral* and *central* manifestations of neuroglycopenia [85]. It is then possible to follow Marks and Rose [80] in recognizing three clinical syndromes: *acute*, *subacute* and *chronic* neuroglycopenia. Subacute and chronic neuroglycopenia are the result of failure of early warning autonomic responses to a falling blood glucose and may occur as a result of preceding experience of hypoglycaemia. The results do not necessarily imply a different duration of the particular episode.

Acute neuroglycopenia

Early symptoms include lassitude, light headedness or a feeling of unease. A pricking sensation in the skin precedes a cold sweat, and tremor develops, together with mild tachycardia and awareness of a forceful heart beat. Sounds are heard as from a distance and the eyes become unfocused. The sense of time is impaired, so that it seems to pass more quickly. Patients often feel passive, detached and sleepy, but prolonged hypoglycaemia becomes progressively more unpleasant, with restlessness, irritability and a drained sensation. Treatment with glucose leads to shivering as the hypothermia of hypoglycaemia is reversed, and recovery may be followed by an occipital or frontal headache.

Subacute neuroglycopenia

The warning symptoms described above may be absent or may not be noticed because of the central consequences of glucose deficiency. Movement and thought are slow, and spontaneous activity is reduced to a minimum. Friends or relatives can often spot the change before the patient does. A form of automatism may develop and has important medico-legal consequences; if disturbed, the patient may become confused, manic or occasionally violent. Further manifestations are almost endlessly variable, and include a variety of focal neurological disorders, of which reversible hemiplegia is the most dramatic. Depending upon the circumstances, patients may recover spon-

taneously from such episodes or progress to coma, sometimes leading to convulsions.

Chronic neuroglycopenia

Some authorities describe changes in personality, the mental changes of dementia or even psychotic behaviour as a syndrome occurring in patients with chronic recurrent hypoglycaemia which although not reversible acutely by restoring normoglycaemia may be relieved by removal of the cause of the recurrent hypoglycaemic episodes (e.g. removal of insulinoma).

The classification of hypoglycaemia can be approached in three stages:

1. *Clinical presentation*; from the history, it should be clear whether the patient has *fasting* or *reactive* hypoglycaemia. Fasting hypoglycaemia, if confirmed, always has an organic basis.
2. *Mechanism*; in the steady state, the amount of glucose secreted by the liver is equal to the amount taken up by the periphery. Hypoglycaemia may result from one – or more often from a combination – of the following mechanisms:
   (a) Excessive or inappropriate action of insulin or insulin-like molecules. Hepatic glucose production is inhibited despite adequate glycogen stores (which can be mobilized by injection of glucagon), while peripheral uptake is enhanced.
   (b) An impaired neuroendocrine response, with an inadequate counter-regulatory response to insulin action.
   (c) Structural damage to the liver, or abnormality of liver enzyme systems involved in glycogenolysis or gluconeogenesis, with resulting failure of hepatic glucose production.
   (d) Inadequate hepatic glucose production because of a failure to mobilize the substrates needed for gluconeo-

Table 10.4 Causes of hypoglycaemia

Type	Cause
Insulinomas	Benign (85%)
	Malignant (15%)
	Pluriglandular syndrome (MEN1)
Other tumours	Mesenchymal tumours
	Primary hepatic carcinoma
	Adrenal carcinoma
	Carcinoids
Endocrine	Pituitary insufficiency
	Isolated ACTH deficiency
	Addison's disease
	Hypothyroidism
Autoimmune	Autoimmune insulin syndrome
Hepatic/renal causes	Hepatocellular disease
	Congestive liver disease
	End-stage renal failure
Postprandial	Idiopathic
	Alcohol-induced
	Late dumping
Drug-induced	Insulin
	Sulphonylureas
	Alcohol
	Quinine
	Salicylates
Miscellaneous	Starvation
	Prolonged exercise
	Septicaemia
	Factitious hypoglycaemia

genesis. The most important of these 3-carbon molecules are lactate, pyruvate, certain amino acids and glycerol.

3. *Cause*; an aetiological classification is given in Table 10.4.

General considerations

Although there are many potential causes of hypoglycaemia, few of these pose any diagnostic difficulty. Hypoglycaemia is a late manifestation of non-islet cell tumours, usually those secreting insulin-like growth factors, at a stage when the growth is large

and clinically obvious. Severe liver, kidney or heart disease, septicaemia and alcohol abuse are equally self-evident. Drug-induced hypoglycaemia is usually easy to identify from the history, although in one recent report investigations for an insulinoma were begun before it was realized that a pharmacist had accidentally substituted Diabenese (chlorpropamide) for Diamox (acetazolamide), which stood next to it on the shelf [86].

In the otherwise healthy patient, the main problem is to establish whether Whipple's triad is present. Once this has been confirmed the likely diagnosis is insulinoma, although factitious hypoglycaemia and occasional rarities like isolated adrenocorticotropic hormone (ACTH) deficiency still need to be borne in mind.

10.2.3 INSULINOMA

Clinical presentation

Diagnosis is often delayed, sometimes for years, from appearance of the first symptoms. This is partly because early symptoms may be intermittent, with long trouble-free periods in between, and partly because of delay in suspecting the diagnosis. About 50% of patients are first seen by a neurologist or a psychiatrist. Analysis of symptoms in a large series showed that 85% had symptoms of acute neuroglycopenia, with visual manifestations (diplopia and visual blurring) prominent among these. Some 80% had occasional abnormal or bizarre behaviour, and half had experienced hypoglycaemic coma or amnesia. Fits were the presenting feature in 12% of patients [87]. The timing of attacks must be carefully elicited. The great majority occur in the overnight fasted state, but the first symptoms sometimes occur later in the day, and can be precipitated by exercise, alcohol or religious fasts.

As this section will demonstrate, insulinoma is relatively straightforward to diagnose. The main problem is that most people referred for investigation of insulinoma turn out not to have one! There may be a temptation to multiply investigations with a diminishingly small return in an attempt to appease the patient's demands for a firm diagnosis, but there is hardly ever a need to pursue investigation if a properly-conducted 72-hour fast fails to demonstrate Whipple's triad.

About 60% of insulinoma patients are female, with a mean age at diagnosis in the fifties. Presentation before the age of 20 is rare but 10% present over the age of 70. About 10% have the syndrome of multiple endocrine neoplasia (MEN) type 1, and these tend to present in their twenties. The most commonly associated endocrine tumours are of the parathyroid and pituitary. When MEN is present, about 80% of insulinomas are multiple.

The types of tumours in one large series were as follows:

single benign: 80%
multiple benign: 11%
single malignant: 6%.

The remaining 3% were accounted for by multiple malignant tumours and islet hyperplasia [88]. The median size for an insulinoma is 1.5 cm, and the distribution is even through the head and tail of the pancreas. Ectopic insulinomas are very rare indeed – considerably rarer than the number of patients with factitious hypoglycaemia in whom the diagnosis is suspected.

Investigations

The aims of investigation are to demonstrate Whipple's triad [89], to rule out other causes of hypoglycaemia, most notably self-induced (factitious) hypoglycaemia, and to localize the tumour(s) as accurately as possible prior to surgery. Whipple's triad remains the main-stay of diagnosis. This is satisfied when:

Symptoms are associated with fasting or exercise
Hypoglycaemia can be confirmed by a reliable method in conjunction with these symptoms
Symptoms are relieved by administration of glucose.

A fourth criterion – demonstration of inappropriately raised insulin levels during hypoglycaemia – could usefully be added to these.

Biochemical investigation

Fasting blood glucose levels

Procedure

The initial investigation is to obtain three fasting paired blood samples for glucose and insulin assay.

Interpretation

Demonstration of a blood glucose below $3 \, mmol \, l^{-1}$ with non-suppressed insulin levels is diagnostic of an insulinoma. Service and colleagues consider that an insulinoma is virtually certain when fasting hypoglycaemia is present in association with an insulin level about $10 \, uU \, l^{-1}$, and likely if the level does not suppress below $6 \, uU \, l^{-1}$ [90]. It should, however, be remembered that few hospital biochemistry laboratories run regular insulin assays, so that quality control may be less good than with more routine tests. Further, insulin assays, especially from kits, rarely perform well at the lower end of the range.

These cautions can be ignored if insulin levels are unequivocally elevated during hypoglycaemia, but may prove important in borderline cases.

Supervised prolonged fast

Procedure

If hypoglycaemia is not clearly demonstrated on a fasting sample, the next step is hospital admission for a supervised fast. This should always be performed on an endocrine ward with experienced staff. Patients are allowed non-calorie containing drinks, and should be as active as possible. Blood samples for glucose, insulin and (if possible) C-peptide, are taken 6 hourly. In addition to sending a laboratory sample for glucose measurement, the nurses should check the glucose reading with a reflectance meter at each time point, and should reduce the sampling frequency to 2 hourly if the level falls below $3 \, \text{mmol} \, l^{-1}$.

Interpretation

The results of blood tests done on the ward must not be communicated to the patient. It is not enough to demonstrate hypoglycaemia during a fast; neuroglycopenia must also be present. This is because blood glucose levels can fall below $2.6 \, \text{mmol} \, l^{-1}$ in healthy pre-menopausal women who fast for 36–72 hours, without symptoms [91], whereas men maintain higher glucose levels. As and when symptoms develop a doctor should be called. Symptoms and signs are carefully recorded, further blood samples are taken, and glucose administered. Textbooks suggest that an EEG should be recorded when symptoms develop and during glucose administration, but this counsel of perfection can rarely be achieved.

If no symptoms have developed within 48 hours, the fast should be prolonged to a maximum of 72 hours. In a series of 90 patients investigated at the Mayo Clinic, Whipple's triad was confirmed in 92% within 48 hours and in 98% within 72 hours [92].

Other useful investigations

The patient should have a full blood count, biochemical screen including liver function tests and calcium levels, cortisol and thyroxine measurement, and X-rays of the chest together with a lateral skull film to show the pituitary fossa.

C-peptide estimation

Autonomous insulin secretion can be demonstrated by measurement of C-peptide levels. C-peptide is secreted from the pancreatic beta cells on a molar basis with insulin, but is absent from commercial insulin preparations and thus provides an invaluable marker of endogenous insulin production.

Interpretation

If C-peptide levels rise in parallel with insulin during the supervised fast, exogenous insulin administration can be ruled out. Some patients have induced hypoglycaemia by surreptitious ingestion of sulphonylurea drugs (in which case C-peptide levels will rise), and this can be checked by chromatography of plasma or urine. It is traditional to send a serum sample for measurement of insulin antibodies, as a check on exogenous insulin administration, but this has little value if highly purified human insulin has been used.

The C-peptide suppression test

This may be useful when non-suppression of endogenous insulin secretion has not been demonstrated by other means. There is a small risk of precipitating severe hypoglycaemia during the procedure, and appropriate precautions are necessary.

Procedure

The patient should be in the post-absorptive or fasted state, and the plasma glucose should be greater than $3 \, \text{mmol} \, \text{l}^{-1}$ at the outset. To perform the test, insulin is infused at the rate of $0.1 \, \text{U} \, \text{kg}^{-1}$ for 60 minutes, and glucose and C-peptide are measured every 10 minutes; the test is stopped if symptoms of hypoglycaemia develop.

Interpretation

Healthy subjects suppress C-peptide to below $1.2 \, \text{ng} \, \text{ml}^{-1}$, whereas insulinoma patients almost invariably remain well above this level [90].

Proinsulin

Proinsulin measurement has been advocated in the diagnosis of insulinoma. Proinsulin is normally secreted by the beta cell at a ratio of one molecule for ten of insulin.

Interpretation

With insulinomas this ratio decreases, so that in 80% of patients proinsulin constitutes more than 20% of the total [93]. The potential value of the test is limited by unavailability of reliable proinsulin assays, and because limited clinical experience has been acquired in interpretation of the test.

Obsolete investigations

A wide variety of tests have found advocates at different times. Although the glucose tolerance test may be abnormal, and the incidence of gastric ulcer is increased, the OGTT and barium meal have no value as routine tests. The fish insulin or Turner–Harris suppression test could be considered as a predecessor of the C-peptide suppression test, and is based on the same principle.

Interpretation

Since fish insulin lowers plasma glucose without interfering with the radioimmuno-assay for human insulin, infusion of fish insulin allows non-suppression of endogenous insulin secretion during hypoglycaemia to be demonstrated.

The tolbutamide test is still used in some centres. Intravenous infusion of tolbutamide stimulates insulin secretion and thus lowers plasma glucose.

Interpretation

Patients with insulinomas produce more insulin, and do not suppress endogenous insulin secretion appropriately following the infusion. Glucose levels therefore remain lower and insulin levels higher in the insulinoma patient [92]. The test is potentially hazardous, and despite the clinical experience that has been acquired in its use it is generally considered obsolete. This judgement applies to a number of other tests of insulin secretion, including the leucine and glucagon stimulation tests [92].

Tumour localization

An experienced surgeon will be able to locate the great majority of insulinomas by palpation [94], but preoperative investigation increases the chance of success, allows multiple tumours to be spotted, and may help to avoid the disaster of closing the abdomen on a functioning islet tumour. Angiography has a reportedly high success rate if the techniques of stereoscopy, magnification and subtraction are used. Islet cell tumours show up as homogeneous, highly vascular and sharply delimited. Samples for insulin assay can be taken through the cannula used for injection of dye. Since insulin secretion from healthy islet tissue is suppressed, it is often possible to demonstrate a clear gradient leading away from the tumour bed [95]. The alternatives are ultrasound and computerized tomography (CT), which have the great advantage of being non-invasive.

Preoperative investigation

There is a traditional belief that plasma glucose levels will rise as soon as the insulinoma is removed, but the increase is variable and often delayed. If the location of the tumour is not obvious, sequential blood samples can be taken from the pancreatic vein and assayed for insulin using a rapid method which gives approximate results in some 50 minutes. There is little justification for 'blind' hemi-pancreatectomy if this expedient fails.

Successful resection of an insulinoma is well worth while. In one series of 95 patients, 54% of tumours were removed by enucleation and 38% by partial pancreatectomy. The overall cure rate was 84% [87].

Factitious hypoglycaemia

This bizarre and unexplained condition constitutes the main alternative diagnosis in patients in whom an insulinoma is suspected. The literature reports the triumphant unmasking of many ingenious deceivers, but a number have undoubtedly been subjected to fruitless and sometimes heroic surgery. Those responsible are generally too modest to report their experience! Unfortunately, the need for suspicion complicates investigation and is often resented, since it 'can lead to great unpopularity with the nursing and junior medical staff who may suspect the clinician of being unreasonable in view of the patient's obviously genuine illness' [80]. The C-peptide suppression test and drug screens for sulphonylureas should, however, identify patients who have managed to give themselves insulin or sulphonylureas in the course of a supervised fast.

Endocrine causes

Hypoglycaemia may occur in hypopituitarism, and is a prominent component of pituitary coma. Mild hypoglycaemia may occur with Addison's disease or hypothyroidism, but should cause little diagnostic difficulty.

Isolated ACTH deficiency may cause more problems, and is demonstrated by failure of ACTH and cortisol to rise during induced hypoglycaemia, with a preserved adrenocortical response to exogenous ACTH.

REFERENCES

1. WHO Study Group (1985) *Diabetes Mellitus*, Technical Report no. 727, World Health Organization, Geneva.
2. O'Sullivan, J.B. (1984) Subsequent morbidity among gestational diabetic women. In *Carbohydrate Metabolism in Pregnancy and the Newborn* (ed. H.W. Sutherland and J.M. Stowers), Churchill Livingstone, Edinburgh, p. 174.
3. O'Sullivan, J.B. (1982) Body weight and subsequent diabetes mellitus. *J. Am. Med. Ass.*, **248**, 949.
4. Goldfine, I.D., Kahn, C.R., Roth, J. *et al.* (1973) *Biochem. Biophys. Res. Comm.*, **53**, 852.
5. Kahn, C.R., Megyesi, K., Bar, R.S. *et al.* (1977) *Ann. Intern. Med.*, **86**, 205.
6. American Diabetes Association (1987) A consensus statement on self-monitoring of blood glucose. *Diabetes Care*, **10**, 95–9.
7. Bergman, M., Migake, C. and Felig, P. (1989) Misdiagnosis of gestational diabetes and hypoglycemia using portable blood glucose meters. *Archs Intern. Med.*, **149**, 2602–3.
8. Weiner, C.P., Faustick, M.W., Burns, J., Fraser, M., Whitaker, L. and Klugman, M. (1987) Diagnosis of gestational diabetes by capillary blood samples and a portable reflectance meter. Derivation of threshold values and prospective validation. *Am. J. Obstet. Gynec.*, **156**, 1085–9.
9. MacDonald, A.W., Fisher, G.F. and Burnham, C.B. (1965) Reproducibility of the oral glucose tolerance test. *Diabetes*, **14**, 473–80.
10. Hatem, M., Anthony, F., Hogston, P., Rowe, D.J.F. and Dennis, K.J. (1988) Reference values for 75 gm oral glucose tolerance test in pregnancy. *Br. Med. J.*, **296**, 676–8.
11. O'Sullivan, J.B. and Mahan, C.M. (1964)

Criteria for the oral glucose tolerance test in pregnancy. *Diabetes*, **13**, 278.

12. Carpenter, M.W. and Coustan, D.R. (1982) Criteria for screening tests for gestational diabetes. *Am. J. Obstet. Gynec.*, **768**, 144.

13. Weiner, C.P. (1988) Effect of varying degrees of 'normal' glucose metabolism on maternal and perinatal outcome. *Am. J. Obstet. Gynec.*, **159**, 862–70.

14. Weiner, C.P. (1989) Screening for gestational diabetes. *Am. J. Obstet. Gynec.*, **161**, 1423–4.

15. Palmer, J.P. and McCulloch, D.K. (1991) Prediction and prevention of IDDM – 1991. *Diabetes*, **40**, 943–7.

16. Harrison, L.C. (1992) Islet cell antigens in insulin-dependent diabetes: Pandora's box revisited. *Immunol. Today*, **13**, 348–52.

17. Baekkeskov, S., Aanstoot, H.J., Christgau, S., Reetz, A., Solimena, M., Cascalho, M., Folli, F., Richler-Olesen, H. and de Camilli, P. (1990) Identification of the 64K autoantigen in insulin-dependent diabetes as the GABA-synthesising enzyme glutamic acid decarboxylase. *Nature*, **347**, 151–6.

18. Boitard, C., Bonifacio, E., Bottazzo, G.F., Gleichmann, H. and Molenaar, J. (1988) Immunology and diabetes workshop: Report on the Third International (Stage III) Workshop on the standardisation of cytoplasmic islet cell antibodies. *Diabetologia*, **31**, 451–5.

19. Bingley, P.J., Bonifacio, E. and Gale, E.A.M. (1993) Can we really predict IDDM? *Diabetes*, **42**, 213–20.

20. Van Dieijen-Visser, M.P., Seynaeve, C. and Brombacher, P.J. (1986) Influence of variations in albumin or total protein concentration on serum fructosamine concentration. *Clin. Chem.*, **32**, 1610.

21. McCance, D.R., Coulter, D., Smye, M. and Kennedy, L. (1987) Effect of fluctuations in albumin on serum fructosamine assay. *Diabetic Med.*, **4**, 434–6.

22. Fluckiger, R., Woodtli, T. and Berger, W. (1987) Evaluation of the fructosamine test for measurement of plasma protein glycation. *Diabetologia*, **30**, 648–52.

23. Baker, J.R., Metcalf, P.A. and Scott, D.J. (1984) Serum fructosamine concentrations in patients with Type II (noninsulin dependent) diabetes mellitus during changes in treatment.

Br. Med. J., **288**, 1484–6.

24. John, W.G. and Jones, A.E. (1985) Affinity chromatography: a precise method for glycosylated albumin estimation. *Ann. Clin. Biochem.*, **22**, 79–83.

25. Keen, H. and Chlouverakis, A. (1963) An immunoassay for urinary albumin at low concentrations. *Lancet*, **ii**, 913–36.

26. Viberti, G.C., Hill, R.D. and Jarrett, R.J. (1982) Microalbuminuria as a predictor of clinical nephropathy in insulin-dependent diabetes mellitus. *Lancet*, **i**, 1430–2.

27. Close, C.F., Scott, G., Keen, H. and Viberti, G.C. (1986) Bedside estimation of microalbuminuria. *Lancet*, **i**, 268–9.

28. Gatling, W., Knight, C. and Hill, R.D. (1985) Screening for early diabetic nephropathy: which sample to detect microalbuminuria. *Diabetic Med.*, **2**, 451–5.

29. Mogensen, C.E. (1976) Progression of nephropathy in long term diabetics with proteinuria and effect of initial antihypertensive treatment. *Scand. J. Clin. Lab. Invest.*, **36**, 383–8.

30. Jones, R.H., Hayakawa, H., MacKay, J.D., Parsons, V. and Watkins, P.J. (1979) Progression of diabetic nephropathy. *Lancet*, **i**, 1105–6.

31. Mogensen, C.E. (1982) Long term antihypertensive treatment inhibits progression of diabetic nephropathy. *Br. Med. J.*, **285**, 685–8.

32. Sorsby, A. (1972) The incidence and causes of blindness in England and Wales (1963–1968). *Reports on Public Health and Medical Subjects*, **28**, 33–51.

33. Foulds, W.S., McCuish, A., Barrie, T., Green, F., Scobie, I.N., Ghafour, I.M., McClure, E. and Barber, J.H. (1983) Diabetic retinopathy in the west of Scotland. Its detection and prevalence and the cost effectiveness of a proposed screening programme. *Health Bull. Edinburgh*, **41**, 318–26.

34. Kohner, E.M. (1984) Photocoagulation in the prevention of blindness and due to diabetic retinopathy: A review. *J. R. Soc. Med.*, **77**, 227–33.

35. Kohner, E.M. and Dollery, C.T. (1970) Fluorescein appearances in diabetic retinopathy. *Br. Med. Bull.*, **26**, 166–8.

36. Cunha-Vaz, J.G., Gray, J.R., Zeimer, R.C. *et al.* (1985) Characterisation of early stages of

diabetic retinopathy by vitreous fluorophoto-metry. *Diabetes*, **34**, 53–6.

37. Chahal, P., Fallon, T.J., Jennings, S.J. *et al.* (1986) Vitreons fluorophotometry in patients with no or minimal diabetic retinopathy. *Diabetes Care*, **9**, 134–9.

38. Klein, R., Klein, B.E., Moss, S.E. *et al.* (1984) The Wisconsin epidemiological study of diabetic retinopathy II. *Archs Ophthalmol.*, **102**, 520–6.

39. Klein, R., Klein, B.E., Moss, S.E. *et al.* (1984) The Wisconsin epidemiological study of diabetic retinopathy III. *Archs Ophthalmol.*, **102**, 527–32.

40. Pirart, J. (1978) Diabetes mellitus and its degenerative complications: a prospective study of 4400 patients observed between 1947 and 1973. *Diabetes Care*, **1**, 168-88.

41. Deckert, T., Poulsen, J.E. and Larson, M. (1978) Prognosis of diabetes with diabetic onset before the age of 31. *Diabetologia*, **14**, 371–7.

42. McCance, D.R., Atkinson, A.B., Hadden, D.R., Archer, D.B. and Kennedy, L. (1989) Long-term diabetic control and diabetic retinopathy. *Lancet*, **ii**, 824–6.

43. The Steno Study Group (1985) Two-year experience with continuous subcutaneous insulin in relation to retinopathy and nephropathy. *Diabetes*, **34**, Suppl. 3, 74.

44. The Kroc Collaborative Study Group (1985) The Kroc Study patients at two years: A report on further retinal changes. *Diabetes*, **34**, Suppl. 1, 39A.

45. Galton, D.J. (1965) Diabetic neuropathy and haemochromatosis. *Br. Med. J.*, **i**, 1169.

46. Chokroverty, S., Reyes, M.G., Rubino, F.A. and Tonaki, H. (1977) The syndrome of diabetic amyotrophy. *Ann. Neurol.*, **2**, 181–94.

47. Kikta, D.G., Breuer, A.C. and Wilbourn, A.J. (1982) Thoracic root pain in diabetes: The spectrum of clinical and electromyographic findings. *Ann. Neurol.*, **11**, 80–5.

48. Odel, H.M., Roth, G.M., Keating, F.R. and Autono, I.C. (1955) Neuropathy stimulating the effects of sympathectomy as a complication of diabetes mellitus. *Diabetes*, **4**, 92–8.

49. Watkins, P.J. (1973) Facial sweating after food: A new sign of diabetic autonomic neuropathy. *Br. Med. J.*, **i**, 583–7.

50. Lamontagne, A. and Buchthal, F. (1970) Electrophysiological studies in diabetic neuropathy. *J. Neurol. Neurosurg. Psychiat.*, **33**, 442–52.

51. Archer, A.G., Watkins, P.J., Thomas, P.K., Sharma, A.K. and Payan, J. (1983) The natural history of acute painful neuropathy in diabetes mellitus. *Archs Neurol.*, **46**, 491–9.

52. Lawrence, D.G. and Locke, S. (1961) Motor nerve conduction velocity in diabetes. *Archs Neurol.*, **5**, 37–42.

53. Fraser, D.M., Campbell, I.W., Ewing, D.J., Murray, A. and Nielson, J.M.M. (1977) Peripheral and autonomic nerve function in newly diagnosed diabetes mellitus. *Diabetes*, **26**, 546–50.

54. Gregersen, G. (1968) A study of the peripheral nerves in diabetic subjects during ischaemia. *J. Neurol. Neurosurg. Psychiat.*, **31**, 175–81.

55. Thomas, P.K. and Eliasson, S.G. (1984) Diabetic neuropathy. In *Peripheral Neuropathy* (ed. P.J. Dyke, P.K. Thomas, E.H. Lambert and R. Bunge), W.B. Saunders, Philadelphia, pp. 1773–810.

56. Dyke, P.J., O'Brien, P.C., Bushek, W., Oviatt, K.F., Schilling, K. and Stevens, J.C. (1976) Clinical versus quantitative evaluation of cutaneous sensation. *Archs Neurol.*, **33**, 651–5.

57. Dyke, P.J., Karnes, J., O'Brien, P.C. and Zimmerman, I.R. (1984) Detection thresholds for cutaneous sensation in humans. In *Peripheral Neuropathy* (ed. P.J. Dyke, P.K. Thomas, E.H. Lambert and R. Bunge), W.B. Saunders, Philadelphia, pp. 1102–38.

58. Williams, G., Gill, J.S., Aber, V. and Mather, H.M. (1982) Variability in vibration perception threshold among sites. *Br. Med. J.*, **285**, 916–18.

59. Fowler, C.J., Carrol, M.B., Burns, D., Howe, N. and Robinson, K. (1987) A portable system for measuring cutaneous thresholds for warming and cooling. *J. Neurol. Neurosurg. Psychiat.*, **509**, 1211–15.

60. Ewing, D.J. and Clarke, B.F. (1982) Diagnosis and management of diabetic autonomic neuropathy. *Br. Med. J.*, **285**, 916–18.

61. Smith, S. (1982) Reduced sinus arrhythmias in diabetic autonomic neuropathy; diagnostic value of an age related normal range. *Br. Med. J.*, **285**, 1599–601.

62. Martyn, C.N. and Ewing, D.J. (1986) Pupil cycle time; a simple way of measuring an autonomic reflex. *J. Neurol. Neurosurg. Psychiat.*, **49**, 771–4.

63. Smith, S.A. (1988) Pupillary function in autonomic failure. In *Autonomic Failure* (ed. R. Bannister), Oxford University Press, Oxford, pp. 410–11.

64. De Vos, A., Marcus, J.T., Reulen, J.P.H., Peters, H.F.M., Heiman, J.J. and Van der Veen, E.A. (1989) The pupillary light reflex in diabetes mellitus. Evaluation of a newly developed infrared light reflection method. *Diabetes Res.*, **10**, 191–5.

65. Clarke, C.F., Piesowcz, A.T. and Spathis, G.S. (1985) Pupillary size in children and adolescents with Type 1 diabetes mellitus. *Diabetic Med.*, **2**, 378–82.

66. Gilbey, S.G., Sutton, R.A., Thompson, S. and Watkins, P.J. (1985) A new simple non-invasive method for assessing gastric empty-ing and its application in diabetic autonomic neuropathy. *Diabetic Med.*, **2**, 378–82.

67. Bradley, W.E. (1980) Diagnosis of urinary bladder dysfunction in diabetes mellitus. *Ann. Intern. Med.*, **92**, 323–6.

68. Ewing, D.J. and Clarke, B.F. (1986) Auto-nomic neuropathy: its diagnosis and prog-nosis. *Clin. Endocrinol. Metab.*, **15**, 855–88.

69. Kirby, R.S. and Fowler, C.J. (1988) Bladder and sexual dysfunction in autonomic failure. In *Autonomic Failure* (ed. R. Bannister), Oxford University Press, Oxford, pp. 424–7.

70. Low, P.A. (1984) Quantisation of autonomic responses. In *Peripheral Neuropathy* (ed. P.J. Dyke, P.K. Thomas, E.H. Lambert and R. Bunge), W.B. Saunders, Philadelphia, pp. 1138–65.

71. Low, P.A., Caskey, P.E., Tuck, R.R., Fealey, R.D. and Dyke, P.J. (1983) Quantitative sudo-motor axon reflex in normal and neuropathic subjects. *Ann. Neurol.*, **14**, 573–80.

72. Kennedy, W.R., Sakuta, M., Sutherland, D. and Goetz, F.C. (1984) Quantification of the sweating deficiency in diabetes mellitus. *Ann. Neurol.*, **15**, 482–8.

73. Ryder, R.E.J., Marshall, R., Johnson, K., Ryder, A.T., Owen, D.R. and Hays, T.M. (1988) Acetylcholine sweatspot test for autonomic denervation. *Lancet*, **i**, 1303–5.

74. Genovely, H. and Pfeifer, M.A. (1988) R–R variation: the autonomic test of choice in diabetes. *Diabetes Metab. Rev.*, **4**, 255–71.

75. Ewing, D.J., Martyn, C.N., Young, R.J. and Clarke, B.F. (1985) The value of cardiovascular autonomic function tests: ten years' experi-ence in diabetes. *Diabetes Care*, **8**, 491–8.

76. Ewing, D.J. (1988) Recent advances in the non-invasive investigation of autonomic neuropathy. In *Autonomic Failure* (ed. R. Bannister), Oxford University Press, Oxford, pp. 667–89.

77. Gregersen, G. (1957) Diabetic neuropathy: Influence of age, sex, metabolic control and duration of diabetes on motor conduction velocity. *Neurology*, **17**, 973–80.

78. McNair, P. (1988) Bone mineral metabolism in human Type I (insulin dependent) diabetes mellitus. *Dan. Med. Bull.*, **35**, 109–21.

79. Hui, S.C., Epstein, S. and Johnston, Jr, C.C. (1985) A prospective study of bone mass in Type 1 diabetes mellitus. *J. Clin. Endocrinol. Metab.*, **60**, 74–80.

80. Marks, V. and Rose, F.C. (1981) *Hypogly-caemia*, 2nd edn, Blackwell, Oxford.

81. Heller, S.R., Herbert, M., MacDonald, I.A. and Tattersall, R.B. (1987) Influence of sym-pathetic nervous system on hypoglycaemic warning symptoms. *Lancet*, **ii**, 359–63.

82. Pramming, S., Thorsteinnson, B., Thielgaard, A., Pinner, E.M. and Binder, C. (1986) Cog-nitive function during hypoglycaemia in Type I diabetes. *Br. Med. J.*, **292**, 647-50.

83. Amiel, S.A., Pottinger, R., Archibald, H.R., Chusney, G., Cunnah, D., Prior, P.F. and Gale, E.A.M. (1991) Effect of antecedent glucose control on cerebral function during hypoglycaemia. *Diabetes Care*, **14**, 109–18.

84. Simonson, D.C., Tamborlane, W.V. and DeFronzo, R.A. (1985) Intensive insulin therapy reduces counterregulatory hormone responses to hypoglycaemia in patients with Type 1 diabetes. *Ann. Intern. Med.*, **103**, 184–90.

85. Bolli, G. and Gale, E.A.M. (1992) Hypogly-caemia. In *International Textbook of Diabetes* (ed. K.G.M.M. Alberti, R.A. DeFronzo, H. Keen and L.P. Krall), Wiley, Chichester.

86. Hooper, P.L., Tello, R.J., Burstein, P.J. and Abrams, R.S. (1990) Pseudoinsulinoma – the

Diamox–Diabenese switch. *New Engl. J. Med.*, **323**, 488.

87. Service, F.J., van Heerden, J.A. and Sheedy, P.F. (1983) Insulinoma. In *Hypoglycaemic Disorders* (ed. F.J. Service), G.K. Hall, Boston.

88. Service, F.J. and Nelson, R.L. (1980) Insulinoma. *Compr. Ther.*, **6**, 70–4.

89. Whipple, A.O. (1938) The surgical therapy of hyperinsulinism. *J. Int. Chir.*, **3**, 237–76.

90. Service, F.J. *et al.* (1977) C-peptide suppression test for insulinoma. *J. Lab. Clin. Med.*, **90**, 180–6.

91. Merimee, T.J. and Tyson, J.E. (1974) Stabilization of plasma glucose during fasting. *New Engl. J. Med.*, **291**, 1275–8.

92. Service, F.J. (1983) Clinical presentation and laboratory evaluation of hypoglycaemic disorders in adults. In *Hypoglycaemic Disorders* (ed. F.J. Service), G.K. Hall, Boston.

93. Turner, R.C. and Heding, L.G. (1977) Plasma proinsulin, C-peptide and insulin in diagnostic suppression tests for insulinomas. *Diabetologia*, **13**, 571–7.

94. Daggett, P.R. *et al.* (1981) Is preoperative localisation of insulinomas necessary? *Lancet*, **i**, 483–6.

95. Turner, R.C. (1978) Localisation of insulinomas. *Lancet*, **i**, 515–18.

11

Dyslipidaemias and their investigation

I. JIALAL

11.1 INTRODUCTION: LIPOPROTEIN STRUCTURE AND METABOLISM

Lipoproteins are separated and identified by techniques exploiting differences in lipoprotein size, density, electric charge and apoprotein composition. The major classes of plasma lipoproteins are shown in Table 11.1.

Each type of lipoprotein particle consists of a macromolecular complex of lipid and protein. The proteins are termed apoproteins and the major lipid constituents are cholesterol, cholesteryl esters, triglycerides and phospholipids. The neutral lipids, cholesteryl esters and triglycerides are located in the hydrophobic core of the particle, and this core is surrounded by a polar surface coat containing phospholipids, unesterified cholesterol and apoproteins, all of which stabilize the lipoprotein particles to keep them in solution in plasma. The major apoproteins and their physiological functions are shown in Table 11.2.

Chylomicrons, the largest lipoprotein particles, are synthesized in the intestinal wall in response to dietary fat. They transport dietary triglycerides, which constitute over 90% of their weight. They also carry dietary cholesterol. Chylomicrons contain apo B-48,

apo A-I and apo A-IV, all of which are made in the intestine, and apo E and apo Cs that are made in the liver and transferred to the chylomicrons from high density lipoprotein (HDL). After secretion into the lymphatic system, chylomicrons enter the general circulation via the thoracic duct. In the circulation they are exposed to lipoprotein lipase (LPL), an enzyme on the surface of capillary endothelial cells. Following activation by apo C-II on the surface of chylomicrons, LPL hydrolyses the core triglycerides to fatty acids, and these fatty acids enter adipocytes and muscle cells where they are oxidized or re-esterified into triglycerides. After hydrolysis of most triglycerides, a residual particle, called a chylomicron remnant, returns to the circulation. Chylomicron remnants are removed by the liver by a specific receptor-mediated process that recognizes apoprotein E. A scheme depicting chylomicron metabolism is shown in Fig. 11.1.

Very low density lipoproteins (VLDL) are secreted by the liver and transport endogenously synthesized triglycerides and cholesterol. VLDL contain about 50% triglyceride. Their major apoproteins are apo B-100, apo E and apo Cs (C-I, C-II, C-III). Like chylomicrons, VLDL particles are carried to tissue

Table 11.1 Composition and properties of major lipoproteins

	Chylomicrons	VLDL	IDL	LDL	HDL
Origin	Gut	Liver	VLDL	VLDL and IDL	Liver, gut, intravascular metabolism
Density (g ml^{-1})	0.94	0.94–1.006	1.006–1.019	1.019–1.063	1.063–1.21
Electrophoretic mobility	Origin	Pre-beta	Beta–pre-beta	Beta	Alpha
Particle size (nm)	75–1200	30–80	25–35	18–25	5–12
Major apoproteins	B-48, C, E	B-100, C, E	B-100, E	B-100	A-I, A-II, C, E
Protein (%)	1%	10%	15%	20%	50%
Major lipid (%)	Triglyceride (90%)	Triglyceride (55%)	Cholesterol (35%)	Cholesterol (50%)	Phospholipid (25%), cholesterol (20%)
Function	Transport dietary triglycerides	Transport endogenous triglycerides	Transport of cholesterol esters; LDL precursor	Transport of cholesterol esters	Reverse cholesterol transport

Table 11.2 Physiological functions of major apoproteins

1. Co-factor for an enzyme

Apo C-II	Lipoprotein lipase
Apo A-I	Lecithin cholesterol acyltransferase

2. Structural protein (biosynthesis)

Apo B-48	Chylomicrons
Apo B-100	VLDL and LDL
Apo A-I	HDL

3. Ligand for cellular receptor

Apo B and Apo E	LDL receptor
Apo A-I	? HDL receptor
Apo E	Chylomicron remnant receptor

capillaries where apo C-II activates LPL, and VLDL core triglycerides are hydrolysed and enter tissue cells. A portion of VLDL remnants, including intermediate density lipoproteins (IDL), is taken up and catabolized by the liver. Hepatic uptake of VLDL remnants appears to be mediated by receptors that recognize their apo E. The remaining VLDL remnants are converted to low density lipoprotein (LDL) by removal of the residual triglyceride and apo E. LDL contains essentially cholesterol ester as its core lipid, and apo B-100 as its only surface apoprotein.

LDL carries approximately two-thirds of the plasma cholesterol, and provides cholesterol for membrane biosynthesis and steroidogenesis. LDL can be catabolized by cells via a receptor-dependent and non-receptor-dependent mechanism. At least 70% of the LDL is removed from the circulation by cells through specific endocytosis, termed the LDL-receptor pathway. This pathway was elucidated by the pioneering studies of Brown and Goldstein. Its principal function is to provide cholesterol to cells and to maintain cellular cholesterol homeostasis. The LDL

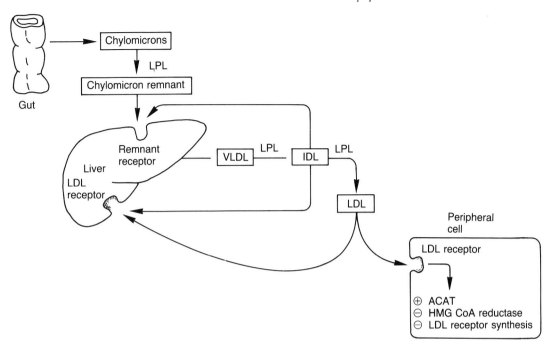

Fig. 11.1 Overview of lipoprotein metabolism.

receptor recognizes apo B-100 and apo E, the latter with higher affinity. Thus it removes both VLDL remnants and LDL. The LDL receptor gene has been localized to the short arm of chromosome 19 and codes for a protein of 839 amino acids, to which carbohydrate is added in the Golgi complex such that the mature receptor is a glycoprotein. The ligand-binding domain of the LDL receptor is a cysteine-rich, negatively charged domain of 292 amino acids at the amino terminal. A membrane spanning domain of 22 amino acids is important in anchoring the receptor in the cell membrane. A cytoplasmic domain of 50 amino acids at the carboxyl terminal end is important for the correct localization of the receptor in the coated pit regions of the cell membrane. LDL is taken up by the LDL receptor via a process of adsorptive endocytosis; in this process, endocytotic vesicles are formed that fuse with cellular lysosomes. Following internalization, the receptor dissociates from LDL and recycles to the cell surface. The LDL protein is hydrolysed by proteases to amino acids, and the cholesteryl esters are hydrolysed by an acid lipase. The accumulating free cholesterol in the cell regulates two microsomal enzymes; it suppresses HMG CoA reductase, the rate limiting enzyme in cholesterol synthesis, and it activates acyl CoA-cholesteryl acyl transferase (ACAT), facilitating cholesterol esterification. Also, the unesterified cholesterol shuts off LDL-receptor synthesis. The liver clears 60%–70% of the LDL by this LDL-receptor pathway. The remaining LDL is taken up and degraded by a low affinity or scavenger pathway that includes macrophages of the reticulo-endothelial system.

HDL is a heterogenous group of particles composed of 50% protein and 50% lipid, by weight. They are the smallest of all lipo-protein particles and carry about 20% of the plasma cholesterol. Although the major apo-protein of HDL is A-I, it also has other apo-proteins including A-II, Cs, and E. Its major classes are HDL2 (1.063–1.125) and HDL3 (1.125–1.21). It has been hypothesized that HDL is involved in 'reverse cholesterol trans-port', i.e. the removal of cholesterol from peripheral tissues and transport to the liver for excretion. Nascent HDL particles resem-bling stacked discs consist largely of phos-pholipids and apoproteins, and are secreted by both the liver and intestine. On entry into the circulation they gain additional apopro-teins (C and E), phospholipids and cholesterol from the hydrolysis of the surface-coat con-stituents of VLDL and chylomicrons. After picking up unesterified cholesterol, the par-ticles mature to the spherical HDL particles by conversion of the cholesterol to cholesteryl ester by lecithin cholesterol acyl transferase (LCAT); apo A-I is an important co-factor for LCAT. HDL also exchange lipid with other lipoproteins through the action of cholesteryl ester transfer protein (CETP). CETP transfers cholesteryl esters from HDL to chylomicrons

VLDL and IDL. Thus, whereas HDL particles may promote reverse cholesterol transport of tissue cholesterol, the route to the liver may be direct or it may be indirect via transfer of cholesteryl ester to VLDL, IDL and LDL; these lipoproteins in turn may then deliver cholesterol to the liver via the LDL or rem-nant pathway.

11.2 THE HYPERLIPOPROTEINAEMIAS: PATHOPHYSIOLOGY, PRESENTATION AND DIAGNOSIS

The hyperlipoproteinaemias can usually be identified by measuring the plasma chol-esterol and triglyceride levels after a 12–14 hour fast. The precautions undertaken prior to blood sampling will be discussed later when the investigation of hyperlipoprotein-aemia is reviewed. Arbitrarily, hyperlipo-proteinaemia denotes either an increased cholesterol, triglyceride or both (>90th or 95th percentile for a respective population). In most routine laboratories, in addition to plasma cholesterol and triglyceride, the HDL-cholesterol levels are also assayed.

Table 11.3 Familial hyperlipoproteinaemias

Genetic disorder	Phenotype	Biochemical defect	Clinical presentation	Plasma cholesterol	Plasma triglycerides
Familial LPL deficiency	I	Absence of LPL activity	Eruptive xanthoma; hepatosplenomegaly; pancreatitis	↑	↑ ↑ ↑
Familial apo C-II deficiency	I or V	Absence or abnormal structure of apo C-II	Pancreatitis	↑	↑ ↑ ↑
Familial hypercholesterolaemia	IIa or IIb	Deficiency of LDL receptors	Tendinous and tuberous xanthoma; premature atherosclerosis	↑ ↑ ↑	↑ or N
Familial dysbetalipoproteinaemia	III	Abnormal apo E and defect in triglyceride-rich metabolism	Tubero-eruptive and planar xanthoma; premature athersclerosis	↑ ↑	↑ ↑
Familial combined hyperlipidaemia	IIa, IIb, or IV	Unknown	Premature atherosclerosis	↑ or N	↑ or N
Familial hypertriglyceridaemias	IV and V	Unknown	Eruptive xanthoma; hepatosplenomegaly; pancreatitis	N ↑	↑ (IV) ↑ ↑ ↑ (V)

Since chylomicrons are not present in the fasting state, and the cholesterol content of VLDL approximates one-fifth of the plasma triglycerides, the LDL-cholesterol (LDL-Chol) can be computed as follows provided the plasma triglycerides are not greater than $400 \, \text{mg dl}^{-1}$ ($4.5 \, \text{mmol l}^{-1}$):

$$\text{LDL-Chol} = \text{Total Chol} - \text{HDL-Chol} - \frac{\text{Trig}}{5}$$

The most important clinical consequences of hyperlipoproteinaemia include premature atherosclerosis, pancreatitis and xanthoma formation. A lipoprotein disorder can either be inherited (primary hyperlipoproteinaemia) or caused by other disease states or medications (secondary hyperlipoproteinaemia). Hyperlipoproteinaemia can result from either increased synthesis or diminished removal of plasma lipoproteins or their constituents.

There are several classifications of lipoprotein disorders, none of which is entirely satisfactory. For the purpose of this chapter the phenotypic classification is adopted, since it remains most practical for routine use, as long as it is understood that it describes only abnormalities of plasma lipoproteins and not specific diseases. However, where possible the specific monogenic familial disorders will be discussed as representative of the different phenotypes. A summary of the salient characteristics of the major primary hyperlipoproteinaemias is shown in Table 11.3.

11.2.1 TYPE I HYPERLIPOPROTEINAEMIA

LPL deficiency

LPL deficiency is a rare autosomal recessive disorder. It presents in childhood with attacks of abdominal pain, pancreatitis, eruptive xanthoma, hepatosplenomegaly and lipaemia retinalis. These patients are not prone to premature atherosclerosis. Because of LPL deficiency patients develop chylomicronae-

mia. The disorder manifests with a marked elevation of triglycerides, which may exceed $10\,000 \, \text{mg dl}^{-1}$ ($112.0 \, \text{mmol l}^{-1}$); cholesterol levels can be markedly increased due to the cholesterol content of chylomicrons. If lipoprotein levels are measured both LDL and HDL-cholesterol levels are low. The diagnosis is strengthened by the refrigerator test (plasma at 4°C for 18 hours), when one sees a creamy layer on a clear infranate.

Lipoprotein electrophoresis on paper or agarose will reveal a dense band of chylomicrons at the origin. The diagnosis is established by assaying LPL levels in post-heparin plasma, adipose tissue or muscle biopsy. The parents are obligate heterozygotes for the LPL defect but are often clinically normal; sometimes they have mild hypertriglyceridaemia or hypercholesterolaemia. The severe hypertriglyceridaemia and its attendant turbidity will render some laboratory tests, such as amylase, erroneous. In an attempt to avert pancreatitis, plasma triglycerides should be kept below $1000 \, \text{mg dl}^{-1}$ by restricting fat intake to below $20 \, \text{g}$ per day. Medium-chain triglycerides can be used as one source of dietary fat because they do not form chylomicrons.

Measurement of LPL activity

This can be measured either in post-heparin plasma or in tissues. The measurement of LPL activity in plasma after a bolus injection of heparin requires the selective inhibition of hepatic lipase. This can be accomplished by pre-incubation of the plasma with protamine. Several types of assay are available at present, all of which are based on the hydrolysis of triolein emulsions stabilized with detergents, gum arabic or phospholipids.

Procedure

Heparin in a dose of $100 \, \text{IU kg}^{-1}$ is given intravenously and post-heparin plasma is collected 5–15 minutes later.

Interpretation

LPL activity is extremely sensitive to alterations in diet, habitual physical activity, smoking habits and alcohol intake. Post-heparin PLP activity reflects the enzyme activity from adipose tissue and muscle, and the normal values for LPL activity in normal men range from 35 ± 20 to 310 ± 103 nmol min^{-1} ml^{-1}.

Apoprotein C-II deficiency

Apoprotein C-II deficiency is a much rarer autosomal recessive disorder caused by an absence of apo C-II, the essential co-factor for LPL; this results in a functional deficiency of LPL and accumulation of chylomicrons and VLDL. The clinical presentation is similar to LPL deficiency except that hypertriglyceridaemia is less severe, pancreatitis is less common, and eruptive xanthomata usually are not observed. The reasons for these differences are not known.

The diagnosis requires the demonstration of deficient LPL activity in post-heparin plasma, but the appearance of LPL activity when either normal serum or purified apo C-II is added to assay medium.

The diagnosis is confirmed by demonstration of absent or defective apo C-II by electrophoretic techniques and/or functional assays. The treatment is similar to LPL deficiency except that normal serum transfusion may be helpful to avert imminent pancreatitis.

11.2.2 TYPE II HYPERLIPOPROTEINAEMIA

Familial hypercholesterolaemia

Familial hypercholesterolaemia (FH) is the result of a mutation of the LDL receptor that prevents its normal function. It is transmitted as an autosomal dominant trait and occurs in 1 in 500 persons. Both the heterozygote and homozygous forms of the disease are recognized. In heterozygotes the increased cholesterol is often detectable at birth or shortly thereafter and reaches levels of 350–500 mg dl^{-1} (9.1–12.9 mmol l^{-1}). Characteristic physical findings include xanthoma, especially over the extensor tendons of the hands and Achilles tendons. Patients may also develop arcus cornealis and xanthelasmas, but neither lesion is specific for FH. Manifestations of coronary artery disease begin to appear in men by the third or fourth decade and occur about 10 years later in women. The age of onset of these symptoms is highly variable and in part relates to the presence of other risk factors. FH homozygotes occur with a frequency of one in one million and manifest cholesterol levels exceeding 600 mg dl^{-1} (1.55 mmol l^{-1}). Homozygous children develop cutaneous xanthoma at various sites in the first few months of life in addition to tendon xanthoma. These xanthoma are located in the webs between the fingers, and at the knees, elbows and buttocks. Atherosclerosis in the homozygote is very severe and affects the aortic root as well as the carotid, coronary and major peripheral arteries. Cholesterol is also deposited in the aortic valve and may produce symptomatic aortic stenosis.

Numerous mutations of the LDL receptor have been described, which can be classified into four functional categories:

1. Class 1 mutation: receptors are not synthesized.
2. Class 2 mutation: receptors are synthesized in the rough endoplasmic reticulum but are blocked or dramatically slowed in transit from the endoplasmic reticulum to the Golgi and the cell surface.
3. Class 3 mutation: receptors properly traverse the Golgi and reach the cell surface but they fail to bind LDL.
4. Class 4 mutation: receptors are capable of binding LDL normally but are not clustered in coated pits, resulting in an internalization defect.

Since heterozygotes inherit one normal and one mutant allele they produce only half the normal number of receptors and hence their cultured cells degrade only half the normal amount of LDL. However, the cultured cells of homozygotes bind and degrade little or no LDL since they have two mutant alleles. The increased LDL-cholesterol in patients with FH not only is due to impaired catabolism of LDL via the LDL receptor but also to increased conversion of IDL to LDL because less of the latter is removed directly from the circulation.

Hypercholesterolaemia in heterozygous FH is usually severe, being $>350\,mg\,dl^{-1}$ $(9.1\,mmol\,l^{-1})$. Plasma triglycerides are either normal (type IIa) or increased slightly (type IIb) and plasma HDL-cholesterol levels generally are decreased. It should be pointed out that the majority of patients with a type IIa phenotype do not have FH. Instead their elevated LDL-cholesterol is a primary disorder of undetermined causes. The secondary causes of an increased cholesterol will be discussed later. The presence of tendon xanthoma strongly supports the diagnosis of FH, although not all FH patients have xanthoma. Since FH is inherited as a dominant trait it is important to screen first-degree relatives of the propositus since one parent will be affected and statistically 50% of the siblings and off-spring will also be affected. The finding of severe hypercholesterolaemia $(>600\,mg\,dl^{-1}$ or $15.5\,mmol\,l^{-1})$ and cutaneous xanthoma in a child strongly suggests the diagnosis of homozygous FH. Receptor studies in skin fibroblasts or lymphocytes can be diagnostic but are available only in specialized research laboratories.

Since the major thrust of this review is on the investigation of hyperlipoproteinaemia the therapy of FH will not be discussed. Suffice to say that the heterozygote requires both diet and drug therapy with bile acid resins, niacin and HMG-CoA reductase inhibitors. The combination of bile acid resins and reductase inhibitors is particularly efficacious.

Primary moderate hypercholesterolaemia

Primary moderate hypercholesterolaemia is the most common pattern of an isolated increase in LDL-cholesterol. In this condition, LDL-cholesterol levels range from 160 to $220\,mg\,dl^{-1}$ $(4.1–5.7\,mmol\,l^{-1})$. It is believed to be due to a complex interaction of genetic and environmental factors, and it has been referred to as 'polygenic' hypercholesterolaemia. Moderate elevations of LDL-cholesterol probably result from a variety of causes. Patients with moderate hypercholesterolaemia are at increased risk for premature atherosclerosis. Compared to patients with familial hypercholesterolaemia, they have less severe hypercholesterolaemia, absence of xanthoma, and a low frequency of first-degree relatives with elevated plasma cholesterol. This last feature helps to differentiate these patients from those with familial combined hyperlipidaemia. Recently, a mutation in the receptor-binding region of apoprotein B has been described as one cause of moderate hypercholesterolaemia.

11.2.3 TYPE III HYPERLIPOPROTEINAEMIA: FAMILIAL DYSBETALIPOPROTEINAEMIA

Familial dysbetalipoproteinaemia is also referred to a remnant removal disease or broad beta disease. It is a rare disorder with a frequency of 1 in 1000 persons. Although the disorder is genetically transmitted, additional factors are usually required for clinical expression of hyperlipoproteinaemia. Type III hyperlipoproteinaemia is characterized by the accumulation in plasma of chylomicrons, VLDL remnants and IDL, resulting in a combined increase in cholesterol and triglycerides.

This disorder is not expressed before early adulthood. Clinically, two forms of xanthoma are observed in these patients, xanthoma striata palmaris, which develops in the creases of the palms and fingers where it imparts a yellowish discoloration, and tubero-eruptive xanthoma, which occurs at the elbow, knees and buttocks. As a consequence of accumulation of lipoprotein remnants, severe atherosclerosis of the coronary arteries, aorta and peripheral arteries is the rule during later life. Not infrequently the disorder is associated with obesity, abnormal glucose intolerance and hyperuricaemia.

The defect in type III hyperlipoproteinaemia is intimately related to apo E polymorphism. Apo E is present at a single genetic locus with three common alleles in the population: E2, E3 and E4. These alleles encode three E apoproteins: apo E2, apo E3 and apo E4. Six major apo E phenotypes present in the population include homozygotes for E2, E3 and E4 and heterozygotes for E2/3, E2/4 and E3/4. Type III hyperlipoproteinaemia is associated most often, but not exclusively, with the E2/2 genotype. Since apo E appears to mediate binding of VLDL and chylomicron remnants to their hepatic receptors, remnants accumulate because the E2/2 isoform does not bind adequately. Whereas the apo E2/2 genotype has a frequency of 1 in 100, the frequency of the type III syndrome is 1 in 1000, or even less common; this difference in frequency suggests that other factors such as obesity, diabetes or hypothyroidism are required to induce the clinical syndrome by possibly leading to an overproduction of VLDL. Very rarely, patients with type III hyperlipoproteinaemia may also have familial apo E deficiency in which no apo E can be detected in plasma.

The presence of type III hyperlipoproteinaemia is suggested by an elevation of cholesterol (300–600 mg dl^{-1} or 7.8–15.5 mmol l^{-1}) and triglycerides (400–700 mg dl^{-1} or 4.5–7.9 mmol l^{-1}) to a similar degree. Plasma is usually turbid on standing at 4°C overnight and shows a thin layer of chylomicrons over a turbid infranatant. Agarose gel electrophoresis usually reveals a broad beta band spanning both the beta and pre-beta regions due to migration of remnants between the beta and pre-beta position. Levels of LDL-cholesterol and HDL-cholesterol are often decreased. To confirm the diagnosis, ultracentrifugation is required to isolate VLDL and compute the VLDL-cholesterol/total plasma triglyceride ratio; a ratio ⩾0.30 usually indicates the presence of type III hyperlipoproteinaemia. In addition, in specialized laboratories the isoforms of apo E can be determined by isoelectric focusing. Although dietary therapy can dramatically improve the hyperlipoproteinaemia, therapy with fibrates or niacin is usually required to normalize the lipid profile.

11.2.4 TYPE IV HYPERLIPOPROTEINAEMIA: PRIMARY ENDOGENOUS HYPERTRIGLYCERIDAEMIA

This disorder is commonly transmitted as an autosomal dominant trait and results in elevated VLDL triglycerides. In this case it is called familial hypertriglyceridaemia. This disorder, which manifests mainly in adulthood, does not appear to have any unique clinical or biochemical features. There is uncertainty whether patients with familial hypertriglyceridaemia are predisposed to coronary artery disease. Certainly, risk for coronary heart disease is not as great as in genetic disorders characterized by increased cholesterol levels. Obesity, abnormal glucose tolerance, hyperinsulinism, hypertension and hyperuricaemia are often associated with this disorder. Some affected individuals appear to have a defect leading to enhanced hepatic triglyceride synthesis with secretion of triglyceride-enriched large VLDL; however, the nature of the primary defect is not known. In other families a defect in catabolism of VLDL triglycerides appears to be the underlying cause.

Patients with primary endogenous hypertriglyceridaemia have triglyceride levels in the range of 250–600 mg dl^{-1} (2.8–6.8 mmol l^{-1}), with normal or slightly increased cholesterol levels due to the increased VLDL. HDL-cholesterol levels are usually reduced, whereas LDL-cholesterol levels are normal. Agarose gel electrophoresis, if undertaken, will reveal an increase in the pre-beta band. Family members will often manifest a similar pattern of hyperlipoproteinaemia. The term 'sporadic hypertriglyceridaemia' refers to hypertriglyceridaemic persons who do not have affected first-degree relatives with increased lipids.

The hypertriglyceridaemia can be aggravated by several factors, such as poorly controlled diabetes, alcohol ingestion, hypothyroidism, weight gain, oestrogen, diuretics, steroids and beta-adrenergic blocking agents. The result can be a severe hypertriglyceridaemia (>1000 mg dl^{-1}) with increase in both VLDL and chylomicrons (type V pattern). Severe hypertriglyceridaemia puts subjects at an increased risk of pancreatitis and the development of eruptive xanthoma. Treatment of the type IV hyperlipoproteinaemia is dietary, with weight control, alcohol restriction, and, in high-risk patients, niacin or fibrate therapy.

11.2.5 TYPE V HYPERLIPOPROTEINAEMIA

This disorder is characterized by fasting chylomicronaemia and elevated VLDL levels. While the familial nature is well recognized, the pattern of inheritance is not clear. Moreover, no specific molecular defect has been identified. Both increased VLDL production and decreased clearance contribute to the expression of the disease. The chylomicronaemia is the consequence of the increased VLDL levels, probably saturating the common clearance of the triglyceride-rich lipoproteins.

Patients with the type V phenotype present in mid-adulthood and are often obese. The clinical presentation includes pancreatitis, eruptive xanthoma, hepatosplenomegaly, lipaemia retinalis, polyneuropathy, a sicca-like syndrome and an organic brain syndrome (memory deficiency etc.). Hyperuricaemia and abnormal glucose tolerance are not infrequent accompaniments. These patients do not appear to be at increased risk for coronary artery disease. The type V disorder is suggested by fasting chylomicronaemia and elevated VLDL levels manifesting as severe hypertriglyceridaemia (>1000 mg dl^{-1} or 11.3 mmol l^{-1}). Agarose gel electrophoresis of a serum sample reveals an increased band at the origin (chylomicrons) and an increased pre-beta band (VLDL). Plasma stored at 4°C will reveal a creamy layer over a turbid infranate. Although plasma cholesterol levels are increased, the increase occurs entirely in triglyceride-rich lipoproteins; both HDL and LDL levels are moderately decreased. Aggregation of severe hypertriglyceridaemia in the family suggests the type V disorder. With a few exceptions, LPL activity in post-heparin plasma is normal in patients with type V hyperlipoproteinaemia. Therapy should start with identification and control of aggravating factors (obesity, alcohol, diabetes and oestrogens). If these measures are not satisfactory, then drug therapy with either fibrates or niacin may prove helpful. In refractory cases fish oil supplements may prove useful in lowering triglyceride levels.

11.2.6 FAMILIAL COMBINED HYPERLIPIDAEMIA

Familial combined hyperlipidaemia (FCHL), also referred to as familial multiple lipoprotein-type hyperlipidaemia, is so named because patients and their affected first-degree relatives may at various times manifest hypercholesterolaemia, hypertriglyceridaemia or both abnormalities. It appears to be inherited in an autosomal dominant mode. To date, however, the underlying defect has not been discovered. In FCHL there appears to be hepatic overproduction of apo B-containing lipoproteins that results in an increase in apo B levels of VLDL, IDL and LDL particles. The variability in lipoprotein pattern suggests that concomitant modifications, either genetic or acquired, in lipoprotein metabolism determine which lipoprotein is present in excess.

Patients usually present with hyperlipidaemia in the third or fourth decade and have an increased propensity for premature coronary artery disease. They rarely have tendon xanthoma. The disorder may be accompanied by obesity, hyperuricaemia and abnormal glucose tolerance. These individuals may manifest with type IIa (1/3), IIb (1/3) or IV (1/3) patterns of hyperlipoproteinemia. The lipid elevations are rarely marked. HDL-cholesterol levels are usually low.

The diagnosis depends on the demonstration of multiple lipoprotein phenotypes in first-degree relatives of the patient. Many patients with this disorder have varying lipoprotein patterns over time. Immunoassay of apoprotein B, if available, may reveal increased levels. In addition, a subset of patients with normal lipid levels and increased apo B levels have been described, and this group has been termed hyperapobetalipoproteinaemia.

11.2.7 FAMILIAL HYPERALPHALIPOPROTEINAEMIA

This condition is characterized by an elevation of plasma HDL-cholesterol (>70 mg dl^{-1} or 1.8 mmol l^{-1}) resulting in a mild hypercholesterolaemia. In some pedigrees it appears to be transmitted as an autosomal dominant trait. The mechanism of the increased HDL-cholesterol has not been determined. However, an increased HDL-cholesterol can be secondary to regular alcohol ingestion, phenytoin therapy and oestrogen therapy.

While the HDL-cholesterol level is increased, both LDL-cholesterol and VLDL-cholesterol levels are normal. The condition is benign and the reason for distinguishing it from other forms of hypercholesterolaemia is that it requires no treatment. In fact, the familial form appears to impart a longer life expectancy.

11.2.8 ELEVATED LIPOPROTEIN (a)

Lipoprotein (a) (Lp(a)) is another risk factor for coronary artery disease, first detected in 1963. It contains the unique apoprotein apo (a) linked by a disulphide bridge to LDL to form Lp(a). Protein and c DNA sequencing show close homology with plasminogen. Lp(a) contains 37 copies of Kringle 4 plasminogen and 1 copy of Kringle 5. This similarly may herald the long-sought connection between serum lipoproteins and the clotting system. However, whereas the mechanism of the atherogenicity of Lp(a) is as yet unknown, elevated levels are strongly associated with coronary atherosclerosis. At levels greater than 30 mg dl^{-1} the relative risk of coronary disease increases twofold; when both LDL-cholesterol and Lp(a) levels are elevated the relative risk increases fivefold. However, before Lp(a) becomes part of the routine screening the assay needs to be standardized, its metabolism understood, and therapeutic measures that successfully lower its levels must be available.

11.3 SECONDARY HYPERLIPOPROTEINAEMIAS

An important aspect in the work up of a patient with hyperlipoproteinaemia is to rule out a secondary cause. These conditions can either cause a hyperlipoproteinaemia or unmask a hyperlipoproteinaemia in a genetically predisposed individual. Table 11.4 depicts the more common causes of either a predominantly increased cholesterol or triglyceride level.

Table 11.4 Causes of secondary hyperlipidaemia

1. *Predominantly hypertriglyceridaemia*
   Obesity
   Diabetes mellitus
   Alcoholism
   Renal failure
   Lipodystrophy
   Glycogen storage disease
   Dysglobulinemias
   Oestrogen therapy
   Steroid therapy
   Beta blocker therapy
   Isotretinoin therapy

2. *Predominantly hypercholesterolaemia*
   Hypothyroidism
   Cholestasis
   Nephrotic syndrome
   Dysglobulinaemias
   Acute intermittent porphyria
   Anorexia nervosa
   Hepatoma
   Anabolic steroids
   Progestins
   Diuretics
   Cyclosporin

It should be pointed out that there is significant overlap in the increased lipids that result from most of these secondary disorders. For example, chronic renal failure, hypothyroidism and diabetes can cause a combined hyperlipoproteinaemia. The risk of coronary artery disease in some of the secondary hyperlipoproteinaemias may be less marked than in the primary ones because of the shorter duration. A discussion of the detailed mechanisms whereby these disorders or therapies induce hyperlipoproteinaemia is beyond the scope of this review, and the reader is referred to the further reading. Suffice to say that in obstructive jaundice there is a distinct lipoprotein abnormality that resembles LCAT deficiency; the bulk of the free cholesterol and phospholipids present in these patients is due to the presence of an abnormal lipoprotein termed LP-X. In addition to a careful history and physical examination, certain laboratory tests are useful in excluding a secondary cause of hyperlipoproteinaemia. These include a urinalysis (protein and glucose), plasma urea and creatinine, thyroxine and TSH, glucose, albumen, globulins, bilirubin, alkaline phosphatase, transaminases and serum protein electrophoresis. Correction of the underlying disorder usually corrects or significantly ameliorates the lipoprotein abnormality, except when the secondary disorder exacerbates a primary hyperlipoproteinaemia.

11.4 LABORATORY ASSESSMENT OF HYPERLIPOPROTEINAEMIA

Either plasma or serum can be used to measure lipoprotein levels. Plasma is preferred because samples can be cooled rapidly. Values obtained in plasma for both cholesterol and triglycerides are approximately 3% lower than in serum. At least two lipid estimates, preferably a week apart, should be made before an individual is diagnosed as having hyperlipoproteinaemia, since plasma lipids show biological variation from day to day. Three measurements are helpful to establish a baseline before a patient is started on drug therapy. Drug therapy should rarely, if ever, be started from a single measurement. Precautions that need to be undertaken prior to blood sampling include:

1. 12–14 hour fast (not necessary if assaying for total cholesterol or HDL-cholesterol only).
2. Avoiding alcohol on evening prior to sampling.
3. Having been on habitual weight-maintaining diet for at least 2–3 weeks.
4. Deferring lipid analysis for 2–3 weeks after a minor illness and for 3 months after a major illness, surgery or trauma. Cholesterol may be measured within 24 hours of onset of chest pain in myocardial infarction.

5. Posture should be standardized, e.g. most convenient to take the sample after the patient has been seated for 5–10 minutes.
6. Discontinuing drugs that affect lipid metabolism for at least 3 weeks, if possible.

Routine lipid analyses that are useful in delineating the majority of hyperlipoproteinaemias include plasma cholesterol, triglycerides and HDL-cholesterol. The HDL-cholesterol is determined after precipitation of apo B-containing lipoproteins by polyanions and divalent cations. Accuracy for these assays should be within 5% of the reference value and precision should be better than 4% for plasma cholesterol and triglycerides, and 6% for HDL-cholesterol. If the plasma triglyceride is below $400 \, \text{mg} \, \text{dl}^{-1}$ ($4.5 \, \text{mmol} \, \text{l}^{-1}$) and a type III hyperlipoproteinaemia is not suspected, LDL-cholesterol can be calculated with reasonable accuracy according to Friedwald's formula:

$$LDL\text{-}Chol = Total \, Chol - HDL\text{-}Chol - Trig/5$$

Although lipoprotein electrophoresis is not necessary to diagnose the different hyperlipoproteinaemias, its two most useful applications appear to be to identify the broad beta band in type III hyperlipoproteinaemia and to confirm the presence of chylomicrons. If a sample with fasting hypertriglyceridaemia ($>350 \, \text{mg} \, \text{dl}^{-1}$ or $4.0 \, \text{mmol} \, \text{l}^{-1}$) is encountered the refrigerator test may prove useful in determining if VLDL, chylomicrons or both are increased. This test requires 4 ml plasma to be stored in a glass tube at 4°C for 18 hours. It is interpreted as follows:

1. Turbid infranate with creamy layer on top: increased VLDD plus increased chylomicrons.
2. Clear infranate with creamy layer on top: increased chylomicrons.
3. Even turbidity throughout sample: increased VLDL.

It should be pointed out that electrophoresis is more sensitive than visual inspection of plasma for detection of chylomicrons. Whereas increased apo B and decreased apo A-I and decreased apo A-I/apo B ratio have been shown to be good discriminators in identifying coronary artery disease, the addition of these assays to the present lipoprotein repertoire requires as an essential first step the standardization of the techniques. To confirm type III hyperlipoproteinaemia, ultracentrifugation is required to quantitate VLDL-cholesterol. Apoprotein E phenotyping by isoelectric focusing, if available, may also help to confirm a diagnosis of type III hyperlipoproteinaemia.

To confirm type I hyperlipoproteinaemia, determination of plasma LPL activity following an injection of heparin or adipose tissue LPL levels is required.

Although determination of LDL-receptor status in fibroblasts in culture grown from skin explants or in lymphocytes may help to confirm a diagnosis of homozygous familial hypercholesterolaemia, they may not clearly differentiate heterozygotes from normal.

FURTHER READING

1. Albers, J.J., Brunzell, J. and Knopp, R.H. (1989) Apoprotein measurements and their clinical application. *Clin. Lab. Med.*, **9**, 137–51.
2. Bachorik, P. (1989) Measurement of total cholesterol, HDL-cholesterol and LDL-cholesterol. *Clin. Lab. Med.*, **9**, 61–72.
3. Bierman, E.L. and Glomset, J.A. (1985) Disorders of lipid metabolism. In *Textbook of Endocrinology*, 7th edn. (ed. J.D. Wilson and D.W. Foster), W.B. Saunders, Philadelphia, pp. 1108–36.
4. Bilheimer, D.W. (1989) Disorders of lipid metabolism. In *Textbook of Internal Medicine* (ed. W.N. Kelley), J.B. Lippincott, Philadelphia, pp. 2258–69.
5. Brewer, H.B., Gregg, R.E., Hoeg, J.M. and Fojo, S.S. (1988) Apoproteins and lipoproteins in human plasma: an overview. *Clin. Chem.*, **34**, 4–8.
6. Brown, W.V. and Ginsberg, H. (1987) Classification and diagnosis of the hyperlipidemias.

Contemp. Issues Endocrinol. Metab., **3**, 143–68.

7. Brown, M.S. and Goldstein, J.L. (1984) How LDL receptors influence cholesterol and atherosclerosis. *Sci. Am.*, **251**, 58–66.

8. European Atherosclerosis Society (1988) The recognition and management of hyperlipidaemia in adults: a policy statement of the European Atherosclerosis Society. *Eur. Heart J.*, **9**, 571–600.

9. Gordon, D.J. and Rifkind, B.M. (1989) High density lipoproteins – the clinical implications of recent studies. *New Engl. J. Med.*, **321**, 1311–16.

10. Gotto, A.M. (1988) Etiology, diagnosis and treatment of the lipid transport disorders. *Prog. Cardiol.*, **16**, 23–49.

11. Grundy, S.M. (1984) Pathogenesis of hyperlipoproteinemia. *J. Lipid Res.*, **25**, 1611–18.

12. Grundy, S.M., Greenland, P., Herd, A. *et al.* (1987) Cardiovascular and risk factor evaluation of healthy American adults. *Circulation*, **73**, 1340–62.

13. Hoeg, J.M., Gregg, R. and Brewer, B. (1986) An approach to the management of hyperlipoproteinemia. *J. Am. Med. Ass.*, **255**, 512–21.

14. Kane, J.P. and Malloy, M.J. (1988) When to treat hyperlipidaemia. *Adv. Intern. Med.*, **33**, 143–64.

15. Lavie, C.J., Gau, G., Squires, R. and Kottke, B.A. (1988) Management of lipids in primary and secondary prevention of cardiovascular diseases. *Mayo Clin. Proc.*, **63**, 605–21.

16. Morrisett, J.D., Guyton, J., Gaubatz, J. and Gotto, A.M. (1987) Lipoprotein (a): structure, metabolism and epidemiology. In *Plasma Lipoproteins* (ed. A.M. Gotto), Elsevier, Amsterdam, pp. 129–52.

17. Naito, H.K. (1987) Serum apolipoprotein measurements: an improved discriminator for assessing coronary heart disease risk. *Comp. Ther.*, **13**, 43–52.

18. Patsch, W. Patsch, J. and Gotto, A.M. (1989) The hyperlipoproteinemias. *Med. Clin. North Am.*, **73**, 859–93.

19. Scanu, A.M. (1988) Lipoprotein (a). *Archs Path. Lab. Med.*, **112**, 1045–7.

20. Schaefer, E.J. and Levy, R.I. (1985) Pathogenesis and management of lipoprotein disorders. *New Engl. J. Med.*, **312**, 1300–10.

21. Scriver, C.R., Beaudet, A.L., Sly, W.S. and Valle, D. (ed.) (1989) *The Metabolic Basis of Inherited Disease. Part 7. Lipoprotein and Lipid Metabolism Disorders*, 6th edn, McGraw-Hill, New York, pp. 1129–304.

22. The Expert Panel (1988) Report of the National Cholesterol Education Programm Expert Panel on detection, evaluation and treatment of high blood cholesterol in adults. *Archs Intern. Med.*, **148**, 36–69.

12

Growth disorders

A.M. COTTERILL and M.O. SAVAGE

12.1 INTRODUCTION

The investigation of growth disorders begins with the appreciation by the clinician that the growth pattern of a child or adolescent is deviating from accepted physiological limits. A basic knowledge of normal growth is therefore needed to form the background of this assessment. Section 12.2 describes normal childhood and pubertal growth, and Section 12.3 deals with clinical growth assessment. The differential diagnosis of short stature is described in Section 12.4, followed by an account of laboratory and radiological investigations in Section 12.5. Tall stature is briefly discussed in Section 12.6, although assessment of excess growth hormone (GH) secretion is covered in Chapter 2.

12.2 NORMAL GROWTH

Normal linear growth results from an interplay of intrinsic and extrinsic factors on the genetically determined capacity for growth of body cells. Adult height depends on the rate and duration of linear growth. Factors that influence growth vary at different ages; for example foetal growth is known to be independent of pituitary function. Growth in infancy is related to similar control mechanisms, with nutrition playing a major role.

GH is responsible for childhood growth, provided thyroid function is normal, and growth during adolescence depends on GH and sex steroid secretion, which are both needed for the attainment of full adult height [1].

These control factors have been used to develop a model of growth (Fig. 12.1) known as the infancy–childhood–puberty (ICP) model [2], which has been applied to different causes of growth failure [3].

12.2.1 GROWTH AT PUBERTY

Pubertal development is associated with a rapid increase in height velocity known as the adolescent growth spurt. Any factor that suppresses growth during adolescence will compromise adult height. The amplitude of the growth spurt is greater in boys, where peak height velocity may reach 10.5 cm per year, compared with 9.0 cm per year in girls. Pubertal growth also occurs two years later in boys (Fig. 12.2), further contributing to the difference in adult height of 12.6 cm between males and females.

12.3 CLINICAL GROWTH ASSESSMENT

The assessment of growth and recognition of abnormal growth is based on accurate

228

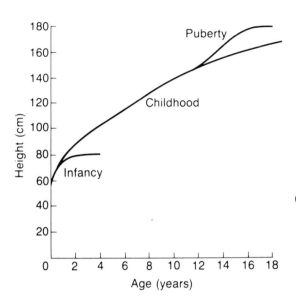

Fig. 12.1 The ICP model for attained height in boys: 50th percentile values (from [3]).

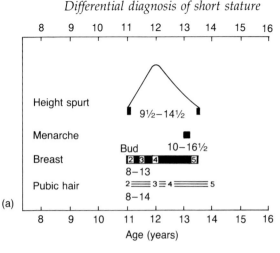

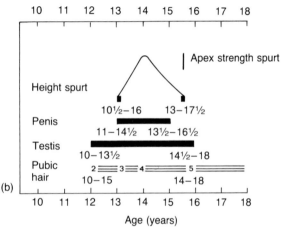

Fig. 12.2 Diagrams of the sequence of events at adolescence in (a) girls and (b) boys. The range of ages within which some of the events may occur is given by the figures placed directly below them (from [4]).

measurement techniques [5]. These need to be standardized [6], and essential equipment is listed in Table 12.1.

The heights of the child's parents should be plotted on the centile chart with a correction for sex, adding 12.6 cm to the mother's height if the child is male and subtracting the same figure from the father's height for a girl. In this way, the patient's height can be compared with parental centiles. Prediction of final adult height [7] can be calculated most accurately from height and bone age, best assessed using the Tanner–Whitehouse 2 method [8].

12.4 DIFFERENTIAL DIAGNOSIS OF SHORT STATURE

The essence of clinical short stature assessment is the diagnosis of disorders in which treatment will cause acceleration of growth and substantially improve final height. The majority of children referred for short stature are apparently healthy and the clinician needs

to be aware of treatable disorders that may not be clinically obvious, such as occult chronic systemic disease [9,10]. The assessment of upper to lower segmentations, revealing disproportionate stature, suggests skeletal dysplasias. The principal causes of short stature are listed in Table 12.2.

229

Table 12.1 Essential equipment for growth assessment

Height stadiometer[a]
Sitting height table[a]
Infant measuring table[a]
Weight scales
Orchidometer
Bone age atlas[b]
Standard percentile charts for height, height
    velocity, weight[b]

[a] Available from Holtain Ltd, Crymmych, Pembs, UK.
[b] Recommended atlases are Tanner–Whitehouse 2, and Greulich and Pyle.

Table 12.2 Principal causes of short stature

Normal height velocity
Genetic short stature
Constitutional growth delay
Low birth weight

Subnormal height velocity
Skeletal disorders (metaphyseal dysplasia)
Dysmorphic syndromes, e.g. Noonan, Aarskog
    syndromes, pseudohypoparathyroidism
Turner syndrome
Endocrine disorders
    GH insufficiency
    Hypothyroidism
    Cushing's disease
Chronic systemic disease
    Coeliac disease, Crohn's disease, ulcerative
        colitis
    Cystic fibrosis, asthma
    Cyanotic congenital heart disease
    Renal failure, renal tubular defects
    Inflammatory joint disease
Emotional deprivation

Table 12.3 Screening tests for short stature

Full blood count
ESR
Creatinine
Electrolytes
RBC folate
Liver function tests
Karyotype (in girls) for Turner syndrome
Midstream urine culture
T4
TSH

Table 12.4 Definitive tests to exclude chronic non-endocrine causes of short stature

Jejunal biopsy
Barium meal and follow through
Colonoscopy
Sweat sodium concentration
Chest X-ray
Echocardiogram
Tests of renal function
Metabolic amino acid screen
Tests of immune function

ably performed at the first outpatient vist. These tests are listed in Table 12.3.

If this is done, at the second visit the results will be available, which, together with the child's height velocity, calculated from measurements at both visits, should orientate the clinician towards either reassurance of the patient and parents or to more definitive studies such as jejunal biopsy, barium meal and follow through, or assessment of GH secretion (Table 12.4).

12.5 INVESTIGATION OF SHORT STATURE

12.5.1 LABORATORY TESTS

Every child with abnormal growth needs a number of screening tests, which are prefer-

12.5.2 RADIOLOGICAL INVESTIGATIONS

The majority of patients referred for short stature have no radiological abnormality. Delayed skeletal maturation, shown on bone assessment of the X-ray of the left hand and wrist, is common and non-specific. It does, however, give some indication of the physical maturity of the patient and can be used in the calculation of predicted adult height. Lateral skull X-ray, showing the pituitary fossa, is almost always normal and is not indicated in the asymptomatic child. In the child with headaches, vomiting, visual disturbance or proven hypopituitarism, however, it is essential to carry out X-rays and Goldman perimetry of visual fields.

High resolution computerized tomography (CT) scan or nuclear magnetic resonance (NMR) imaging of the pituitary fossa is normal in most children with short stature and in most patients with idiopathic GH insufficiency [11]. In hypopituitarism, one of these imaging techniques is indicated to exclude a structural abnormality of the pituitary region such as craniopharyngioma or a developmental lesion such as septo-optic dysplasia [12].

Skeletal X-rays are indicated in children with disproportionate short stature. Abnormalities of the skull, spine or long bones may have specific radiological features which will classify the disorder and give a prognosis for growth as well as genetic counselling (Fig. 12.3).

Radiological investigations which may be helpful in patients with growth disorders are shown in Table 12.5.

12.5.3 ASSESSMENT OF GH SECRETION

Physiological tests

Basal concentration

As GH levels in normal subjects return to undetectable levels between peaks, a basal sample is unlikely to exclude GH deficiency and is therefore not recommended.

Exercise test

The importance of this test is to standardize the amount of work the patient performs. A

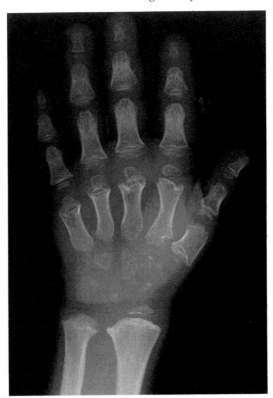

Fig. 12.3 Skeletal changes consistent with pseudoachondroplasia in a child with disproportionate (short-limbed) short stature.

Table 12.5 Radiological studies in assessment of short stature

Pituitary fossa
Left hand and wrist for bone age
High resolution CT scan of pituitary region
NMR of pituitary region
Skeletal survey (limited)

bicycle ergometer is recommended for this reason. Physical exertion should be between 150 and 300 $kilopond\,m^{-1}\,min^{-1}$, i.e. approximately 50% of maximal working capacity [13]. The child is fasted and exercises for 10 minutes. Blood samples for GH are taken at

–30, 0, 10 and 20 minutes [14]. In our experience the GH values often fall into an equivocal range, seldom formally confirming or excluding GH insufficiency.

Studies of GH pulsatility

Pulsatile GH release occurs throughout 24 hours but increases within 1–2 hours of sleep onset. Overnight venous sampling at 15–20 minute intervals can detect pulsatile GH secretion and samples obtained in this way can exclude or confirm severe GH insufficiency [15]. A good correlation exists between peak pulsatile GH values and those during insulin-induced hypoglycaemia [16].

The concept of 'neurosecretory dysfunction' i.e. 'normal' GH values on pharmacological testing in a short child with subnormal physiological release [17] is in our opinion a true phenomenon. In this situation, overnight sampling can confirm GH insufficiency, although in the absence of other pathology, this can be assumed from a subnormal height velocity.

Pharmacological tests

There are many different pharmacological tests of GH secretion. Most require an intact hypothalamo–pituitary axis. Pharmacological testing carries a false negative rate of about 15% [16]. For this reason many authorities recommend performing a second test.

Insulin tolerance test

Insulin-induced hypoglycaemia stimulates pituitary GH and adrenocorticotrophic hormone (ACTH) reserve. A reproducible and standardized hypoglycaemic stress is produced when the patient's blood glucose falls to less than $2.2\,mmol\,l^{-1}$ ($40\,mg\,100\,ml^{-1}$) and the patient is seen to sweat [18]. In response to this stimulus GH, ACTH, corticosteroids, prolactin and catecholamines should be secreted. In GH insufficiency, the GH response to hypoglycaemia is impaired. Normal plasma thyroxin and cortisol concentrations should be documented before performing the test.

The insulin dose is $0.1\,U\,kg^{-1}$ (in young children) or $0.15\,U\,kg^{-1}$ in older children and adults. The test is safe, providing there is adequate supervision; however, we do not perform it in patients under 5 years of age due to insulin sensitivity in the young child and the potential difficulty with venous access. GH levels, sampled for 90 minutes, should rise to above $40\,mU\,l^{-1}$ ($20\,ng\,ml^{-1}$). Levels between 20 and $40\,mU\,l^{-1}$ may indicate partial GH insufficiency. Twenty-five per cent dextrose ($0.2\,g\,kg^{-1}$ or $0.8\,ml\,kg^{-1}$) should be drawn up ready for use and given if consciousness is impaired. At the end of the test the children are given a meal and observed for 2–3 hours to confirm complete recovery.

Glucagon test

Glucagon stimulates GH and ACTH reserve. This test is used in children under 5 years of age or when the insulin test is contraindicated, e.g. in epilepsy or untreated ACTH deficiency. We have found the paediatric protocol of glucagon $100\,\mu g\,kg^{-1}$ i.m. [19] to produce significant hypoglycaemia in young children. Consequently, we use a lower dose of $15\,\mu g\,kg^{-1}$ i.m., which produces sufficient GH stimulation. Samples are taken for 180 minutes for GH and cortisol.

Arginine test

Intravenous infusion of arginine stimulates GH release. In children the dose is $0.5\,g\,kg^{-1}$ up to a maximum dose of 30 g over 30 minutes. Blood is sampled for GH every 30 minutes for 2 hours.

Clonidine test

This has gained favour as an alternative to the insulin test in children [20]. It does not

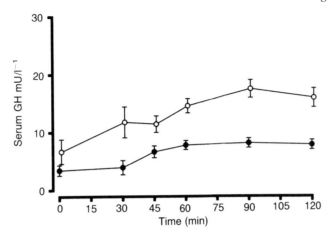

Fig. 12.4 Enhancement of the growth hormone response to insulin-induced hypoglycaemia after stilboestrol priming. (○), primed; (●), unprimed, mean ± SD (from [21]).

cause hypoglycaemia and may only induce mild drowsiness. The locus and mechanism of its action are not clear. However, the ACTH–cortisol axis is not stimulated. The dose is $0.15\,mg\,m^{-2}$ surface area given orally. Samples are taken for 3 hours.

Sex steroid priming of GH stimulation tests

Both endogenous and exogenous sex steroids are known to enhance basal and stimulated GH release. As may children demonstrate a transient GH deficiency before puberty, the enhancing effect of sex steroids on GH release has been used to differentiate these children from those with true GH insufficiency. We currently administer stilboestrol 1 mg twice daily for 2 days before the GH stimulation test [21] (Fig. 12.4) in patients with a bone age of greater than 10 years.

I.m. depot testosterone 125 mg may also be used if stilboestrol induces vomiting such that the priming dose cannot be given orally.

Growth hormone releasing hormone test

Characterization of the hypothalamic peptide growth hormone releasing hormone (GHRH) has introduced an additional tool in the assessment of GH secretion. Bolus injection of GHRH in a dose of 1–$3\,\mu g\,kg^{-1}$ selectively promotes GH release in normal male subjects [22]. The majority of patients with GH insufficiency will show a GH response to GHRH. However, the longer the duration of GH insufficiency, the poorer the response to GHRH [23].

GH responses to GHRH in GH insufficient children are lower than those in normal adults [24] (Fig. 12.5).

However, because of the marked intra- and inter-subject variability in response, the GHRH test cannot be considered a diagnostic test of GH insufficiency.

Urinary growth hormone

Measurement of urinary GH excretion has recently gained prominence as a potential means of assessing integrated GH secretion, either overnight or during 24 hours [25]. There are practical advantages over sampling plasma, however, the accuracy and physiological significance of urinary GH excretion have yet to be established.

Overnight urinary GH, measured by immunoradiometric assay, was shown to identify children with GH insufficiency [26]. There

233

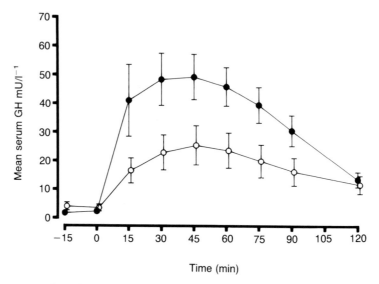

Fig. 12.5 Mean serum GH after 100 µg GHRH (1–29) NH$_2$ in 16 normal adult males and 18 short idiopathic GH deficient children (peak serum GH during insulin-induced hypoglycaemia <10 mU l^{-1}). (○), short; (●), normal, mean ± SD (from [24]).

was a strong correlation between urinary GH concentrations and peak GH levels during stimulation.

Plasma IGF-I concentration

The insulin like growth factors (IGF-I and IGF-II) both have growth promoting actions. They circulate bound to at least three specific plasma binding proteins (IGF-BP1, IGF-BP2 and IGF-BP3). IGF-I and IGF-BP3 are GH dependent. IGF-BP3 binds the majority of the circulating pool of the IGFs, binding either IGF-I or IGF-II with equal affinity. IGF-BP3 exists in equimolar concentration to the combined molar concentration of IGF-I and IGF-II [27].

In the past, studies have examined the possibility of using either plasma IGF-I or IGF-II levels as a screening test for GH deficiency. The idea is attractive because at present one can look at GH status either non-physiologically using pharmacological stimuli to produce easily quantifiable and repeatable results, or using difficult and time consuming methods one can obtain poorly repeatable assessments of the physiological secretion of GH. Thus, measurements of IGF-I concentrations could represent an easy way of assessing in a standard fashion the GH status of a subject without the use of pharmacological stimuli.

Although IGF-I or IGF-II levels generally reflect GH status there are a number of reports of either normal IGF-I or IGF-II levels in the presence of GH deficiency [28–30]. Thus, individually IGF-I or IGF-II are not reliable in identifying GH deficiency. When both IGF-I and IGF-II levels are low, however, one can make a confident diagnosis of GH deficiency [31].

Unfortunately, the matter is complicated by the fact that because of low sensitivity of the IGF-I radioimmunoassay, it is not possible to differentiate between low levels of IGF seen in early childhood and the low levels due to GH deficiency.

Recently it has been proposed that IGF-BP3

Table 12.6 Principal causes of tall stature

Genetic tall stature
Constitutional advanced growth
Cerebral gigantism (Sotos' syndrome)
Arachnodactyly and gigantism (Marfan's syndrome)
Chromosomal syndromes
Endocrine disorders
  Gigantism
  Sexual precocity
  Eunuchoidism
  Hyperthyroidism

Table 12.7 Investigations indicated in tall stature

Skull X-ray
Bone age
T4
TSH
Basal GH concentrations
Karyotype

could be used to screen for GH deficiency because this binding protein exists in equimolar concentration to IGF-I and IGF-II. If IGF-BP3 levels are low one may more easily diagnose GH deficiency [27]. This remains to be proven in field conditions.

12.6 TALL STATURE

Most children who are referred for tall stature have variations of the physiological growth pattern. The main causes of tall stature are given in Table 12.6.

Investigations indicated in patients with tall stature are shown in Table 12.7.

REFERENCES

1. Tanner, J.M. (1986) Normal growth and techniques of growth assessment. *Clin. Endocrinol. Metab.*, **15**, 411–51.
2. Karlberg, J. (1989) On the construction of the infancy–childhood–puberty growth standard. *Acta Paediat. Scand.* (suppl.), **356**, 26–37.
3. Tse, W.Y., Hindmarsh, P.C. and Brook, C.G.D. (1989) The infancy–childhood–puberty model of growth: clinical aspects. *Acta Paediat. Scand.* (suppl.), **356**, 38–43.
4. Tanner, J.M. (1962) *Growth at Adolescence*, 2nd edn, Blackwell, Oxford.
5. Brook, C.G.D. (1982) *Growth Assessment in Childhood and Adolescence*, Blackwell, Oxford.
6. Cameron, N. (1978) The methods of auxological anthropometry. In *Human Growth* (ed. F. Falkner and J.M. Tanner), Plenum Press, New York, pp. 35–87.
7. Tanner, J.M., Landt, K.W., Cameron, N., Carter, B.S. and Patel, J. (1983) Prediction of adult height from height and bone age in childhood. *Archs Dis. Childh.*, **58**, 767–76.
8. Tanner, J.M., Whitehouse, R.H., Marshall, W.A., Healy, M.J. and Goldstein, H. (1975) *Assessment of Skeletal Maturity and Prediction of Adult Height (TW2 method)*, Academic Press, London.
9. Preece, M.A., Law, C.M. and Davies, P.S.W. (1986) The growth of children with chronic paediatric disease. *Clin. Endocrinol. Metab.*, **15**, 453–77.
10. Savage, M.O. (1987) Growth and its defects. In *Recent Advances in Medicine*, vol. 20 (ed. A.M. Dawson and G.M. Besser), Churchill Livingstone, London, pp. 69–83.
11. Kendall, B. (1983) Current approaches to hypothalamicpituitary radiology. *Clin. Endocrinol. Metab.*, **12**, 535–66.
12. Leaf, A.A., Ross, R.J.M., Jones, R.B., Besser, G.M. and Savage, M.O. (1989) Response to growth hormone-releasing hormone as evidence of hypothamic defect in optic nerve hypoplasia. *Acta Paediat. Scand.*, **78**, 416–19.
13. Lacey, K.A., Hewison, A. and Parker, J.M. (1973) Exercise as a screen test for growth hormone deficiency in children. *Archs Dis. Childh.*, **57**, 944–7.
14. Hughes, I.A. (1986) *Handbook of Endocrine Tests in Children*, John Wright and Sons, Bristol.
15. Albertsson-Wikland, K. and Rosberg, S. (1988) Analysis of 24-hour growth hormone profiles in children: relation to growth. *J. Clin. Endocrinol. Metab.*, **67**, 493–500.
16. Brook, C.G.D., Hindmarsh, P.C., Smith, P.J.

and Stanhope, R. (1986) Clinical features and investigations of growth hormone deficiency. *Clin. Endocrinol. Metab.*, **15**, 479–93.

17. Spiliotis, B.E., August, G., Hung, W., Sonis, W., Mendelson, W. and Bercu, B.B. (1984) Growth hormone neurosecretory dysfunction: a treatable cause of short stature. *J. Am. Med. Ass.*, **251**, 2223–30.

18. Hall, R. and Besser, G.M. (1989) *Fundamentals of Clinical Endocrinology*, 4th edn, Churchill Livingstone, Edinburgh.

19. Vanderscheuren-Lodeweyckx, M., Wolter, R., Malvaux, P., Eggermont, E. and Eeckels, R. (1974) The glucagon stimulation test: effect on plasma growth hormone and on immunoreactive insulin, cortisol and glucose in children. *J. Pediat.*, **85**, 182–7.

20. Gil-Ad, I., Topper, E. and Laron, Z. (1977) Oral clonidine as a growth hormone stimulation test. *Lancet*, **ii**, 278–9.

21. Ross, R.J.M., Grossman, A., Davies, P.S.W., Savage, M.O. and Besser, G.M. (1987) Stilboestrol pretreatment of children with short stature does not affect the growth hormone response to growth hormone-releasing hormone. *Clin. Endocrinol.*, **27**, 155–61.

22. Grossman, A., Lytras, N., Savage, M.O., Wass, J.A.H., Coy, D.H., Rees, L.H., Jones, A.E. and Besser, G.M. (1984) Growth hormone-releasing factor: comparison of two analogues and demonstration of hypothalamic defect in growth hormone release after radiotherapy. *Br. Med. J.*, **288**, 1785–7.

23. Shriock, E.A., Lustig, R.H., Rosenthal, M., Kaplan, S.L. and Grumbach, M.M. (1987) Effect of growth hormone (GH)-releasing hormone (GRH) on plasma GH in relation to magnitude and duration of GH deficiency in 26 children and adults with isolated GH deficiency or multiple pituitary hormone deficiencies: evidence for hypothalamic GRH de-

ficiency. *J. Clin. Endocrinol. Metab.*, **58**, 1043–9.

24. Besser, G.M. and Ross, R.J.M. (1989) Are hypothalamic releasing hormones useful in the diagnosis of endocrine disorders? In *Recent Advances in Endocrinology and Metabolism*, vol. 3, Churchill Livingstone, Edinburgh, pp. 135–58.

25. Albini, C.H., Quattrin, T., Vandlen, R.L. and McGillivray, M.H. (1988) Quantitation of urinary growth hormone in children with normal and abnormal growth. *Pediat. Res.*, **23**, 89–92.

26. Walker, J.M., Wood, P.J., Williamson, S., Betts, P.R. and Evans, A.J. (1990) Urinary growth hormone excretion as a screening test for growth hormone deficiency. *Archs Dis. Childh.*, **65**, 89–92.

27. Ranke, M.B., Blum, W.F. and Bierich, J.R. (1988) Clinical relevance of serum measurements of insulin-like growth factors and somatomedin binding proteins. *Acta Paediat. Scand.* (suppl), **347**, 114.

28. Hall, K., Enberg, G., Ritzen, M., Svan, H., Fryklund, L. and Takano, K. (1980) Somatomedin A levels in serum from healthy children and from children with growth hormone deficiency or delayed puberty. *Acta Endocrinol., Copenhagen* (suppl.), **94**, 155.

29. Underwood, L.E., D'Ercole, J.A. and van Wyk, J.J. (1980) Somatomedin-C levels.

30. Zapf, J., Walters, H. and Froesch, E.R. (1981) Radioimmunological determination of insulin-like growth factors I and II in normal subjects and in patients with growth disorders and extrapancreatic tumor hypoglycaemia. *J. Clin. Invest.*, **68**, 1321.

31. Rosenfield, R.G., Wilson, D.M., Lee, P.D.K. and Hintz, R.L. (1986) Insulin-like growth factor I and II in evaluation of growth retardation. *J. Pediat.*, **109**, 428.

13

Investigation of testicular disorders

E. UR and P.M. BOULOUX

13.1 THE HYPOTHALAMO-PITUITARY-TESTICULAR AXIS

13.1.1 PHYSIOLOGICAL CONSIDERATIONS

The male gonad has a dual role in human physiology: first, the production of the gametes (spermatogenesis) which constitute the male contribution to fertilization, and second, the synthesis of an endocrine product with diverse androgenic and anabolic effects. These two function are carried out by structurally distinct compartments within the testes, seminiferous tubules and Leydig cells (Fig. 13.1), respectively.

The interstitial Leydig cells are lipid rich and polygonal in shape. They are found in small groups within the intertubular tissue, and constitute up to 10% of total testicular volume. Leydig cells are primarily under the control of pituitary luteinizing hormone (LH) which stimulates the production of testosterone and other androgens and their secretion into the circulation. A small quantity of oestradiol is also produced by the Leydig cells, although this represents only one-quarter of circulating oestradiol, the remainder originating from peripheral aromatization of testosterone and androstenedione.

Most testosterone is bound to sex hormone binding globulin (SHBG), leaving a small, physiologically active, free testosterone fraction. Secretion of testosterone takes place in the form of sharp rhythmic pulses of about 30 minutes' duration. In addition, circulating levels of testosterone show a circadian rhythmicity with a peak at 8 a.m. and a nadir at 2 a.m. Falls in testosterone are associated with the onset of REM sleep. Levels of testosterone are independent of adrenocorticotropic hormone (ACTH) and are not dexamethasone suppressible. Moreover, they do not appear to be influenced by minute to minute changes in LH secretion.

Exercise and other physical and psychological stresses cause a rapid decrease in plasma testosterone. The development of a dissociation between maintained 'normal' levels of LH and the decreased levels of testosterone is also well described in such situations. Testosterone levels rise in boys before there is clinical evidence of puberty. While normal levels may be maintained into extreme old age, as a rule after the age of 50 an increasing proportion of men show a falling off of testosterone levels with a commensurate rise in gonadotropin levels.

Androgen effects are exerted at target organs via stimulation of cytosolic receptors which, when activated, bind to nucleoproteins and initiate DNA transcription. In

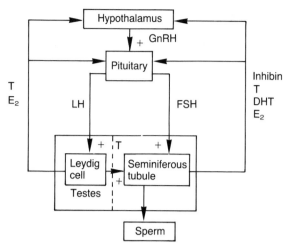

Fig. 13.1 The hypothalamo-pituitary-testicular axis. GnRH, gonadotropin releasing hormone; LH, luteinizing hormone; FSH, follicle stimulating hormone; T, testosterone; DHT, dihydrotestosterone; E_2, oestradiol.

most androgen-responsive target tissues there is local conversion of testosterone to dihydrotestosterone (DHT), a significantly more potent androgenic ligand. This reaction is catalysed by the enzyme 5α-reductase. Testosterone has an affinity 2–10 times less for the androgen receptor (range of Kd 2–12 nmol) than does dihydrotestosterone (Kd 0.5–1.7 nmol) [1–3]. The biological relevance of this is that in some settings the levels of testosterone are adequate to activate its own androgen mediated actions, whereas a biological amplification step (via 5α-reductase conversion to DHT) may be required for other processes. In particular, tissue derived from the urogenital sinus (penis, scrotum) is especially dependent on DHT as its principal androgen.

The seminiferous tubules consist of germ cells and Sertoli cells. Sertoli cells span the thickness of the tubule wall and partition it into basal and adluminal compartments. Spermatogonia in the basal compartment are continuously replenished by mitotic division.

They then migrate to the adluminal compartment where a series of divisions occurs, culminating in the production of spermatids, which are in turn transformed into spermatozoa (spermiogenesis). Sertoli cells supply nutrient to the developing spermatogenic cells. They also secrete a variety of protein growth factors which regulate and co-ordinate sperm development. The production of mature spermatozoa from immature spermatogonia takes 72 days in man and another 14 days are required for the transport of spermatozoa through the epididymis, vas deferens and ejaculatory ducts [4]. During the passage into the epididymis, spermatozoa become motile, and undergo the maturation necessary to acquire the capacity to fertilize.

Spermatogenesis is principally under the control of follicle stimulating hormone (FSH), which acts on Sertoli cells modulating the production of these local factors. Sertoli cells are also known to secrete inhibin, a recently characterized peptide which acts at the pituitary level inhibiting the secretion of FSH. Serum inhibin levels rise during puberty as a consequence of gonadal development. The significance of inhibin in relation to disorders of gonadal function such as infertility is unknown.

13.2 CLINICAL ASSESSMENT OF TESTICULAR DYSFUNCTION

Aspects of the medical history and physical examination will often lead to an aetiological diagnosis. With the infertile male, the medical history should focus on the presence of any recent or chronic medical illness, previous infections of the genito-urinary tract and surgical procedures. Febrile illness due to viral or bacterial infection occurring within a few months may temporarily suppress semen quality. Chronic illness with weight loss, renal failure and liver disease will perturb the hypothalamo-pituitary-

Table 13.1 Physical examination of the hypogonadal male

Height, weight, body proportions
Voice, fat distribution
Muscle mass
Body hair distribution
Gynaecomastia
External genitalia
Varicocele, cryptorchidism, vas deferens and
   epididymis
Testis size (use Prader orchidometer) and
   consistency
Rectal examination and prostatic size and
   consistency

testicular axis. Sinopulmonary infections should alert the clinician to underlying cystic fibrosis, immotile cilia syndrome and Young's syndrome [5]. A history of mumps orchitis may be relevant. Previous tuberculosis or venereal infection may be the cause of vas deferens blockage. Exposure to insecticides, drugs or irradiation, and gossypol are associated with infertility. A large number of drugs causing hyperprolactinaemia may suppress gonadal function. Chronic high alcohol intake is toxic to the testis, particularly spermatogenesis, and may affect testis and pituitary

function indirectly through liver disorders [6]. Heavy cigarette smoking is associated with reduced sperm quality [5]. Opiates suppress the hypothalamo-pituitary-testicular axis centrally, and androgen abuse (e.g. body builders) inhibits spermatogenesis [7]. High intratesticular temperatures suppress spermatogenesis, and the patient should be questioned about hot baths, tight underwear and saunas. Physical examination should elucidate the details shown in Table 13.1.

13.3 INVESTIGATION OF THE HYPOTHALAMIC-PITUITARY-TESTICULAR AXIS

13.3.1 ROUTINE SEMINAL ANALYSIS

Semen is collected following a minimum of two days' abstention. The specimen must be freshly produced and is collected in a sterile container (Table 13.2). Patients who do not wish to obtain a sample by masturbation may be provided with a special condom (Mylex, Chicago) which, unlike regular condoms, does not contain spermicidal agents.

Because of the inherent variability in sperm production, ideally, two or three samples should be examined several weeks apart.

Table 13.2 Semen sample collection

1. The sample container should be sterile and wide mouthed. If a plastic container is used it should be checked for possible toxic effects on the spermatozoa.
2. Patient should abstain from ejaculation for 2–7 days.
3. Sample should be collected in a room near the laboratory. If collected at home, it should be delivered to the laboratory within one hour of ejaculation.
4. The patient should carefully wash his hands and genital region, rinse the soap away and dry with a fresh towel.
5. The patient should pass urine and then collect semen by masturbation.
6. The sample must be complete and include the first portion of the ejaculate.
7. The sample must be protected from extremes of temperature (not $< -20°C$ or $> 40°C$) during transportation to laboratory.

Volume and viscosity are assessed by drawing semen into a measuring tube via a pipette. Motility and the presence of leukocytes and bacteria are assessed by immediate microscopic examination. The significance of leukocytes in semen is unclear [8], although Wolff *et al.* [9] have shown a significant relationship between increased leukocyte concentration and a decrease in sperm count motility and velocity. Peroxidase staining can distinguish between granulocytes, lymphocytes and other round cells (e.g. spermatogonia). Recent use of specific monoclonal antibodies against granulocytes, T and B lymphocytes and macrophages may permit rapid screening of semen samples and clearly distinguish leukocytes from immature germ cells [10,11]. Sperm density can be estimated with a haemocytometer, although it is preferable to use a Makler semen-counting chamber. In patients with small-volume ejaculate or a history of pelvic surgery, it is important to look at the first 10 ml of urine voided immediately after ejaculation in order to exclude retrograde ejaculation into the bladder.

Routine parameters are [12]:

---

1. Semen pH 7.2–7.8
2. Ejaculate volume (normal 2–5 ml)
3. Sperm concentration (normal $>20 \times 10^6 \, ml^{-1}$)
4. Motility (normal $>50\%$)
5. Morphology (normal $>50\%$ oval forms)
6. White blood cells <1 million per ml
7. Zinc (total) 2.4 μmol per ejaculate
8. Citric acid (total) 52 μmol per ejaculate
9. Fructose 13 μmol or more per ejaculate
10. MAR test: fewer than 10% spermatozoa with adherent particles
11. Immunobead test: fewer than 10% spermatozoa with adherent particles.

Multivariate discriminant analysis using conventional semen parameters has shown that sperm concentration and morphology are the variables that provide the most consistent and valuable information to discriminate between fertile and infertile men [13–15]. In particular, sperm morphology is most useful in predicting success in IVF [16].

13.3.2 SPERM CULTURE

This should be part of the initial seminal analysis, provided the sample has been collected correctly. The uniform growth of more than 1000 aerobic pathogens such as *E. coli*, *Bacillus proteus*, Klebsiella, or group D streptococcus, usually in association with raised leukocyte counts, is indicative of accessory gland infection [17].

13.4 SPECIALIZED TESTS

13.4.1 TESTS OF SEMINAL VESICULAR FUNCTION

This is of value in men with azoospermia. Fructose is usually produced by the seminal vesicles and transported into the vas deferens by the ejaculatory ducts. Absence of fructose may indicate congenital absence or obstruction of the seminal vesicles and vas deferens. The presence of a normal fructose content indicates a block proximal to the seminal vesicles and is an indication for vasography. The diagnosis of congenital agenesis of the vas deferens can, however, be made by a careful physical examination and the laboratory findings of low semen volume with acidic pH and absence of spermatozoa.

13.4.2 TESTS OF PROSTATIC FUNCTION

An alkaline pH may signify prostatitis. Acid phosphatase, zinc and citric acid are seminal markers of prostatic function, and L-carnitine and alpha glucosidase are markers of epididymal function. In general, infection of the genito-urinary tract leads to a fall in concentration of these markers.

13.4.3 SEMEN IMMUNOLOGY

There is an immune basis for infertility in up to 10% of cases. Normally, spermatozoa are anatomically separated from the immune system. However, contact can occur after injury or surgery, precipitating the production of autoantibodies. These can be measured in the seminal plasma and serum (antisperm antibodies). Iso-antibodies, raised by the female against the partner's sperm, can be assessed in the cervical mucus by a number of techniques (Table 13.3).

The autoantibodies coat the surface of the sperm and are most frequently associated with persistent infertility after technically successful vasectomy reversal. The most commonly used tests to detect this condition are the immunobead test and the mixed antiglobulin reaction (SpermMAR). Sperm antibodies interfere with sperm motility, decrease penetration through cervical mucus and reduce fertilizing capacity as measured by the HOPT test [18].

Table 13.3 Assessment of antisperm iso-antibodies

Gelatin agglutination test (GAT)
Tray agglutination test (TAT)
Sperm immobilization test–Isojima (SIT-I)
Micro-immobilization test
Mixed erythrocyte–spermatazoa antiglobulin
   reaction (MAR)

Immunobead test

Immunobeads are polyacrylamide beads coated with antihuman immunoglobulins which adhere to motile spermatozoa that have surface antibodies. The test is useful for screening as well as to monitor the effects of therapy [18,19].

SpermMAR test

The mixed antiglobulin reaction uses Latex particles coated with antihuman immunoglobulin. A comparison of the characteristics of the two tests is shown in Table 13.4.

This test is more sensitive than the immunobead test [20]; in addition the SpermMAR test for IgG and IgA is more practical to perform on smaller volumes of fresh untreated semen.

13.4.4 THE POST-COITAL TEST

In the post-coital test (PCT), cervical mucus at mid-cycle is aspirated within two hours of intravaginal ejaculation. At least five motile sperm should be seen in each high power field. The cervical mucus in mid-cycle is assessed for amount, clarity, cellularity, spinnbarkeit, and fern formation.

13.4.5 THE SPERM–CERVICAL MUCUS PENETRATION TEST

The sperm–cervical mucus penetration test (S–CMPT) [12] assesses sperm invasion into

Table 13.4 Comparison of immunobead and SpermMAR tests

Immunobead test	SpermMAR
Motility decreases rapidly	Motility remains good
Sperm preparation ('washing') time consuming	No sperm preparation needed
Semen volume, 0.5–2 ml	Semen volume required, 10 µl
Shelf life, 1 month	Shelf life, 1 year
IgG, IgA, IgM	IgG and IgA

the mucus *in vitro*. This is subsequently compared with the activity of a known fertile male donor. The crossover nature of this test allows the determination of defects in the woman's mucus or the man's sperm. When an interaction occurs between sperm and hostile cervical mucus glycoprotein containing antisperm antibodies, the affected sperm show abnormal shaking without progressive movement in the mucus. This phenomenon can be assessed by the sperm–cervical mucus contact (SCMC) test. The SCMC test should be performed in couples with abnormal PCT, enabling abnormalities in the sperm and cervical mucus to be assessed independently *in vitro*. A poor score is present in patients with decreased mobility, increased abnormal spermatozoa and the presence of antisperm antibodies.

13.4.6 HUMAN SPERMATOZOA–ZONA FREE HAMSTER *IN VITRO* PENETRATION TEST (HOPT)

This is a test of capacitation of human sperms. Spermatozoa are washed free of seminal plasma and incubated in capacitating culture medium. Zona free hamster eggs are then incubated with capacitated sperms for several hours. The hamster oocytes are then evaluated for swollen sperm heads within the vitellus.

13.4.7 TESTICULAR BIOPSY

The indications for testicular biopsy are few; it is usually performed where a neoplasm is suspected. It is also indicated in patients with obstructive azoospermia to confirm quantitatively normal spermatogenesis before definitive surgical reanastomosis or epididymal aspiration of spermatozoa for IVF are performed.

13.4.8 BASAL ENDOCRINE TESTS OF HYPOTHALAMO-PITUITARY-TESTICULAR AXIS

Blood should be sampled at 9 a.m. for testosterone, oestradiol, LH/FSH, prolactin, free thyroxine (FT4) and SHBG. In general, basal investigations are adequate to reach a probable aetiological diagnosis [21,22]. Low concentrations of FSH, LH and testosterone indicate hypothalamo-pituitary disease, whereas high concentrations of LH and FSH with low values of testosterone indicate primary testicular failure. Isolated rises in FSH associated with azoospermia indicate Sertoli cell damage, and isolated LH rise suggests Leydig cell damage or insensitivity to the action of testosterone. Low gonadotropins with a raised testosterone and oestradiol may occur in Leydig cell tumours of the testes.

The glycoprotein SHBG binds circulating androgens, and influences free androgen levels. It has two binding sites: one specifically binds the steroid hormone, the other binds to sites on the plasma membrane. Binding to the cell membrane leaves it capable of binding the androgen. If a steroid then binds to the SHBG-membrane receptor complex, a second messenger system is activated [23]. Thus, it is possible for sex steroids to activate intracellular second messengers through their binding to SHBG in addition to direct binding of androgen to the intracellular steroid receptor. A number of factors can influence SHBG (Table 13.5).

13.5 DYNAMIC HORMONE TESTS

13.5.1 CLOMIPHENE STIMULATION TEST

Clomiphene is a non-steroidal compound with weak oestrogenic effects which binds to oestrogen receptors. Hypothalamic feedback control of the pituitary-gonadal axis by

Table 13.5 Factors affecting the concentration of SHBG

Increased SHBG
Oestrogens
Thyroid hormone
Phenytoin
Anorexia nervosa
Ageing in men
Decreased SHBG
Androgens
Obesity
Glucocorticoids

androgens is mediated by oestradiol, which is derived from central aromatization of testosterone. Thus, when clomiphene competitively occupies hypothalamic oestrogen receptors, the apparent oestradiol deficiency will lead to gonadotropin releasing hormone (GnRH) stimulation and LH/FSH release.

Procedure

The clomiphene stimulation test is performed by administering clomiphene at a dose of $3\,mg\,kg^{-1}$ in divided doses (maximum 100 mg bd) over the course of seven days. Clomiphene may cause mild visual disturbances or depression (occasionally this is severe enough to warrant discontinuation of the test). Blood is taken for LH/FSH determination at days 0, 4, 7 and 10. Normally LH/FSH levels should increase twofold over basal [24].

Interpretation

Lack of response suggests gonadotropin deficiency due to pituitary or hypothalamic disease. The measurement of testosterone in this test is not helpful as clomiphene will elevate SHBG and thus testosterone via its oestrogenic effects.

13.5.2 HUMAN CHORIONIC GONADOTROPIN STIMULATION TEST

Human chorionic gonadotropin (HCG) has similar biological actions to LH, although it has a considerably longer half-life. It stimulates Leydig cells via LH receptors and thus promotes testicular androgen and to a lesser extent oestrogen secretion. In the HCG stimulation test, HCG administration is used in order to determine the presence of functioning Leydig cells [25,26].

Procedure

HCG is given intramuscularly at a dose of 2000 IU on days 0 and 2. Serum testosterone is monitored on days 0, 2 and 4.

Interpretation

A physiological response is a rise in testosterone to outside the normal range. This confirms the presence of a testis. Where there is no palpable testis in the scrotum, such a result would suggest an intra-abdominal or inguinal gonad. In cases of gonadotropin deficiency, where there is no primary testicular abnormality, the low basal testosterone should triple after HCG. The failure of testosterone to rise after HCG suggests the absence of functioning testicular tissue.

13.5.3 FLUOXYMESTERONE SUPPRESSION TEST

Fluoxymesterone is an orally active androgen used to investigate the pituitary-gonadal axis in order to assess for possible autonomous secretion of testosterone, LH or FSH. Fluoxymesterone is contraindicated in patients with prostatic carcinoma. In about 2% of subjects, intrahepatic cholestatic jaundice may occur, which resolves upon discontinuing the drug.

Procedure

In the fluoxymesterone suppression test, 10 mg of fluoxymesterone are administered orally 6-hourly for 10 days. Serum testosterone, LH and FSH are measured on days 0, 4, 7 and 10.

Interpretation

Normally, all three hormones should be suppressed following administration of fluoxymesterone. When failure of suppression occurs, this suggests autonomous secretion of gonadotropin (for example, gonadotropinoma) or testosterone (for example, testosterone secreting testicular tumour).

13.5.4 GONADOTROPIN RELEASING HORMONE TEST

GnRH acts directly on the anterior pituitary and stimulates secretion of both LH and FSH.

Procedure

The GnRH test is administered in non-fasting individuals, unless combined, as it often is, with other dynamic tests of pituitary function such as an insulin tolerance test and a thyrotropin releasing hormone (TRH) test. An intravenous cannula is inserted at 8.30 a.m. GnRH at a dose of 100 µg is administered intravenously at 9 a.m. Blood for serum LH and FSH levels is taken at 0, 20 and 60 minutes [27].

Interpretation

The normal response is a rise in LH and FSH. Peak levels may be seen either at 20 or 60 minutes (Table 13.6).

Interpretation

The GnRH response will be subnormal in primary pituitary disease and normal or ex-

Table 13.6 LH/FSH response to GnRH (100 µg i.v.)

Time	Serum LH (mUl^{-1})	Serum FSH (mUl^{-1})
20 minutes	13–58	1–7
60 minutes	11–48	1–5

aggerated in patients with hypothalamic disorders.

13.6 SPECIFIC PATHOLOGIES OF THE HYPOTHALAMO-PITUITARY-TESTICULAR AXIS

13.6.1 CLINICAL FEATURES AND CLASSIFICATION OF MALE HYPOGONADISM

Male hypogonadism is best classified according to the site of the lesion in the hypothalamo-pituitary-testicular hierarchy. Thus we may distinguish disorders consequent to primary gonadal failure, where there are high levels of gonadotropins as a result of the loss of feedback signal (hypergonadotropic hypogonadism), from those due to a loss of gonadotropic drive (hypogonadotropic hypogonadism) (Table 13.7).

Clinical features depend upon the state of development at the time of onset. Androgen deficiency in the first trimester of foetal life will result in ambiguous genitalia (see Chapter 6). Where hypogonadism begins prior to the onset of puberty, there is poor development of secondary sexual characteristics associated with a eunuchoid habitus. There is no pubertal androgen-stimulated growth spurt, but long bones continue to grow under the influence of GH in the absence of epiphysial fusion.

Hypogonadism which develops after the onset of puberty may present with diminution of libido or erectile failure. Chronic and severe androgen deficiency will result in loss of secondary sex hair.

Table 13.7 Classification of male hypogonadism

Hypothalamic-pituitary (hypogonadotropic)	Hypopituitarism, pituitary tumour Kallmann's syndrome Hyperprolactinaemia Severe systemic disease Oestrogen-secreting tumour
Testicular	Congenital 　Klinefelter Acquired 　Orchitis 　Trauma 　Drugs 　Autoimmune disorders 　Systemic disease
Defects of androgen action	Testicular feminization Incomplete androgen resistance 　Type I (Reifenstein) 　Type II (5α-reductase deficiency)

13.6.2 HYPOGONADOTROPIC HYPOGONADISM

Kallmann syndrome

This form of selective hypogonadotropic hypogonadism occurs both sporadically and in an inherited form. The condition is generally inherited as an X-linked trait, although autosomal forms are also documented.

The primary defect is a result of defective migration of GnRH-producing neurons from the primitive olfactory placode to the arcuate nucleus. This results in failure of GnRH secretion into the hypothalamo-hypophyseal portal vessels. In normal individuals, this production mediates the pulsatile LH secretion which precipitates sexual maturation at puberty. Characteristically, affected individuals are hypogonadal with low levels of LH and FSH.

Clinically, the syndrome is associated with partial or complete anosmia as well as other midline abnormalities, and in the X-linked form a 50% incidence of unilateral renal agenesis [28]. In adulthood, the diagnosis is straightforward once structural hypothalamic and pituitary abnormalities are excluded, most readily by computerized tomography (CT) or magnetic resonance imaging (MRI). The presenting features are micropenis, undescended testicles and delayed puberty. Formal smell testing may be undertaken in order to confirm associated anosmia.

In early puberty the diagnosis is more difficult to make, and is suggested by the clinical features of hypogonadism and the presence of a family history as well as anosmia. However, it is often necessary to undertake a number of dynamic stratagems in order to differentiate cases of Kallmann from patients with delayed puberty (Table 13.8).

Investigations

Overnight sampling may be undertaken looking for the characteristic nocturnal LH pulses of puberty. Clomiphene citrate, which normally induces LH secretion by blocking gonadal feedback, has no such effect in Kallmann syndrome. In prepubertal individ-

Table 13.8 Dynamic stratagems in the diagnosis of Kallmann's syndrome

---

Absence of LH pulses during overnight sampling
Absence of LH rise in response to clomiphene citrate administration
Attenuated testosterone response to HCG
Attenuated prolactin response to TRH
Attenuated LH response to GnRH

---

uals the administration of 2000 IU of HCG results in significantly lower levels of testosterone, as measured after 4 days, in hypogonadotropic patients as compared with normal subjects.

In pubertal individuals, the test is modified by administering two doses of 2000 IU HCG and measuring the testosterone response after 4 and 15 days. Prolactin responses to TRH and LH responses to GnRH are also found to be attenuated. Most centres use a combination of these tests in order to increase diagnostic specificity.

Klinefelter syndrome

This is the most common chromosomal cause of androgen deficiency and infertility. It has an incidence of 1 in 500 males and manifests clinically with variable degrees of seminiferous tubule failure and decreased Leydig cell function. The underlying defect is the presence of one or more additional X chromosomes as revealed by karyotypic analysis: a consequence of maternal non-disjunction.

Apart from some degree of intellectual impairment, there are usually no symptoms prior to the onset of puberty. Patients present as tall phenotypic males with gynaecomastia, a eunuchoid habitus and small firm testes. Histologically, these show severely sclerosed tubules which are lined only by Sertoli cells. More often than not there is a total failure of spermatogenesis. Leydig cells are plentiful but ultrastructurally lack components of the cellular secreting apparatus.

Investigations

Basal endocrinology will reveal a low testosterone in the presence of high gonadotropins, placing the lesion at the level of the testes. Diagnostic confirmation is achieved by chromosomal analysis which will demonstrate the presence of one or more Barr-bodies (inactivated X chromosomes).

13.6.3 DISORDERS OF ANDROGEN SENSITIVITY

Upon entering a target cell, testosterone is converted by 5α-reductase to DHT, which binds to a receptor protein and enters the nucleus in order to effect transcription of the proteins that mediate the androgen effect (Fig. 13.2).

There are a number of clinical syndromes associated with abnormalities of androgen activity on a cellular level.

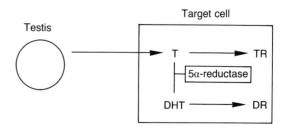

Fig. 13.2 Intracellular actions of testosterone. T, testosterone; DHT, dihydrotestosterone; TR, testosterone/receptor protein complex; DR, dihydrotestosterone/receptor protein complex.

Testicular feminization syndrome

These patients are phenotypically normal women who lack pubic and axillary (androgen-dependent) hair and internal female genitalia. Genotypically they are 46, XY carrying an X-linked recessive gene which renders target organ insensitivity to androgen. This is a consequence of qualitative (e.g. resulting from mutations within the nine exons that make up the gene) or quantitative (e.g. absent) changes in the androgen receptor.

Feminization occurs as a result of the unopposed action of adrenal and testicular oestrogens. Crypto-orchid testicles may be found in the inguinal canal or the abdomen and need to be removed because of the danger of malignant change in 10% of cases. Patients present as females with amenorrhoea and infertility, frequently with a labial or inguinal mass, and a history of an affected sister, aunt or cousin. A phenotypic female with primary amenorrhoea, breast development, scant or absent pubic and axillary hair, a shallow vagina and absent cervix and an XY karyotype has complete resistance (Table 13.9).

Before puberty, the differential diagnosis includes defects of testosterone biosynthesis and 5α-reductase deficiency.

Investigations

Individuals with testicular feminization syndrome have a markedly elevated plasma testosterone with no evidence of virilization. LH levels are also elevated but FSH is normal. In the prepubertal patient, the family history, phenotype, endocrine evaluation including the C19 and C21 responses to HCG and ACTH, determination of androgen receptor activity, and if necessary metabolic responses to testosterone are used to establish the diagnosis. DNA analysis using the PCR/sequencing strategy will play an increasingly important role in future.

Reifenstein's syndrome

These patients have incomplete androgen resistance as a consequence of partial androgen receptor activity deficiency. They have a 46, XY genotype with normal Wolffian structures but ambiguous external genitalia with wide variation in the degree of masculinization: a function of the degree of andro-

Table 13.9 Features of complete androgen resistance

XY karyotype
X-linked recessive inheritance
Genitalia: female with blind vaginal pouch
Wolffian ducts usually absent; less commonly; rudimentary or
    hypoplastic
Mullerian duct derivatives absent
Gonads: testes
Scant or absent public and axillary hair; 'hairless woman'
Plasma LH raised, testosterone raised, increased oestradiol (for men)
FSH often normal or slightly raised
Androgen receptor studies:
    Low or undetectable amount of normal receptor
    Unstable receptor
    Receptor positive form (abnormal receptor)
    Molecular genetic demonstration of absent or mutant gene

gen resistance. Plasma LH, testosterone and oestradiol levels are markedly elevated.

5α-Reductase deficiency

This genetically acquired condition, associated with a 46, XY karyotype results in male pseudohermaphroditism as a consequence of the absence of DHT (which is responsible for the masculinization of the external genitalia) but not testosterone (which brings about the development of Wolffian duct derivatives). Affected individuals are born with ambiguous external genitalia: a small hypospadic phallus, inguinal testes and a blind vaginal pouch.

At puberty, virilization occurs under the control of testosterone: the phallus enlarges and the testes enlarge and descend into the labia. In view of this virilization, gender identity often changes from female to male at puberty.

Investigations

These reveal that plasma testosterone concentrations are normal but DHT levels are very low. The high testosterone/DHT ratio is even more exaggerated following HCG stimulation. The 5α-reductase deficiency can be detected in cultured skin fibroblasts, thus confirming the diagnosis.

13.6.4 DELAYED PUBERTY

Delayed puberty is defined as the presence of testes less than 2.5 cm in axial length at the age of 14. This definition designates pubertal development less than 2.5 standard deviation below the mean and will include 0.6% of the normal population who have constitutional developmental delay. These individuals may often be distinguished by the presence of a family history of delayed but spontaneous puberty among parents or siblings. They also show maintenance of a normal growth velocity for their bone age.

Nevertheless, this diagnosis is often not readily established and it may become necessary to undertake investigation in order to exclude hypogonadism (see Table 13.7). The main difficulty in differential diagnosis is in distinguishing between constitutional delay and hypothalamic hypogonadism (particularly in the absence of anosmia). A series of dynamic stratagems must be employed (see Table 13.8).

13.6.5 GYNAECOMASTIA

Gynaecomastia is characterized by the bilateral or unilateral concentric increase of breast glandular and stromal tissue in the male. The most common differential diagnosis for breast enlargement is the deposition of fat tissue, but in unilateral cases, particularly when the glandular tissue is eccentric, it is important to exclude carcinoma of the male breast. This can be readily excluded by mammography and/or biopsy.

The principal causes of gynaecomastia and their pathophysiologies are listed in Table 13.10.

Most of these aetiologies have in common a relative imbalance between oestrogen and androgen concentrations brought about by a variety of mechanisms. Drug-induced causes should be excluded on the basis of history. It should be noted that patients may be reluctant to attest to the use of marijuana, amphetamines and methadone. Therefore, a urinary drug screen in order to detect these compounds in appropriate patients may be a worthwhile first-line test. Once this has been carried out, investigation of gynaecomastia is relatively straightforward as it essentially involves only basal hormonal estimations.

Investigations

There is usually no elevation of oestrogens *per se*, although it is important to exclude feminizing oestrogen secreting adrenal and

Table 13.10 Classification of gynaecomastia

↓ Free testosterone:
   Primary gonadal failure
   ↑ SHBG, e.g. hyperthyroidism, liver disease

↑ Oestrogen:
   Feminizing adrenocortical adenoma
   Leydig cell tumour

↑ Gonadotropins → Leydig cell stimulation → ↑ oestrogen relative to
(e.g. Klinefelters,   testosterone
   puberty)

HCG-producing tumours → Leydig cell stimulation (trophoblast/
   non-trophoblast)

↑ Prolactin: mammotrophic action

Drugs:
   Phenothiazines (↑ prolactin)
   Spironolactone (↓ androgen production)
   Cimetidine (antagonises androgen activity)

↑ Breast tissue sensitivity – familial/idiopathic gynaecomastia

Leydig cell tumours. Low levels of testosterone will be found in primary gonadal failure. An elevated SHBG may be found as a consequence of thyrotoxicosis. HCG secreting neoplasms may be detected by determination of serum HCG by β-subunit radioimmunoassay. Serum prolactin elevation in the absence of an obvious pharmacological aetiology must be followed up by visual field determination and assessment of the pituitary gland by means of high resolution CT. If clinical findings are suggestive of a Klinefelter phenotype (for example, the presence of bilaterally small testes and the persistence of pubertal gynaecomastia) a buccal smear or karyotypic analysis must be undertaken. Abnormalities of liver and thyroid function may be readily excluded by biochemistry. It is important to bear in mind that many causes will remain idiopathic.

13.6.6 MALE INFERTILITY

One in ten couples seeks medical attention for infertility. Of those, 40% of cases can be attributed to male factors. These factors and their frequency of occurrence are listed in Table 13.11.

At least one year of regular unprotected intercourse should have elapsed before investigations are undertaken. Although this chapter deals only with male aspects, both partners should be seen and investigated. In 20% of cases, factors can be attributed to both partners.

Diminished libido and defective technique should be established on the basis of history. Structural abnormalities such as varicocele (the single most common factor) should be sought by physical examination. This is best done with the patient standing up.

Investigations

All subjects with infertility should have semen analysis and, if normal, a post-coital test and semen immunology studies, as described above. If physical examination and baseline endocrinology suggest hypogonadism, investigations should be carried out in order to

Table 13.11 Classification of male infertility

Structural abnormalities
Varicocele (40%)
Ductal obstruction (10%)
Retrograde ejaculation
Seminal vesicle/prostatic disease
Anatomic defects of penis e.g. hypospadias

Endocrine disorders
Hypothalamic-pituitary (5%), e.g. Kallmann's syndrome, pituitary
   tumours
Testicular (10%), e.g. Klinefelter's syndrome, cryptorchidism,
   seminiferous tubule failure
Hyper/hypothyroidism
Hyperprolactinaemia

Sexual dysfunction/Poor coital technique

Antibodies to sperm or seminal plasma (5%)

exclude the diagnoses listed in Table 13.7. Disorders of thyroid and adrenal function may be excluded by biochemical assessment. Prolactin determination is also mandatory as hyperprolactinaemia may cause otherwise silent infertility. In these circumstances, the elevated prolactin may be the only abnormal finding in what is an eminently treatable condition. In the presence of normal size testes, azoospermia or oligospermia should be investigated by vasography and testicular biopsy in order to establish the diagnosis of ductal obstruction.

REFERENCES

1. Grino, P.B., Griffin, J.E. and Wilson, J.D. (1990) Testosterone at high concentrations interacts with the human androgen receptor similarly to dihydrotestosterone. *Endocrinology*, **126**, 1165–72.
2. Wilbert, D.M., Griffin, J.E. and Wilson, J.D. (1983) Characterization of the cytosol androgen receptor of the human prostate. *J. Clin. Endocrinol. Metab.*, **56**, 113–20.
3. Kovacs, W.J., Griffin, J.E., Weaver, D.D. *et al.* (1984) A mutation that causes lability of the androgen receptor under conditions that normally promote transformation to the DNA-binding state. *J. Clin. Invest.*, **73**, 1095–104.
4. Heller, C.G. and Clermont, Y. (1964) Kinetics of germinal epithelium in man. *Recent Prog. Horm. Res.*, **20**, 545–71.
5. Handelsman, D.J., Conway, A.J., Boylan, L.M. *et al.* (1984) Testicular function in potential sperm donors: Normal ranges and the effects of smoking and varicocele. *Int. J. Androl.*, **7**, 369–82.
6. Boyden, T.W. and Pamenter, R.W. (1983) Effects of ethanol on the male hypothalamo-pituitary-gonadal axis. *Endocr. Rev.*, **4**, 389–95.
7. Wilson, J.D. (1988) Androgen abuse by athletes. *Endocr. Rev.*, **9**, 181–99.
8. Barratt, C.L.R., Bolton, A.E. and Cooke, I.D. (1990) Functional significance of white blood cells in the male and female reproductive tract. *Hum. Reproduction*, **5**, 639–48.
9. Wolff, H., Politch, J.A., Martinez, A. *et al.* (1990) Leukocytospermia is associated with poor semen quality. *Fertil. Steril.*, **53**, 528–36.
10. El-Demiry, M.I.M., Young, H., Elton, R.A. *et al.* (1986) Leukocytes in the ejaculate of fertile and infertile men. *Br. J. Urol.*, **58**, 715–20.
11. Wolff, H. and Anderson, D.J. (1988) Immuno-

histologic characterization and quantification of leukocyte subpopulations in human semen. *Fertil. Steril.*, **49**, 497–504.

12. World Health Organization (1992) *Laboratory Manual for the Examination of Semen and Sperm–Cervical Mucus Interaction*, 3rd edn, Cambridge University Press, Cambridge.

13. Sherins, R.J., Brightwell, D. and Sternthal, P.M. (1977) Longitudinal analysis of semen of fertile and infertile men. In *The Testes in Normal and Infertile Men* (ed. P. Troen and Nankin), Raven Press, New York, pp. 473–88.

14. Wicklings, E.J., Freischem, C.W., Langer, K. and Neislag, E. (1983) Heterologous ovum penetration test and seminal parameters in fertile and infertile men. *J. Androl.*, **4**, 261–71.

15. Wang, C., Chan, S.Y.W., Ng, M. *et al.* (1988) Diagnostic value of sperm function tests and routine semen analyses in fertile and infertile men. *J. Androl.*, **9**, 384–9.

16. Oehninger, S., Acosta, A.A., Morshedi, M. *et al.* (1988) Corrective measures and pregnancy outcome in *in-vitro* fertilization in patients with severe sperm morphology abnormalities. *Fertil. Steril.*, **50**, 283–7.

17. Comhaire, F., Verschraegen, G. and Vermeulen, L. (1980) Diagnosis of accessory gland infection and its possible role in male infertility. *Int. J. Androl.*, **3**, 32–45.

18. Bronson, R.A., Cooper, G.W. and Rosenfeld, D.L. (1984) Sperm antibodies: their role in infertility. *Fertil. Steril.*, **42**, 171–6.

19. Clark, G.N., Elliott, P.J. and Smailer, C. (1985) Detection of sperm antibodies in semen using the immunobead test: A survey of 813 consecutive patients. *Am. J. Reproductive Immunol. Microbiol.*, **7**, 118–23.

20. Ackerman, S., McGuire, G., Fulgham, D.L. and Alexander, N.J. (1988) An evaluation of a commercially available assay for the detection of antisperm antibodies. *Fertil. Steril.*, **49**, 732–4.

21. Swerdloff, R.S., Wang, C. and Kandeel, F.C. (1988) Evaluation of the infertile couple. *Endocrinol. Metab. Clin. North Am.*, **17**, 301–37.

22. Swerdloff, R.S., Wang, C. and Sokol, R.Z. (1991) Endocrine evaluation of the infertile male. In *Infertility in the Male* (ed. L.I. Lipshultz and S.S. Howards), C.V. Mosby, St Louis, pp. 179–210.

23. Rosner, W. (1990) The functions of corticosteroid-binding globulin and sex-hormone binding globulin: Recent advances. *Endocr. Rev.*, **11**, 80–91.

24. Anderson, D.C., Marshall, J.C., Young, J.L. *et al.* (1972) Stimulation tests of pituitary-Leydig cell function in normal male subjects and hypogonadal men. *Clin. Endocrinol.*, **1**, 127–40.

25. Grant, D.B., Laurence, B.M., Atherden, S.M. *et al.* (1976) HCG stimulation test in children with abnormal sexual development. *Archs Dis. Childh.*, **51**, 596–601.

26. Toublanc, J.E., Canlorbe, P. and Job, J.C. (1975) Evaluation of Leydig cell function in normal pubertal and prepubertal boys. *J. Steroid Biochem.*, **6**, 95–9.

27. Mortimer, C.H., Besser, G.M., McNeill, A.S. *et al.* (1973) Luteinizing hormone and follicle stimulating hormone releasing hormone test in patients with hypothalamic-pituitary-gonadal dysfunction. *Br. Med. J.*, **4**, 73–7.

28. Bouloux, P.M.G., Munroe, P., Kirk, J. and Besser, G.M. (1992) Sex and smell: An enigma resolved. *J. Endocrinol.*, **133**, 323–6.

14

The diagnosis of adrenal failure

P.J. TRAINER and L.H. REES

14.1 INTRODUCTION

The principal function of the adrenal glands, which weigh 5–7 g each, is the production and secretion of three classes of hormones. Glucocorticoids are synthesized in the zona fasciculata and reticularis of the inner cortex under regulation by adrenocorticotropic hormone (ACTH). The most important glucocorticoid in man is cortisol, and approximately 15–20 mg is secreted per day, under basal conditions. Mineralocorticoids, of which aldosterone is the principal, are released from the zona glomerulosa of the adrenal cortex under the regulation of the renin–angiotensin system. In response to stimulation by preganglionic cholinergic nerves, the adrenal medulla, which accounts for about 10% of the gland, secretes the catecholamines: adrenalin, noradrenalin and dopamine. Destruction of the adrenal medulla has been shown to result in a lower catecholamine response to stress, but this is not of any apparent clinical consequence and there is no need for replacement therapy.

Destruction of 90% of both adrenal glands is necessary before glucocorticoid and mineralocorticoid deficiency become significant [1].

14.2 DIAGNOSIS OF ADRENOCORTICAL INSUFFICIENCY

The clinical signs and symptoms at presentation of hypoadrenalism vary depending on the aetiology and the degree of decompensation. The classical symptomatology of hyperpigmentation, postural hypotension, lethargy, weight loss, nausea, vomiting, diarrhoea and abdominal pain may be of such insidious onset that long delays can occur before medical help is sought or the diagnosis considered. Some patients may have sufficient adrenal function to remain relatively symptom free for a long time, only to have a hypoadrenal crisis precipitated by what would normally be a trivial illness.

Neonatal hypoadrenalism, usually secondary to congenital adrenal hyperplasia or hypoplasia, can present with either a salt losing crisis or, typically, at one week of age when the transplacental supply of maternal cortisol is exhausted, with hyperpigmentation and failure to thrive.

14.2.1 DISEASE CLASSIFICATION
(see Table 14.1)

Adrenal insufficiency can be primary, namely disease of the adrenal glands, or secondary to ACTH deficiency, due to hypothalamo-

252

Table 14.1 The aetiology of primary adrenal failure

Autoimmune

Infection
Tuberculosis
Fungal infection
Acquired immune deficiency syndrome (AIDS)

Congenital
Adrenal hyperplasia
ACTH resistance

Hereditory
Adrenoleucodystrophy
Adrenomyeloneuropathy

Drugs inhibiting cortisol synthesis
Aminoglutethamide
Metyrapone
*o,p'*DDD
Ketoconazole
Suramin

Drugs increasing cortisol clearance
Barbiturates
Phenytoin
Rifampicin

Other
Haemorrhage (Friderichsen–Waterhouse syndrome)
Metastatic tumour (commonly lung)
Amyloidosis
Sarcoidosis
Bilateral adrenalectomy
Anti-coagulant therapy

pituitary failure. Hyperpigmentation, initially found in skin creases and buccal mucosa, results from the grossly elevated plasma ACTH levels seen in primary adrenal failure consequent upon the feedback stimulation of the pituitary. Secondary adrenal failure does not cause insufficiency of mineralocorticoid production, and hence mineralocorticoid replacement is appropriate only in primary adrenal failure.

14.2.2 DIAGNOSTIC PITFALLS

A potentially serious source of diagnostic confusion in the acutely ill patient with hyponatraemia is the syndrome of inappropriate anti-diuretic hormone secretion (SIADH). However, the measurement of serum and urine osmolality and confirmation of the SIADH allows the instigation of fluid restriction, the opposite therapy to that required for hypoadrenalism.

14.3 DIAGNOSTIC TESTS OF ADRENAL FAILURE

14.3.1 BIOCHEMICAL FEATURES

Hyponatraemia, hyperkalaemia and elevation of plasma urea are the most common biochemical abnormalities in hypoadrenalism, with hypercalcaemia being present in approximately 6% and, rarely, a low plasma magnesium [2].

Hypoglycaemia is a recognized feature of a hypoadrenal crisis and probably occurs as the result of impaired gluconeogenesis; it is particularly common in children presenting with hypoadrenalism.

Anaemia, with an associated eosinophilia, is common at presentation and rapidly resolves with treatment, the eosinophilia within hours.

14.3.2 CORTISOL AND ACTH

If in an emergency situation a hypoadrenal crisis is suspected, the diagnosis can usually be established by obtaining plasma for ACTH and cortisol. Care should be exercised in handling the samples for ACTH (see Chapter 1).

Interpretation

A plasma cortisol $<200\,\text{nmol}\,\text{l}^{-1}$ and an ACTH $>200\,\text{pg}\,\text{ml}^{-1}$ in an ill patient is diagnostic of primary adrenal failure. If doubt exists as to the diagnosis and more detailed investigation is required, patients can be put on dexamethasone, thus avoiding cross-reactivity in cortisol assays, and be thoroughly investigated.

14.3.3 ACTH STIMULATION TESTS

ACTH stimulation tests (AST) are the 'gold standard' for the diagnosis of adrenal insufficiency.

Procedure

The short AST involves the intramuscular administration at 9 a.m. of 250 mcg of soluble synthetic 1–24 ACTH (tetracosactrin, Synacthen) and the measurement of serum cortisol at 0, 30 and 60 minutes.

The long AST is performed in a similar manner except 1 mg of depot ACTH is used and additional samples are taken at 90 and 120 minutes plus 4, 6, 8, 12 and 24 hours. Note that the cortisol response to 1 mg of depot ACTH in the first hour is superimposable on that seen with 250 mcg of soluble ACTH (Fig. 14.1).

Interpretation

A failure to respond to a short AST suggests adrenal failure or atrophy. Primary adrenal failure can only be confidently excluded by a long AST and, therefore, if this is thought to be the diagnosis a short AST is unnecessary. Plasma cortisol should remain low throughout the 24 hours of the long test.

The normal ranges for serum cortisol used in the interpretation of AST need to be established for each laboratory. With our assay in a healthy subject serum cortisol should be $>580\,\text{nmol}\,l^{-1}$ with an increment of >200 $\text{nmol}\,l^{-1}$ 60 minutes after either soluble or depot ACTH and $>1000\,\text{nmol}\,l^{-1}$ 8 hours after depot ACTH [3].

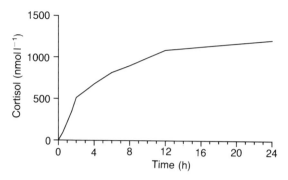

Fig. 14.1 A long Synacthen test in a patient with secondary hypoadrenalism due to pituitary tumour. Intramuscular depot Synacthen (1 mg) was administered at 9 a.m. (zero hours).

14.4 DIAGNOSIS OF SECONDARY ADRENAL FAILURE

14.4.1 ACTH

Measurement of plasma ACTH is obviously of value in the differentiation between primary adrenal disease and secondary hypoadrenalism, a value of $>200\,\text{pg}\,\text{ml}^{-1}$ being indicative of primary adrenal failure. A random plasma ACTH in the normal range does not exclude secondary adrenal insufficiency (see Table 14.2).

14.4.2 LONG AST

Very rarely a patient with secondary adrenal atrophy may not respond to 1 mg of depot ACTH, in which case repeating the same dose for 3 days followed by a repeat short AST on the fourth morning is useful both as a diagnostic and as a therapeutic manoeuvre. In our experience 100% of patients with secondary adrenal failure, including those on exogenous glucocorticoid therapy, have an adequate cortisol response to the short AST stimulation test on day 4, as opposed to primary adrenal failure, where a cortisol increment is still absent. The supraphysiological stimulation of the adrenals by three days of

Table 14.2 The aetiology of secondary adrenal failure

Pituitary
1. Compression
   Functionless
   Prolactinoma
   Growth hormone secreting
   Metastatic (commonly breast or lung)
   Infiltrative (commonly sphenoid ridge meningioma)
   Rathke's pouch cyst
2. Vascular
   Infarction of tumour (pituitary apoplexy)
   Postpartum haemorrhage (Sheehan's syndrome)
   Trauma
3. Other
   Sarcoidosis
   Histocytosis X
   Acute intermittent porphyria
   Haemochromatosis
   Irradiation
   Hypophysectomy
   Exogenous glucocorticoid therapy (including skin creams and
      inhaled steroids)
   ACTH therapy
   Idiopathic
   Isolated ACTH deficiency

Supra-pituitary
1. Tumours
   Craniopharyngioma
   Pinealoma
   Chordoma
   Third ventricle
   Optic chiasm (commonly glioma)
   Metastatic
2. Vascular
   Aneurysms
   Arteriovenous malformations
   Acute epidural and sub-dural haematoma (post-traumatic)
   Subarachnoid haemorrhage
3. Other
   Tuberculosis
   Sarcoidosis
   Histocytosis X
   Anencephaly
   Irradiation
   Exogenous glucocorticoid therapy (including skin creams and
      inhaled steroids)
   ACTH therapy
   Anorexia nervosa
   Isolated CRH deficiency
   Idiopathic

depot ACTH can be of therapeutic value. In patients in whom pituitary secretion of ACTH is recovering from a period of suppression, hypoadrenalism can persist due to adrenal atrophy, which may be reversed by depot ACTH.

In secondary adrenal failure serum cortisol will rise slowly, peaking at the end of the 24 hours rather than at 4–8 hours as seen in the healthy individual.

Interpretation of AST in patients on glucocorticoid

A normal cortisol response to an AST stimulation test does not mean that it is safe to discontinue glucocorticoid therapy, as the principal suppressive effect of glucocorticoid therapy on the hypothalamo-pituitary-adrenal (HPA) axis is at a suprapituitary level. The axis would need to be tested at this level by means of an insulin tolerance test.

The metyrapone test has no place in the investigation of hypoadrenalism.

14.5 TESTS OF THE AETIOLOGY OF ADRENAL FAILURE

14.5.1 PRIMARY ADRENAL FAILURE

Tuberculous adrenalitis

If the chest radiograph demonstrates either new or old evidence of tuberculosis, or in the presence of a strongly positive tuberculin skin test, a course of anti-tuberculous antituberculous chemotherapy is indicated.

A plain abdominal radiograph may show calcification in the area of the adrenal, which supports the diagnosis.

Autoimmune adrenalitis

In the developed world, however, autoimmune disease is the most frequent cause, accounting for 84% of cases of primary ad-

renal failure [4]. It is often a diagnosis of exclusion helped by the presence in serum of adrenal autoantibodies and evidence of other autoimmune diseases. The adrenal glands are small on computerized tomography (CT), in contrast to most other processes such as tuberculosis, which result in enlarged glands with areas of calcification (Fig. 14.2).

Many systemic processes can effect the adrenal glands (Table 14.1) but there are usually other manifestations to guide the direction of investigation.

As the adrenals have a rich vascular supply, secondary metastatic deposits are common and occasionally bilateral, resulting in hypoadrenalism, lung carcinoma being the most common primary. In patients on anticoagulants, particularly the elderly, bilateral adrenal haemorrhage may present with loin pain and symptoms of hypoadrenalism.

14.5.2 SECONDARY ADRENAL FAILURE

CT Scan

In secondary hypoadrenalism, complete dynamic pituitary function tests must be performed as ACTH secretion is usually the last hormone to be affected by any general insult to the pituitary or hypothalamus. CT or magnetic resonance imaging (MRI) of the pituitary and hypothalamus is mandatory in an attempt to clarify the underlying pathological process.

Insulin tolerance test

Indication

The insulin tolerance test (ITT) is indicated in this context as a measure of pituitary ACTH reserve and the integrity of the HPA axis [5,6]. It should be part of the routine postoperative assessment of any patient undergoing hypophysectomy and at regular intervals

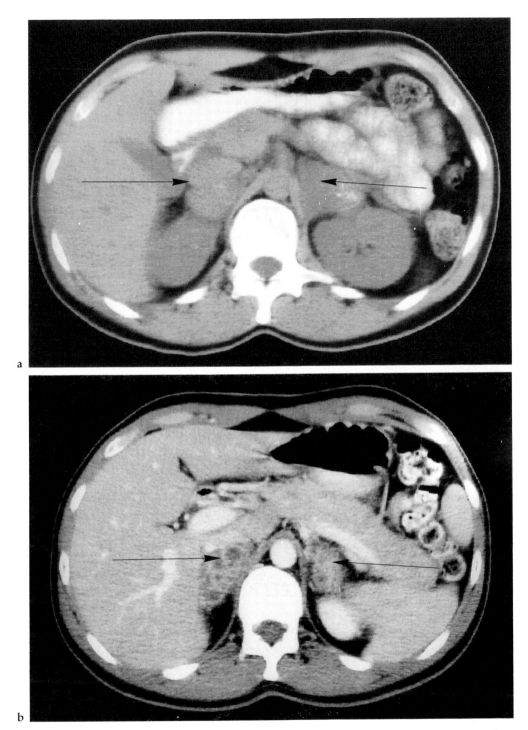

Fig. 14.2 CT scan of the adrenals in a patient with adrenal tuberculosis. The pre-contrast scan (a) shows bilaterally enlarged glands with focal calcification, with patchy enhancement after contrast (b). The areas of non-enhancement are believed to represent focal caseation.

257

following pituitary irradiation, as ACTH deficiency is prone to develop many years after completion of radiotherapy. (For the procedure and contraindications, see Chapter 4.)

Interpretation

In the presence of adequate hypoglycaemia (blood sugar $<2.2 \, \text{mmol} \, l^{-1}$ plus tachycardia and sweating), a peak cortisol response of $<580 \, \text{nmol} \, l^{-1}$ is inadequate. A GH peak of $<20 \, \text{mU} \, l^{-1}$ is further evidence of hypopituitarism, and in a child may be associated with growth failure.

Glucagon test

Indication

The glucagon test is safe to perform when an ITT is contraindicated. Unfortunately nausea is a common side effect of glucagon.

Procedure

1 mg of glucagon (1.5 mg in the obese) is administered subcutaneously and serum cortisol, growth hormone (GH) and blood sugar are measured at 0, 90, 120, 150, 180 and 240 minutes.

Interpretation

The blood glucose usually falls then rises. The criteria for the serum cortisol and GH responses are the same as for an ITT. However, it is a less potent stimulus and prone to produce equivocal results.

14.6 ISOLATED ACTH DEFICIENCY

A rare but increasingly well recognized entity is that of isolated ACTH deficiency. It was first described in 1954 [7] and there are only about 50 well-documented cases in the world literature. The aetiology of isolated ACTH deficiency is uncertain. Postpartum haemorrhage has been held responsible, as has autoimmune lymphocytic hypophysitis. Three children with isolated ACTH deficiency studied by Martin and Martin [8] all had a history of a difficult delivery, raising the possibility of perinatal hypothalamic injury. Lethargy, weakness and wight loss are the commonest presenting complaints with acute hypoadrenalism being a relatively infrequent occurrence. Hypoglycaemia, especially in children, is an important clinical feature in 50% of patients at presentation. Once hypoadrenalism has been demonstrated by a short AST, ACTH deficiency is best documented by performing an ITT. The diagnosis of isolated ACTH deficiency is then confirmed by excluding deficiency of the other anterior pituitary hormones and the absence on CT or MRI scanning of a structural lesion of the hypothalamus or pituitary. Some patients with so-called isolated ACTH deficiency have been demonstrated to have an ACTH response to corticotropin releasing hormone (CRH), indicating the true problem to be hypothalamic CRH deficiency.

14.7 INTERPRETATION OF THYROID FUNCTION TESTS IN HYPOADRENALISM

Thyroid function tests are often abnormal in untreated hypoadrenalism and caution must be exercised with their interpretation. A normal or low serum thyroxine (T4) with a low triiodothyronine (T3) and a normal thyrotropin (TSH) is indicative of the sick euthyroid syndrome and requires no further action other than repeating in the convalescent phase. A more complex problem is that of an elevated serum TSH accompanied by a low T4 and T3. Patients with hypoadrenalism may have the biochemistry of primary thyroid failure but are clinically euthyroid; the biochemical abnormalities resolve on commencing glucocorticoid treatment [9]. Alternatively, as both primary adrenal and thyroid failure can be autoimmune in aetiology they may coexist at the time of diagnosis [10]. It can be very difficult to be certain on clinical grounds that an ill patient is euthyroid, and therefore if doubt exists in a patient with hypoadrenalism and an elevated TSH it is reasonable to commence liothyronine therapy. Liothyronine is preferred, in this context, to T4 as it is of more rapid onset of action and on discontinuation its effects resolve more rapidly. Subsequently, on recuperation, the liothyronine should be discontinued and thyroid function tests followed weekly to see if the TSH rises again, indicating primary thyroid failure.

In all patients with primary thyroid disease a minimum of a 9 a.m. cortisol must be performed to exclude hypoadrenalism – life-threatening adrenal crisis can be induced by T4 therapy in a hypoadrenal patient.

14.8 CONCLUSIONS AND RECOMMENDATIONS

The diagnosis of hypoadrenalism should be considered in a wide variety of clinical situations. In the ill patient withholding treatment to allow investigation is unnecessary and unjustifiable. Once specimens for plasma cortisol and ACTH have been obtained hydrocortisone therapy can be commenced immediately. If further, more detailed, investigation is required subsequently, the patient can be converted to dexamethasone, which will not interfere with cortisol assays.

Short and long ASTs are the mainstay of the diagnosis of hypoadrenalism and the differentiation into primary and secondary causes.

The ITT is a test of ACTH reserve and should not be performed in clearly hypoadrenal patients (cortisol $<150\,\mathrm{nmol\,l^{-1}}$) but is rather of value in the assessment of patients at risk of disruption of the HPA axis.

It is important, when possible, to establish the aetiology of primary and secondary adrenal failure and to treat any underlying pathology. Decompression of the anterior pituitary by excision of a pituitary adenoma regularly results in recovery of ACTH reserve.

Hydrocortisone, the principal glucocorticoid in man, is more reliably absorbed than cortisone acetate and is the treatment of choice for glucocorticoid replacement therapy. Twice daily hydrocortisone administration, two-thirds on waking and the remainder in the early evening, is the most widely used regimen, although some advocate an additional midday dose.

Standard dosage regimens are not ideal as serum cortisol levels are unpredictable and inconsistent. Patients on hydrocortisone replacement therapy should therefore be individually monitored. Serial measurement throughout the day of serum cortisol levels is the best means of assessing hydrocortisone dose. The peak serum cortisol after the morning dose should be between 700 and 1000 $\mathrm{nmol\,l^{-1}}$ and after the evening dose between 500 and 750 $\mathrm{nmol\,l^{-1}}$.

In primary adrenal failure, the dose of fludrocortisone should be adjusted to maintain the plasma renin activity below 1500 $\mathrm{pmol\,l^{-1}\,hour^{-1}}$.

REFERENCES

1. Symington, T. (1969) *Functional Pathology of the Adrenal Gland*, Churchill Livingstone, Edinburgh.
2. Nerup, J. (1974) Addison's disease – clinical studies: a report of 108 cases. *Acta Endocrinol., Copenhagen*, **76**, 127.
3. Galvao-Telves, A., Burke, C.W. and Fraser, T.R. (1971) Adrenal function tested with tetracosactrin depot. *Lancet*, **i**, 557–60.
4. Irvine, W.J., Toft, A.D. and Feek, C.M. (1979) Addison's disease. In *The Adrenal Gland* (ed. V.H.T. James), pp. 131–64, Raven Press, London.
5. Greenwood, F.C., Landon, J. and Stamp,

T.C.B. (1966) The plasma sugar, free fatty acid, growth hormone and cortisol response to insulin in normal control subjects. *J. Clin. Invest.*, **45**, 429–36.

6. Plumpton, F.S. and Besser, G.M. (1969) The adrenocortical response to surgery and insulin induced hypoglycaemia in corticosteroid-treated and normal subjects. *Br. J. Surg.*, **56**, 216–19.

7. Steinberg, A., Shecter, F.R. and Segal, H.I. (1954) True pituitary inotropic deficiency.

J. Clin. Endocrinol., **14**, 1519.

8. Martin, M.M. and Martin, A.L.A. (1971) Idiopathic hypoglycaemia – a defect in hypothalamic ACTH-releasing factor secretion. *Pediat. Res.*, **5**, 396.

9. Gharib, H., Hodgsen, S.F. and Gastineau, C.F. (1972) Reversible hypothyroidism in Addison's disease. *Lancet*, **ii**, 734–6.

10. Schmidt, M.B. (1926) Eine biglandular erkrankung (Nebennieren und Schilddruse) bei morbus Addisonii. *Verh. Dt. Ges. Pathol.*, **21**, 212.

15

Disorders of the sympatho-adrenomedullary system

P.M. BOULOUX

15.1 PATHOLOGY OF THE SYMPATHO-ADRENOMEDULLARY SYSTEM

15.1.1 CATECHOLAMINE DEFICIENCY STATES

The most important condition in this group is autonomic neuropathy, which most frequently supervenes in the context of diabetes mellitus. Inherited conditions, such as the Shy–Drager syndrome, are also associated with dysautonomia, as is the Guillain–Barre syndrome.

Although rare, congenital deficiency of dopamine beta-hydroxylase has been reported [1], and is associated with undetectable circulating adrenaline and noradrenaline but with increased dopamine and DOPA levels.

Patients give a life-long history of severe orthostatic hypotension, ptosis, nasal stuffiness and a failure to show increases in heart rate and cardiac output with stimulation. Treatment with DL-threo-3,4-dihydroxyphenylserine (DL-DOPS) has been shown to be effective in such patients. This compound is taken up by the nerve ending and decarboxylated into noradrenaline, thus bypassing the enzymatic defect. Normal noradrenergic function may be restored on treatment.

15.1.2 CATECHOLAMINE SECRETING TUMOURS

Catecholamine secreting tumours are rare and account for 0.1%–1% of all cases of hypertension [2]; 50% of such tumours are only diagnosed post-mortem [3]. They originate from within the adrenal medulla (phaeochromocytoma), or from extra-adrenal neural crest derivatives (paraganglioma) such as the sympathetic chain. A classification is given in Table 15.1.

The extensive distribution of neural crest derivatives underlies the diverse localization of such tumours: they can occur at the base of the skull, pericardium, atria, para-aortic area (classically the Organ of Zuckerkandl), as well as in the urinary bladder and testicle. Given the potential multicentric origin of tumours, malignant behaviour is difficult to predict from histology alone, and depends upon the demonstration of metastatic disease (usually within lymph nodes, liver and bone).

Although mainly sporadic, heritable lesions are recognized in association with the multiple endocrine neoplasia (MEN) and neurocutaneous syndromes [4,5] (Table 15.2).

261

Table 15.1 Classification of catecholamine secreting tumours

Tumour	Cell of origin
Phaeochromocytoma	Chromaffin cell
Paraganglioma	Chromaffin cell
Ganglioneuroma	Ganglion cell
Ganglioneuroblastoma	Ganglion cell
Sympathoblastoma	Sympathogone
Neuroblastoma	Sympathoblast

Table 15.2 Disorders associated with phaeochromocytoma

Multiple endocrine neoplasia syndromes
MEN2a Medullary carcinoma of thyroid
Hyperparathyroidism (hyperplasia)
Phaeochromocytoma
MEN2b As MEN2a plus Marfanoid phenotype
Visceral neuromas

Neurocutaneous syndromes
Neurofibromatosis
von Hippel Lindau Disease
Ataxia telangiectasia
Tuberose sclerosis
Sturge–Weber syndrome
Multiple neoplasia triad syndrome
Extra-adrenal paragangliomas
Gastric epithelioid leiomyosarcoma
Pulmonary chondromas

In familial cases, there is a higher incidence of bilaterality, multiplicity and multicentricity.

Diagnosis of malignant phaeochromocytomas

This relies on the demonstration of unequivocal metastatic disease. More recently, it has been shown that ploidy of tumour cells, as gleaned from flow cytometry studies, may predict malignant behaviour. Thus, 30%–40% of tumours demonstrating an abnormal DNA flow histogram (suggesting aneuploidy) are malignant [6].

Clinical features

Patients with phaeochromocytoma usually present with a history of poorly controlled and occasionally accelerated hypertension. Detailed history then reveals superimposed episodes of headache, palpitations, pallor and profuse sweating; other presentations are listed in Table 15.3.

Table 15.3 Clinical features of phaeochromocytoma

Symptoms
Headache
Hyperhydrosis
Palpitations
Anxiety
Tremulousness
Nausea, vomiting
Chest and abdominal pain
Weight loss
Dyspnoea
Heat intolerance
Constipation
Acroparaesthesiae
Seizures

Signs
Hypertension (sustained and/or paroxysmal)
Orthostatic hypotension
Bradycardia, tachycardia
Postural tachycardia
Pallor and flushing
Tremor
Raynaud's phenomenon
Thyroid swelling (intermittent)
Pyrexia

Signs of Complications
Left ventricular failure
Pulmonary oedema
Circulatory shock
Cerebrovascular accident
Paralytic ileus

Occasionally, patients present with acute myocardial infarction, or acute renal failure and stroke due to massive catecholamine release; presentations with pseudo-obstruction of the bowel and chronic constipation are well recognized. The 'crises' are usually of uniform composition in individual patients, although they may vary in duration and intensity. The onset is usually sudden and the peak severity reached within a few minutes, with a slower offset, the total duration usually being more than 15 minutes, and shorter than 60 minutes in 80% of cases.

Catecholamine excess may cause cardiac hypertrophy and eventual failure secondary to sustained hypertension. A catecholamine cardiomyopathy is occasionally seen. Cardiac tachyarrhythmias resistant to treatment and reversible changes of transmural myocardial infarction on ECG may also suggest the presence of phaeochromocytoma.

Early diagnosis is of considerable importance, because patients harbouring such tumours are at risk of severe and often unpredictable hypertensive crises, caused by massive tumour catecholamine release. The mechanism of such uncontrolled catecholamine release is uncertain, but is episodic in some individuals and continuous in others. The pressor crises have a significant morbidity and occasional mortality [7]. Although frequently spontaneous, they may be precipitated by various stimuli (Table 15.4).

A number of conditions may mimic phaeochromocytoma clinically; these are referred to as 'pseudophaeochromocytomas' and are listed in Table 15.5.

Hypertension is intermittent in 50% of patients (when it can occur on a background of normotension), and constant in the remainder [8]. In patients with persistent hypertension, the normal circadian blood pressure variation, with nocturnal falls (caused largely by decreased sympathetic tone to resistance vessels and a fall in cardiac output), is retained. This strongly suggests that, despite

Table 15.4 Factors known to precipitate paroxysms in phaeochromocytoma

Spontaneous
Exercise
Bending over
Urination, defecation
Pressure on the abdomen
Induction of anaesthesia
Tumour palpation
Straining, as during parturition

Drugs
  Injection of:
    Histamine
    Tyramine
    Guanethidine
    Glucagon
    Naloxone
    Metoclopramide
    Droperidol
    ACTH
    Cytotoxic drugs
    Saralasin
  Tricyclic antidepressants
  Phenothiazines

Table 15.5 Differential diagnosis

Causes of 'pseudophaeochromocytoma'
Anxiety state
Hyperadrenergic essential hypertension
Menopausal vasomotor instability
Hyperventilation
Excess caffeine intake
Alcohol withdrawal syndrome
Diencephalic seizures (autonomic epilepsy)
Autonomic hyper-reflexia
Thyrotoxicosis

Other causes of paroxysmal hypertension
Acute intermittent porphyria
Acute or chronic lead poisoning
Tabetic crisis
Clonidine, methyldopa withdrawal
Tetanus
Guillain–Barré syndrome
Cord section

263

pathological circulating catecholamine levels, underlying sympathetic nervous regulation of the cardiovascular system is still operative. The unexpected fall in blood pressure following clonidine in patients with phaeochromocytoma further supports this contention.

Occasionally, a paradoxical rise in blood pressure occurs on introducing a beta-blocker in the treatment regimen, alerting the physician to the possibility of underlying phaeochromocytoma.

Tumour secretory products

The dominant tumour secretory products are noradrenaline, adrenaline, dopamine and their precursor DOPA. These vasoactive biogenic amines produce their effect by interacting with alpha (α1 and α2) beta (β1 and β2) or dopamine (d1 and d2) receptors, which are widely distributed in vascular tissues. Many (but not all) biological actions of catecholamines account for the characteristic symptoms and signs of phaeochromocytoma.

The manifestations in individual cases depend to some extent on the dominant type of catecholamine released, and the site and size of the tumour, as well as on the amount and pattern of release. Predominantly noradrenaline secreting tumours (for example, extra-adrenal tumours) activate peripheral α1 and α2 receptors with widespread cutaneous (pallor) and splanchnic vasoconstriction, territories dense in alpha receptors.

Associated pressor crises are accompanied by baroreflex mediated bradycardia. Adrenaline secreting tumours (usually, though not invariably, of intra-adrenal origin) cause both alpha and beta stimulation; pressor crises are associated with increased pulse pressure and tachycardia [9].

Glucose intolerance is associated with adrenaline secreting tumours [10]. Dopamine and dopa secretion may contribute to occasional cases of hypotension seen in phaeochromocytoma. Postural hypotension is more

usually due to shrinkage of the intravascular volume secondary to vasoconstriction, with concomitant failure to compensate fully on orthostatic stimulation [11].

There is no correlation between tumour size and symptomatology. Indeed, the larger tumours are characterized by intratumour catecholamine metabolism, and thus release proportionately less active amines. Paradoxically, small tumours are capable of producing devastating pressor crises.

Dopamine secreting tumours

Pure dopamine secreting tumours are rare. Those reviewed by Proye and colleagues [12] were all malignant, and none of the patients was hypertensive. All patients had an 'inflammatory syndrome' with high ESR, weight loss and fever, and were being investigated for suspected hypernephromas. Mixed noradrenaline and dopamine secreting tumours are more common, but also tend to portend malignancy, although not invariably so.

15.1.3 NON-CATECHOLAMINE TUMOUR PRODUCTS

Catecholamines are not the sole secretory products of phaeochromocytomas. Table 15.6 details neuropeptides extracted from phaeochromocytomas and found in significant circulating concentrations, particularly during crises. These have diverse biological actions, capable of directly or indirectly causing many non-catecholamine mediated effects of phaeochromocytoma. For example, calcitonin gene related peptide (CGRP) and some opioids may cause hypotension and constipation, respectively; tachykinins can account for sweating, and neuropeptide Y will provoke pressor crises partially refractory to alpha adrenoceptor blockade. Parathyroid hormone (PTH) may lead to hypercalcaemia,

Table 15.6 Biologically active non-catecholamine tumour secretory products

Substance	Biological action
Vasoactive intestinal peptide (VIP)	Flushing
Substance P and tachykinins	Sweating
Opioids	Hypotension
Somatostatin	Constipation
Neuropeptide Y	Pallor, vasoconstriction
Endothelin	Vasoconstriction
Calcitonin gene related peptide (GGRP)	Flushing, hypotension
Bombesin	
Gastrin	
Serotonin	
Histamine	Hypotension
Melatonin	
ACTH	Hypertension, Cushing's syndrome
Thyrotropin releasing hormone (TRH)	Hypertension
Insulin	Hypoglycaemia
Calcitonin	
Cholecystokinin	
Renin	Hypertension
Angiotensin converting enzyme	Hypertension
Vasopressin	Hypertension
Growth hormone releasing hormone	
Parathormone	Hypercalcaemia
Chromogranin A, DBH	

and adrenocorticotropic hormone (ACTH) secretion from phaeochromocytomas is a recognized cause of ectopic Cushing's syndrome.

Catecholamines are stored with chromogranin A in secretory vesicles; the co-secreted chromogranin A has a longer half-life than catecholamines (1–2 minutes), and its measurement has been advocated in the detection of phaeochromocytoma.

Diagnosis

Patients requiring investigation

There is considerable controversy as to which hypertensive patients should be investigated biochemically for exclusion of phaeochromocytoma [13]. Young hypertensives, those with a positive family history of phaeochromocytoma or MEN 2, or those with refractory or extremely labile hypertension (especially if accompanied by phaeochromocytoma-associated symptomatology) clearly require investigation. Similarly, patients with hypertension and a neurocutaneous syndrome (such as neurofibromatosis, Sturge–Weber syndrome or von Hippel Lindau disease) should be screened for catecholamine secreting tumours. Hypertension with evidence of glucose intolerance should also prompt an investigation for phaeochromocytoma.

Biochemical diagnosis

Use of catecholamine metabolites (Figs 15.1 and 15.2): the diagnosis of phaeochromocytoma

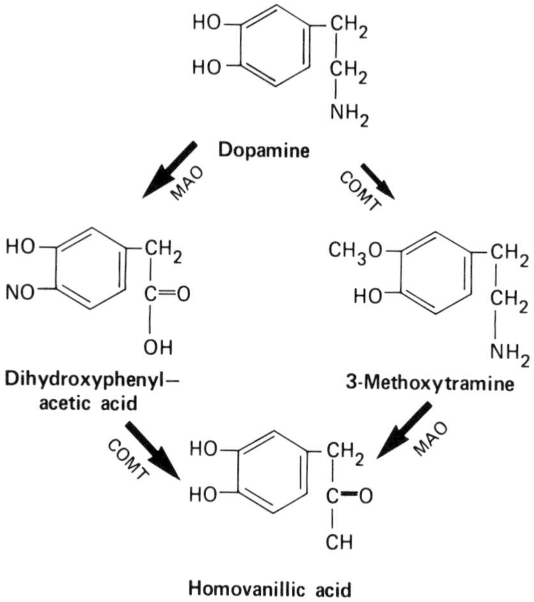

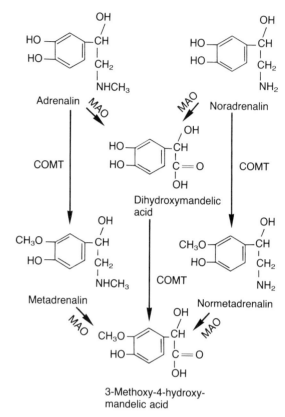

Fig. 15.1 Metabolic pathway of catecholamine degradation. MAO, monoamine oxidase; COMT, catecholamine-*O*-methyl transferase.

Fig. 15.2 Metabolic pathway for degradation of dopamine.

has traditionally depended on the biochemical demonstration of elevated 24-hour (or overnight) urinary catecholamine metabolites, vanillyl mandelic acid (VMA) and metanephrines (MN) measured by the Pisano method [14].

There is now ample evidence that the screening test with the highest sensitivity (90%) and specificity (90%) is urinary MN excretion. Since VMA measurements have approximately 60% sensitivity only, MN should replace VMA excretion as the urinary screening test of choice.

For VMA and MN estimations, patients should be on vanilla- and phenolic acid-free diets for 72 hours prior to urine collection, to reduce the likelihood of false positive results. It should be noted that methylglucamine, a component of many iodinated contrast media, destroys a reagent in the Pisano assay for up to 72 hours and therefore give

rise to a falsely low MN reading. Elevated homovanillic acid excretion is classically seen in cases of neuroblastoma and malignant phaeochromocytomas.

Plasma catecholamine estimations

Highly sensitive and specific plasma catecholamine estimations (radioenzymatic assays and high performance liquid chromatography (HPLC) coupled to electrochemical detection) have recently become more widely available in several laboratories (Fig. 15.3). Blood samples need to be taken under standardized conditions (venous cannulation 30 minutes before sampling supine), heparinized blood

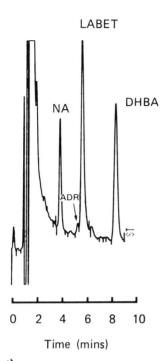

Fig. 15.3 High performance liquid chromatogram of 2 ml extracted plasma from a normal patient. NA, noradrenaline (3.1 nmol l^{-1}); ADR, adrenaline (0.21 nmol l^{-1}). The peak LABET represents interference from labetalol. DHBA is the internal standard.

separated by cold centrifugation and plasma stored at $-80°C$ prior to assay.

Plasma noradrenaline levels consistently exceeding 10 nmol $^{-1}$ (normal range 1.1–3.07 nmol l^{-1}) and adrenaline levels exceeding 1.5 nmol l^{-1} (normal range 0.05–1.07 nmol l^{-1}) give a diagnostic specificity of about 95% and a sensitivity of 85%, particularly when other causes of plasma catecholamine elevation have been ruled out. When blood is sampled during a crisis, plasma catecholamine levels are usually diagnostic beyond doubt. Noise, stress, discomfort, position of body, use of coffee, caffeine, nicotine and food may raise plasma catecholamines.

Because of the potential overlap between plasma noradrenaline levels in essential hypertension and phaeochromocytoma, based on a study of 19 patients with phaeochromocytoma Brown [15] advocates the use of the ratio of 3,4-dihydroxyphenylethylene glycol (DHPG; a noradrenaline metabolite formed in noradrenergic neurons) to noradrenaline in plasma, and finds a ratio <0.5 in phaeochromocytomas and >2.0 in essential hypertension.

DHPG reflects mainly nervous release of noradrenaline, whereas noradrenaline released directly into the bloodstream (as in phaeochromocytoma) is not converted into DHPG. Elevated plasma adrenaline or increased urinary MN excretion generally suggest a tumour of adrenal origin, whereas exclusively noradrenaline secreting tumours suggest either a very large adrenal tumour or a paraganglioma.

Platelet catecholamine estimation

Platelets take up and store catecholamines, and the determination of platelet catecholamines may assist in the diagnosis of phaeochromocytoma when plasma levels are equivocal [16].

Urinary free catecholamines

This is a sensitive indicator of phaeochromocytoma, and may be determined on a 24-hour, 12-hour overnight, or timed collection during a crisis. However, a correction for renal function is required. Measurement of urinary noradrenaline, adrenaline and dopamine by reversed phase HPLC coupled to electrochemical detection has increased the sensitivity of phaeochromocytoma diagnosis to 95%, but with some loss of specificity.

In general, only 50%–70% of tumours produce elevated adrenaline levels, whereas 85% produce elevated noradrenaline levels. Measurement of urinary adrenaline levels is of greatest value in the screening of families for MEN2 and adrenomedullary hyperplasia.

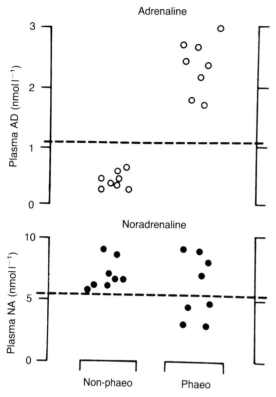

Fig. 15.4 Plasma noradrenalin and adrenalin levels in eight patients with essential hypertension compared to values in eight patients harbouring small intra-adrenal phaeochromocytomas.

Diagnosis of small adrenal lesions

Suppression tests

Very small lesions pose a problem, and minor elevations of circulating adrenaline under basal conditions may be the only indicator of the presence of small intraadrenal tumours (Fig. 15.4). Catecholamine levels are usually sited in an intermediate 'grey' zone and are therefore not diagnostic. A suppression test to see whether these represent physiological elevations or a genuinely autonomous adrenalin tumour secretion is then indicated. The ganglion blocking agent pentolinium can help to distinguish between these two possibilities [18].

Intravenous 2.5–5 mg of pentolinium will suppress plasma catecholamines into the normal range in patients with 'physiological' elevation of adrenaline or noradrenaline but has no effect in cases of tumorous catecholamine elevation, as these lesions are devoid of nicotinic cholinergic neural innervation.

The centrally acting α_2 agonist clonidine has also been used to demonstrate autonomous noradrenaline production by these tumours. Oral clonidine (0.3 mg) suppresses plasma noradrenaline into the low normal range in normal individuals and those with essential hypertension but not in patients with tumorous noradrenaline secretion [19].

In contrast, plasma catecholamines are invariably raised in hypertensive patients harbouring a phaeochromocytoma. This is because in the presence of persistently raised catecholamines, adrenergic receptors down-regulate (desensitization); in order to produce hypertension under these circumstances, plasma catecholamines have to be elevated by several times.

Episodic catecholamine secretors

Episodic catecholamine secretors with a background of normotension pose a difficult problem. If sampling is carried out during normotension, plasma catecholamines may be normal; although 24-hour urinary catecholamine metabolites or timed urinary samples may be elevated under these instances, definitive biochemical diagnosis of catecholamine secretion in such cases may require sampling during a symptomatic crisis.

Where symptomatology strongly suggests the presence of an underlying phaeochromocytoma, but the biochemistry is normal, a provocative test with pharmacological agents such as intravenous tyramine (1 mg), histamine (10 mcg), glucagon (1 mg) or naloxone (10 mg) [20] may be justified. However, this should only be carried out under effective alpha and beta blockade, with plasma catecholamine measurement rather than blood pressure as the response parameter.

The glucagon test using blood pressure and plasma catecholamine measurement is generally considered to be the safest and most accurate provocation test available. A three-fold increase in noradrenaline level over basal level is considered diagnostic, provided that blood is sampled at the time of blood pressure rise.

Localization

Computerized tomography scanning

On obtaining biochemical evidence, tumour localization procedures should be initiated. Computerized tomography (CT) scanning has largely superseded urographic and arteriographic studies for tumour localization [21]. Initially, the adrenal glands are scanned, but if this is negative the rest of the abdomen, including the pelvis, chest and neck, should be scanned. The resolution of fourth generation scanners is in the order of 5 mm.

Because intravenous contrast media can precipitate pressor crises, the examination (as indeed any invasive radiographic procedure) should be conducted only after adequate alpha and beta blockade. A suitable regimen consists of administering the non-selective and non-competitive alpha adrenoceptor antagonist phenoxybenzamine 10–20 mg 6-hourly, followed after the first dose by propranolol 40 mg 8-hourly. The alpha blocking drug must be given first to prevent potential unopposed alpha adrenoceptor stimulation, which would arise if a beta blocker were given first.

Magnetic resonance imaging

Magnetic resonance imaging (MRI) allows some degree of tissue characterization. Most phaeochromocytomas give high T2-weighted signal intensity [22]. The technique is particularly useful in imaging tumours that are in close proximity to major vessels because of the signal void from flowing blood; otherwise it offers no major advantage over CT scanning.

Venous catheterization

This is particularly valuable in patients with strong clinical and biochemical evidence of a phaeochromocytoma but negative CT examination. Blood is sampled from the internal jugular veins, the subclavians, brachycephalic, thymic, superior intercostals, azygous, right atrium, coronary sinus, inferior vena cava, hepatic renal, adrenal, renal, gonadal and internal and external iliac veins. The presence of a noradrenaline hot-spot but normal adrenaline in such instances strongly suggests an extra-adrenal tumour.

The technique is also of value in the investigation of possible bilateral or multiple lesions [23,24]. Because of the frequently multicentric origin of tumours, several sites may need to be sampled. Provided that all likely sites have been sampled (including the coronary sinus), venous sampling is a good way of refuting the diagnosis, particularly when levels of noradrenaline are elevated during sampling.

The interpretation of catheter data is not straightforward, particularly when dealing with adrenal venous samples. As such, there are no 'diagnostic levels' of catecholamines to indicate the presence of a phaeochromocytoma. Generated levels are critically dependent on the adrenal blood flow rate at the time of sampling, position of the catheter tip and direct mechanical stimulation of release by the catheter. The degree of stress experienced by the patient also has an important bearing on interpretation. The absolute levels of noradrenaline and adrenaline are therefore not as helpful as the ratio between the two.

Adrenaline is the dominant catecholamine secreted from the adrenal medulla, both basally and following stress. Under basal sampling conditions, the adrenaline:nor-

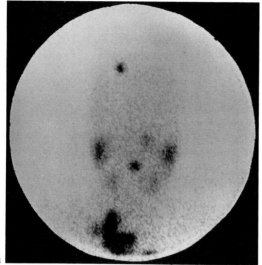

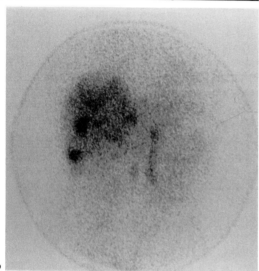

Fig. 15.5 (a) [123]I MIBG scan of head and neck in a patient harbouring a malignant thoracic paraganglioma. There is salivary gland uptake of the radionuclide, and a small skull metastasis is demonstrated. (b) Intrahepatic metastases from a malignant phaeochromocytoma revealed by ^{123}I MIBG scan.

adrenaline ratio is between 4:1 and 10:1. A reversal of this ratio (i.e. more noradrenaline than adrenaline released) is highly significant and indicates the presence of tumour.

Radionuclide scanning

More recently, the radionuclide meta-iodo (^{123}I or ^{131}I)-benzyl guanidine (MIBG) [25,26], a guanethidine analogue taken up by chromaffin cells and incorporated into vesicles, has been used to assist in tumour localization. This is of particular value in the localization of extra-adrenal paragangliomata and metastases (Fig. 15.5a,b).

Normal adrenomedullary tissue can also be visualized in 80%–90% of cases using ^{123}I MIBG.

Approximately 10% of tumours are not demonstrable (false negative) with this technique, but false positives are rare (1%–3%). Specificity is 100% in malignant lesions and in familial tumours [27].

Intraoperative localization with ^{123}I MIBG

Where there are discrepancies between CT scanning of the abdomen and radionuclide imaging (for example, MIBG shows uptake but there is no corresponding mass on CT scanning), a preoperative 4 mCi dose of MIBG may be administered and direct measurement of tissue activity carried out intraoperatively, allowing surgical removal of labelled tumour tissue.

15.2 SUMMARY AND RECOMMENDATIONS

A flow chart giving a strategy for diagnosis, localization and treatment of a suspected phaeochromocytoma is given in Fig. 15.6.

Clinical suspicion of the presence of a phaeochromocytoma should prompt the clinician to demonstrate the presence of pathological excretion of urinary catecholamine metabolites (VMA and MN) or preferably raised urinary free catecholamines. MN excretion appears to have greater sensitivity and is to be preferred over VMA.

If the patient is hypertensive, plasma cat-

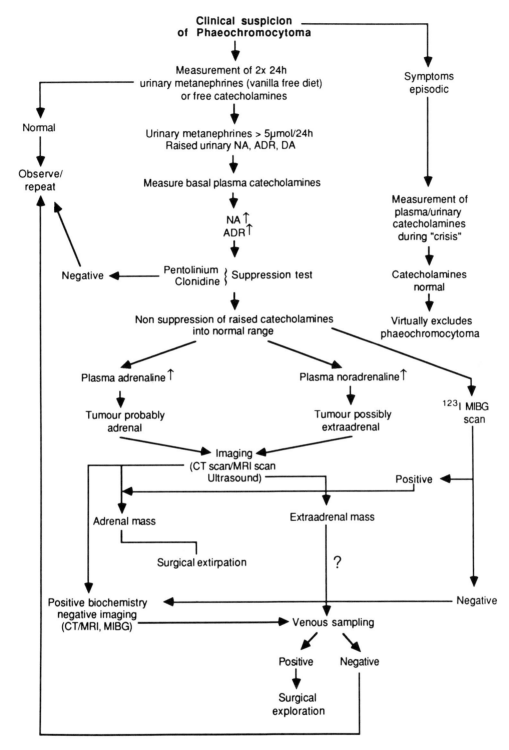

Fig. 15.6 Flow chart for the diagnosis of phaeochromocytoma.

echolamine estimation will be unequivocally raised. Precautions should be taken to collect the plasma sample under basal conditions – patient supine, and cannulated 30 minutes before venous sampling. If plasma catecholamines are elevated, an attempt at suppression with either pentolinium (2.5 mg i.v. with blood sampling at 0 and 10 minutes) or oral clonidine (0.3 mg orally and blood sampling for plasma catecholamines at 0, 60 and 120 minutes) should be performed. Non-suppression into the normal range should prompt a search for a phaeochromocytoma/paraganglioma. Non-suppressible adrenaline suggests the presence of an adrenal lesion, whereas non-suppression of isolated elevated noradrenaline may suggest the presence of an extra-adrenal lesion. The next step is to perform imaging with CT scanning (beware that i.v. contrast can precipitate a pressor crisis, so the patient needs alpha blockade with phenoxybenzamine and beta blockade with propranolol prior to the investigation) or MRI scanning of the adrenals. If a paraganglioma is suspected, imaging of the head and neck, thorax, and entire abdomen right down to the pelvis should be undertaken. [123]I MIBG scanning is particularly useful for localization of extra-adrenal tumours and possible metastases. If the adrenals appear normal, or an extra-adrenal mass is present on imaging but does not take up ^{123}I MIBG, venous catheterization should be undertaken for confirmation of the diagnosis. Finally, blood sampling during a crisis is particularly useful in ruling out a phaeochromocytoma. If the plasma catecholamines are normal during such a crisis, then a phaeochromocytoma/paraganglioma is effectively ruled out. Raised levels may, however, represent a stress response.

REFERENCES

1. Man in't Veld, A.J., Boomsla, F., Moleman, P. and Schalekamp, M.A.D.H. (1987) Congenital dopamine-beta-hydroxylase deficiency. A novel orthostatic syndrome. *Lancet*, i, 183–7.

2. Manger, W.M., Gifford, Jr, R.W. and Hoffman, B.B. (1985) Phaeochromocytoma: A clinical and experimental overview. *Curr. Probl. Cancer*, **9**, 1.

3. Bittar, D.A. (1982) Unsuspected phaeochromocytoma. *Can. Anaesth. Soc. J.*, **29**, 183.

4. Humble, R.M. (1967) Phaeochromocytoma, neurofibromatosis and pregnancy. *Anaesthesia*, **22**, 296.

5. Carney, J.A., Sizemore, G.W. and Tyce, G.M. (1975) Bilateral adrenal medullary hyperplasia in multiple endocrine neoplasia, type 2: the precursor of bilateral phaeochromocytoma. *Proc. Mayo Clin.*, **50**, 3.

6. Hosaka, Y., Rainwater, L.M. and Grant, C.S. (1986) Phaeochromocytoma: Nuclear deoxyribonucleic acid patterns studied by flow cytometry. *Surgery*, **100**, 1003.

7. Modlin, I.M., Farndon, J.R., Shepherd, A. *et al.* (1979) Phaeochromocytoma in 72 patients: Clinical and diagnostic features, treatment and long term results. *Br. J. Surg.*, **66**, 456.

8. Bravo, E.L. and Gifford, R.W. (1984) Phaeochromocytoma: Diagnosis, localisation and management. *New Engl. J. Med.*, **311**, 1298.

9. Page, L.B., Raker, J.W. and Berberich, F.R. (1969) Phaeochromocytoma with predominant epinephrine secretion. *Am. J. Med.*, **47**, 648.

10. Duncan, L.E., Semans, J.H. and Howard, J.E. (1944) Case report. Adrenal medullary tumour (phaeochromocytoma) and diabetes mellitus: Disappearance of disease and removal of the tumour. *Ann. Intern. Med.*, **20**, 815.

11. Brunjes, S., Johns, V.J. and Crane, M.G. (1960) Pheochromocytoma. Postoperative shock and blood volume. *New Engl. J. Med.*, **262**, 393.

12. Proye, C., Fossati, P., Wemeau, J.L., Cecat, P., Marmousez, T.H. and Lagache, G. (1984) Le pheochromocytome dopamino- secretant. *Chirurgie*, **110**, 304–8.

13. Plouin, P.F., Degoulet, P., Tagaye, A. *et al.* (1981) Le depistage du pheochromocytome: Chez quels hypertendus? Etude semiologique chez 2885 hypertendus dont 11 ayant un pheochromocytome. *Nouvelle Presse Med.*, **10**, 869.

14. Freier, D.T. and Harrison, T.S. (1973) Rigorous

biochemical criteria for the diagnosis of phaeo-chromocytoma. *J. Surg. Res.*, **14**, 177.

15. Brown, M.J. (1984) Simultaneous assay of noradrenaline and its deaminated metabolite, dihydroxyphenylglycol, in plasma: A simplified approach to the exclusion of phaeo-chromocytoma in patients with borderline elevation of plasma noradrenaline concentration. *Eur. J. Clin. Invest.*, **14**, 67–72.

16. Zweifer, A.J. and Julius, S. (1982) Increased platelet catecholamine content in phaeo-chromocytoma: A diagnostic test in patients with elevated plasma catecholamines. *New Engl. J. Med.*, **306**, 890.

17. Ganguly, A., Henry, D.P., Yung, H.Y. *et al.* (1979) Diagnosis and localisation of phaeo-chromocytoma. Detection by measurement of urinary norepinephrine excretion during sleep, plasma norepinephrine concentration and computerised axial tomography. *Am. J. Med.*, **67**, 21.

18. Brown, M.J., Allison, D.J., Lewis, P.J. *et al.* (1981) Increased sensitivity and accuracy of phaeochromocytoma diagnosis achieved by plasma adrenaline estimations and a pentolinium suppression test. *Lancet*, **i**, 174.

19. Bravo, E.L., Tarazi, R.C., Fouad, F.M. *et al.* (1981) Clonidine suppression test: A useful aid in the diagnosis of phaeochromocytoma. *New Engl. J. Med.*, **305**, 623.

20. Mannelli, M., Maggi, M., Defeo, H.L. *et al.*

(1983) Naloxone administration releases cat-echolamines. *New Engl. J. Med.*, **308**, 564–5.

21. Sheedy, P.F. II, Hattery, R.R., Stephens, D.H. *et al.* (1983) Computed tomography of the adrenal gland. In *Computed Tomography of the Whole Body*, vol. 2 (ed. J.R. Hagga and F.J. Alfidi), C.V. Mosby, St Louis, p. 681.

22. Fink, I.J., Reinig, J.W., Dwyer, A.J. *et al.* (1985) MR imaging of phaeochromocytoma. *J. Comput. Assisted Tomography*, **9**, 454.

23. Allison, D.J., Brown, M.J., Jones, D.H. *et al.* (1983) Role of venous sampling in locating a phaeochromocytoma. *Br. Med. J.*, **286**, 1122.

24. Jones, D.H., Allison, D.J., Hamilton, C.A. *et al.* (1979) Selective venous sampling in the diagnosis and localisation of phaeochromocytoma. *Clin. Endocrinol.*, **10**, 179.

25. Gasnier, B., Rosin, M.P., Scherman, D. *et al.* (1986) Uptake of meta-iodobenzylgaunidine by bovine chromaffin granule membranes. *Molec. Pharmacol.*, **29**, 275.

26. Guilotteau, D., Baulieu, J.-L., Huguet, F. *et al.* (1984) Meta-iodobenzylguanidine adrenal medulla localisation: Autoradiographic and pharmaceutical studies. *Eur. J. Nucl. Med.*, **9**, 278.

27. Shapiro, B. (1983) Imaging of catecholamine-secreting tumours: uses of MIBG in diagnosis and treatment. *Clin. Endocrin. Metabol.*, **71**, 491–509.

16

Imaging of the pituitary and other parasellar lesions

D.P.E. KINGSLEY

The story of non-invasive imaging of the pituitary and parasellar region commenced with the development of computerized tomography (CT) in the early 1970s. Prior to this, radiological examination necessitated pneumoencephalography or cisternography with air or positive contrast, sometimes aided by angiography. With the early CT scanners, only the large masses were identifiable but an understanding of the imaging appearances often allowed a specific pathological diagnosis to be suggested. Although identification of small lesions awaited the development of the subsequent generation of scanners, by the time magnetic resonance imaging (MRI) became clinically useful the quality of CT was such that the majority of lesions in this region could readily be identified. Early MRI provided adequate anatomical detail but little new information; however, modern scanners not only provide superior anatomical detail, but the resolution and contrast clearly separates anterior from posterior lobes, and may even identify the pars intermedia. This has been particularly useful in pituitary hypoplasia and growth hormone deficiency states.

Imaging of the pituitary region is by conventional radiography – X-ray, CT, MRI and cerebral angiography. Currently, conventional X-rays play virtually no role. Adequate views are often difficult to produce, and even slight canting can make interpretation difficult; even then, a normal radiograph does not exclude a microadenoma. Angiography is indicated to exclude an aneurysm and to evaluate vascular displacement prior to surgery. Further reference to these two techniques will be made infrequently, and evaluation of this region will rely on a description of the techniques and appearances on CT and MRI.

It matters little which of the two techniques is employed in this region as a first study. Each modality has its uses, and in this more than any other region of the cranial cavity is a knowledge of the strong and weak points of each technique important.

16.1 CT TECHNIQUE

The scan technique for examining the pituitary fossa is tailored to the individual case. It is best, therefore, to undertake a plain scan of the head using 5-mm-thick slices from the foramen magnum to the orbital roof with 8-mm-thick or 10-mm-thick slices for the rest of the head. This gives an overview of the brain so that other unsuspected lesions can be excluded. It gives a preliminary evaluation of the sellar region and allows normal anatomy to be identified and any large masses to be excluded.

More detailed examination of the pituitary fossa is usually undertaken using thin slices after the injection of intravenous contrast (35–50 g). The patient may be scanned in two imaging planes, the axial or the coronal. Axial images are most satisfactorily undertaken using a slice thickness of 1–1.5 mm followed by reformatting in the coronal and sagittal planes. Direct coronal imaging can be undertaken using either thin (1–1.5 mm) slices which allow reformatting, or 5 mm slices every 3 mm, providing an overlap. There are proponents of both techniques. Reformatted axial images, if carefully undertaken, can provide the most detailed evaluation of this region, but of necessity the patient must be co-operative and the examination conducted without patient movement. Any minor positional change will result in suboptimal reformats. The quality of the image frequently depends on the thickness of the surrounding bone and the size of the underlying paranasal sinuses. Beam hardening causing black and white streak artefacts across the pituitary fossa is a source of misinterpretation on the reformats, and where low density areas within the pituitary fossa are noted, it is essential to evaluate the axial images individually to exclude such artefact.

Direct coronal CT can, in some cases, provide superior images to the reformatted axial sections, but beam hardening artefact is not infrequent, and dental amalgam can lead to difficulties with scanning in the optimal plane since streak artefact is almost inevitable when a section includes this material. In patients with a significant number of dental fillings, it may be necessary to under-tilt the scan, which results in an image in an oblique coronal plane. This is particularly likely in older patients when cervical spondylosis limits the amount of neck extension. In practice, it is almost impossible to undertake a true coronal image even using the maximum gantry tilt of the CT scanner unless the patient is young and has a very mobile cervical spine.

16.2 MRI TECHNIQUE

The CT image is made up of a matrix of volume elements (voxels). The value of each voxel is proportional to the amount that the X-ray is attenuated in passing through it. Each value can be assigned a colour or a shade on a grey scale to differentiate degrees of X-ray absorption, and this variation results in an image.

MRI is very different. It is similar to CT only in that it uses a colour or grey scale system, but the physical state of each voxel is dependent upon many factors. The principle of MRI is that any atomic nucleus with an unequal number of protons or neutrons can be made to resonate under appropriate circumstances; in most cases, however, there are not enough nuclei of a particular type to provide an adequate signal. The one nucleus that is abundant in biological tissue is hydrogen, and it is the characteristics of this that are being imaged.

The proton behaves in the natural state like a spinning top. In the earth's magnetic field the spins are arranged in a random manner. If the patient is placed inside a magnet of high field strength, the protons align along the magnetic field. Just over 50% of them lie parallel, and just under 50% antiparallel to this field. If energy in the form of a radiowave (radiofrequency or RF pulse) is applied to the system at a frequency which is proportional to the strength of the magnetic field, the protons will resonate and will be tipped out of their axis by an amount which will depend upon the time that the radiowave is applied. When the radiowave is switched off, the protons will return to the magnetic axis in an exponential manner. The rate of decay of the protons can be measured. This so-called T_1 is the longitudinal or spin lattice relaxation time. In a conventional image (inversion recovery), the T_1 decay curve follows the application of an RF pulse sufficient to tip the protons through 180°. Since the signal is only received at right angles to the main field, a 90° pulse must subsequently be applied and the signal collected immediately from protons that have not relaxed completely at the time of data collection.

The second parameter which is important in MRI is the T_2 relaxation time (spin spin relaxation). To understand the principles of this it is important to return to a consideration of the behaviour of the proton in the natural state. The protons are not only randomly placed in the earth's magnetic field with regard to their own north and south poles, but each is also spinning on its own axis and precessing like a gyroscope. When the RF pulse is applied, the protons are not only tilted to an angle, but also the spins are aligned in the same direction. If we consider a pulse sufficient to tilt the protons to 90° at the moment the RF pulse is switched off, all the protons will be pointing in the same direction, and, since the rotation about their axes will be the same, they will be in the same phase. As the process of decay occurs and they return to the plane of the main magnetic field, they are also subject to local forces within their own environment, which will vary the rate each proton spins on its own axis, i.e. it will tend to alter the phase of each proton with respect to its neighbours. They thus tend to get out of phase, which leads to loss of signal in the transverse plane. Capture of the resulting signal is achieved in this spin echo sequence by applying a 180° pulse which causes the phase of each proton to be reversed. Data collection is then undertaken after the same time period as that between 90° and 180°

pulses, at which point, since the differential speed of dephasing of each proton will continue, those that have not lost all signal will return to the same phase and produce an echo.

The conventional sequences are termed spin echo and inversion recovery. The spin echo sequence is most widely used and this consists of a 90° pulse, followed by a 180° pulse, followed after the same time period by data collection. This experiment is repeated again and again in order to acquire sufficient signal to permit an image to be produced. The time between each 90° pulse is termed the repetition time (TR) and the time between the 90° pulse and the data collection is termed the echo time (TE). Altering the TR and TE will increase or decrease the effect of T_1 or T_2 relaxation on the received signal. Signal intensity (contrast) is a product of the number of protons (proton density) as well as T_1 and T_2 relaxation rates. Increasing the TR reduces the effect of the T_1 relaxation time, and increasing the TE increases the effect of the T_2 relaxation time. The effect of the proton density of a given tissue remains relatively constant. Consequently, a T_1-weighted spin echo has a short TR and a short TE; a T_2-weighted spin echo has a long TR and a long TE, and a proton density weighted scan has a long TR and a short TE.

The second common conventional sequence is the inversion recovery, which consists of a 180° pulse which inverts the protons, followed after an interval (TI) by a 90° pulse to tip the protons at right angles to the magnetic field. The inversion recovery sequence is heavily T_1-weighted.

Modern scanners permit the RF pulse to be applied for any desired length of time, which has the effect of tilting the protons to any chosen angle. Varying the tilt angle also alters the T_1 and T_2 weighting and is used in many of the newer sequences.

The pituitary fossa is particularly well suited to investigation with MRI since the optimal imaging planes which are so difficult to achieve with CT are easily performed. Sagittal and coronal planes are anatomically the most appropriate for this region, and axial images are only required, for example, to demonstrate the length of the optic nerve and tract as it passes through the suprasellar cisterns. The natural tissue contrast of MRI differentiates cerebrospinal fluid (CSF) from other solid tissues, and the use of intravenous contrast is therefore rarely required. The main exception to this is for the demonstration of possible microadenomas where the non-contrast scan may be unhelpful. The most appropriate sequence is T_1-weighted. It can be either a conventional short TR/short TE spin echo or a T_1-weighted gradient echo sequence using a flip angle of around 90°. T_2-weighted sequences are more prone to artefact, particularly that due to pulsation of the carotid arteries, and do not provide as clear an anatomical demonstration of this region.

The more recent development of faster sequences on some scanners permits a modified dynamic scan to be undertaken, but this is rarely required except to demonstrate microadenomas that are not resolved on conventional images. Some centres also use three-dimensional imaging, but consistent quality is difficult to achieve. Slice thickness is an important consideration when using two-dimensional studies. With mid- and low-field systems, slices less than 2 mm thick usually require too long a scanning time to acquire sufficient data. Therefore, the optimal slice thickness at this field strength is approximately 3 mm with this technique. Thinner slices can be used with high-field systems.

16.3 NORMAL ANATOMY

The pituitary gland consists of anterior and posterior lobes separated by the pars intermedia. CT usually does not permit separation of these structures on plain or post-contrast

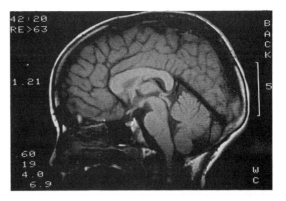

Fig. 16.1 Normal anatomy of the perisellar region, sagittal T_1-weighted MRI scan. The infundibulum is clearly identified extending down to the sella. The neurohypophysis is identified as a high signal posteriorly and is separated from the adenohypophysis anteriorly.

scans, although Bonneville and colleagues claim attenuation values of the neurohypophysis of around 10 Hounsfield units (HU) lower than that of the anterior pituitary [1]. On T_1-weighted MRI sequences, the posterior lobe returns a high signal whereas the anterior lobe has an intensity similar to that of surrounding brain (Fig. 16.1).

The reason for the high signal remains uncertain despite numerous studies attempting to clarify the cause. It is not affected by fat suppression studies [2]. However, it is clear that it is related to a functioning posterior lobe, since it is absent in pituitary aplasia and in some types of diabetes insipidus [3].

The pituitary stalk is clearly identified on post-contrast CT scans either in the axial plane or using reformats [4] (Fig. 16.2), and is frequently seen on the non-contrast study.

It is important to identify this structure extending into the pituitary fossa in patients with an 'empty sella'. Inability to appreciate it immediately in front of the dorsum sellae when the contents of the fossa are of low density is strong evidence of a cystic mass. Unless reformatted CT scans are of superior quality, too much reliance should not be

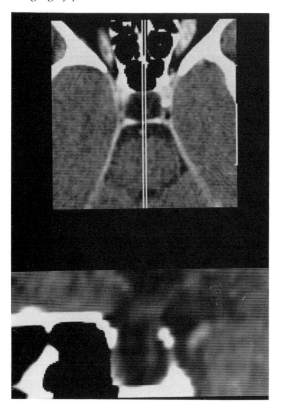

Fig. 16.2 Empty sella, reformatted sagittal CT scan. The pituitary stalk is seen extending down to the floor of the pituitary fossa, which contains CSF. There is only a small amount of pituitary tissue.

placed on identifying the anterior recesses of the third ventricle in this situation.

On MRI, the pituitary stalk returns a signal close to that of adjacent brain. It is clearly seen surrounded by CSF in both coronal and sagittal planes. It usually arises from the pituitary gland at the junction of anterior and posterior lobes, and extends upwards and backwards to the floor of the third ventricle. In a small percentage of normal people, the neurohypophysis does not maintain its normal relationship with the adenohypophysis, but lies below or above it.

The chiasmatic and infundibular recesses of the third ventricle are best seen on sagittal

T_1-weighted scans, and such is usually the quality of these scans that masses of less than 5 mm can usually be appreciated. Therefore, with careful and methodical assessment, tumours in the suprasellar region can usually be excluded with certainty on both CT and MRI.

The optic nerves pass from the optic canals upwards, backwards and medially to the optic chiasm which indents the antero-inferior surface of the third ventricle separating the optic and infundibular recesses. The position of the optic chiasm has been examined in cadavers [5] and on pneumo-encephalography [6], and has been found to be fairly constant. It lies above the dorsum sellae and part of the diaphragma in 79%, anterior to this position either completely over the diaphragma or between diaphragm and sulcus chiasmaticus in 17% (pre-fixed), and behind the dorsum sellae (post-fixed) in 4% [5]. Its position and the tilt of the sella determine the primary direction of expansion of a pituitary mass and whether compression of the optic chiasm occurs early or late [6].

The anterior visual pathway is more clearly seen on MRI, but should be visible on any modern CT scanner if the appropriate thin axial sections are undertaken. The bony margins of the optic canal are more clearly defined on CT, but the optic nerves as they pass through the optic canals are better resolved on MRI, so that minor amounts of swelling can be appreciated at an earlier stage.

At the level of the chiasm, the coronal plane is the most useful since it cuts across rather than along the chiasm, and thus a minor asymmetry of the two sides of the chiasm is more easily appreciated and extension into or displacement of the optic nerves and tracts is usually evident. Extension of a pituitary tumour upwards may lead to elevation and compression of the chiasm, and the relationship of these structures to each other is most clearly appreciated in this plane on MRI. If this is not available, most pathology can be demonstrated on CT, but minor asymmetry may not be appreciated.

The pituitary fossa is bounded on either side by the cavernous sinus. The lateral margin of the fossa cannot usually be clearly separated from this structure either on CT or MRI. The density of the contents of the cavernous sinus and of the adjacent pituitary tissue are similar on both plain and post-contrast CT. MRI has the advantage that the carotid artery can be seen as a signal void and any displacement of this structure indicates lateral extension of an intrasellar mass. It is rare, however, for the separating dura to be identified as a separate structure except with high field strength magnets, and then usually only using thin slices.

16.4 PATHOLOGY

Lesions which arise in the pituitary region may affect the function of the pituitary gland or, if large, cause direct effect on neighbouring structures such as the upper cranial nerves. These conventionally fall into three main groups: (i) tumours, (ii) vascular and ischaemic lesions and (iii) inflammatory processes. Tumours may arise in the pituitary gland itself and extend upwards, backwards and laterally, or they may develop outside the sella where, as well as affecting the neighbouring cranial nerves, they may also compress pituitary tissue.

16.5 PITUITARY TUMOURS

These are conveniently divided into microadenomas and macroadenomas. Microadenomas are defined as tumours of less than 10 mm diameter. Several series of unselected autopsies have demonstrated microadenomas as an incidental and asymptomatic finding in as many as a quarter of the population [7]. Those that become clinically evident are hormone producing and typically

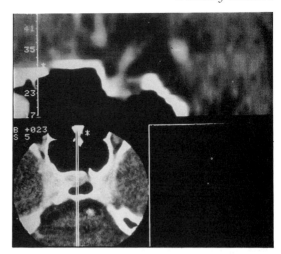

Fig. 16.3 Microadenoma. Reformatted sagittal CT scan showing a non-enhancing mass in the posterior part of the pituitary fossa. Normal enhancing pituitary tissue lies in the anterior part of the sella and the pituitary stalk is displaced forwards.

cause marked elevation of prolactin levels. The diagnosis, however, is mainly a clinical one, and although these lesions can be demonstrated on CT and MRI, management is not dependent upon the radiological appearances of the tumour itself, and imaging is only justified to exclude other lesions.

Plain radiographs have little value and should be discouraged. They causes unnecessary radiation and are frequently inaccurate, with a false positive rate approaching one-third [8–10].

Thin section coronal or reformatted axial CT scans are required. Demonstration of a localized area of relatively low enhancement compared with the surrounding tissue (Fig. 16.3) with a convex upper surface to the gland is suggestive of a microadenoma [11].

Displacement of the pituitary stalk away from this area of hypodensity strengthens the diagnosis. However, careful clinical correlation is required because other lesions, such as cysts of the pars intermedia, epidermoid cysts, metastases and even abscesses,

279

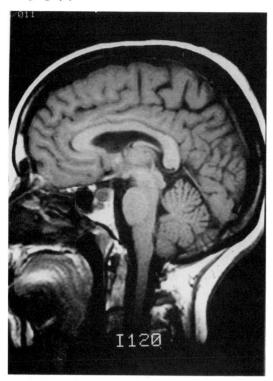

Fig. 16.4 Microadenoma. Sagittal T₁-weighted MRI scan showing a mildly hypointense rounded mass displacing the normal pituitary tissue posteriorly. The neurohypophysis lies in the floor of the sella.

can mimic this tumour [12]. A similar appearance is encountered on MRI, with the tumour being hypointense on T₁- and hyperintense on T₂-weighted sequences in about 90% of patients [13] (Fig. 16.4).

Nevertheless, isointense lesions which do not show differential enhancement after contrast occur in approximately 10% of patients and are more prevalent in Cushing's disease [14]. Intravenous gadolinium-diethylene triaminepenta-acetic acid (DTPA) increases the sensitivity of MRI, with both prolactin and adrenocorticotropic hormone (ACTH) secreting microadenomas [15].

Lesions smaller than 5 mm in diameter may be missed on conventional CT and MRI

but improved sensitivity has been advocated using dynamic CT, with the demonstration of a displaced 'tuft' sign as an indicator of the position of even the smallest tumour [16]. With microadenomas larger than this, the two procedures produce similar results.

Macroadenomas are by definition those larger than 10 mm in diameter. They are usually non-secreting, but some large tumours produce prolactin either primarily or secondarily due to interruption of the pituitary-hypothalamic axis. If evidence of pituitary dysfunction is absent, diagnosis may be delayed until visual problems occur due to compression of the chiasm. In a large series of over 8000 tumours, pituitary adenomas accounted for 8%–12% of intracranial tumours [17].

Tumours of a significant size are usually equally well demonstrated on CT and MRI. On CT, they are either hyperdense or isodense, and enhance markedly after contrast (Fig. 16.5).

Sometimes they contain cysts and, rarely, they are almost entirely cystic. Displacement of the carotid arteries around the mass is better demonstrated on MRI (Fig. 16.6), but can usually be appreciated on CT.

Calcification occurs in less than 1% of adenomas [17]. When present, it is usually relatively insignificant and can only be appreciated on CT.

On T₁-weighted MRI sequences, the intensity is similar to that of brain except where there are cystic/necrotic areas, which are then hypointense. On T₂ and proton density images the signal is close to that of brain, although it may be slightly hyperintense on the T₂-weighted image. Although enhancement occurs, intravenous contrast is hardly justified as it does not improve tumour delineation, nor does it differentiate most types of tumour. However, the main differential of a homogeneous sellar mass is a meningioma of the diaphragma, and the main difficulty arises when the pituitary

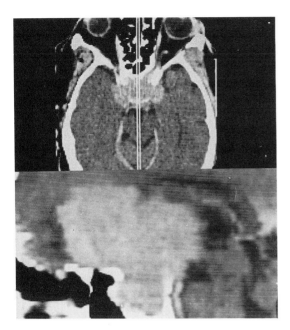

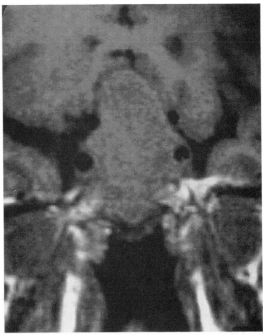

Fig. 16.5 Giant macroadenoma. Reformatted sagittal post-contrast CT scan showing a mass expanding the sella with a large suprasellar extension projecting forwards subfrontally and backwards into the interpeduncular cistern. The optic chiasm cannot be identified and the anterior recesses of the third ventricle are obliterated.

Fig. 16.6 Macroadenoma, coronal T_1-weighted MRI scan. There is a large suprasellar mass with extension on both sides displacing the cavernous carotid arteries laterally.

fossa is not markedly enlarged. In this case, enhancement of the adjacent dura is strongly suggestive of a meningioma.

16.5.1 CRANIOPHARYNGIOMA

This tumour arises within the sella from epithelial remnants of Rathke pouch clefts, but more commonly extends into the suprasellar cistern, where it may obstruct the foramen of Monro, causing hydrocephalus. It can reach a large size, and in 25% of cases it extends along the floor of the anterior cranial fossa, backwards into the interpeduncular fossa or laterally into the middle fossa [18] (Fig. 16.7).

It is the second most common tumour in this region after the pituitary adenoma.

The diagnosis is frequently aided by the demonstration of calcification within the tumour mass, which occurs in over 95% of children. Demonstration of this on MRI requires the presence of a densely calcified mass. Lesser amounts of calcification are far more clearly identified on CT. The tumour may be solid, cystic, or a mixture of both, and these various components can be identified on CT and MRI.

On plain CT, the solid components are usually isodense but enhance after contrast, and even in those that are almost entirely cystic there is usually enhancement of the rim. On MRI, the solid components are iso-intense on the T_1-weighted sequence and are moderately hyperintense on the T_2-weighted sequence. The intensity of cystic components varies with the amount of pro-

281

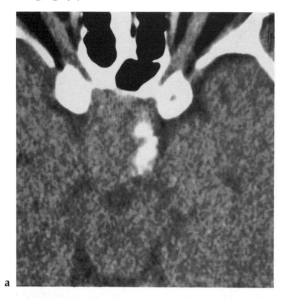

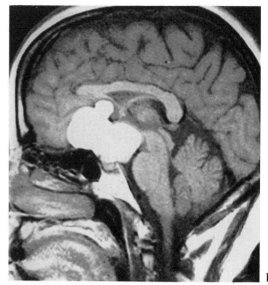

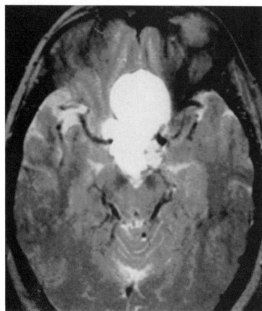

Fig. 16.7 Craniopharyngioma. (a) Axial non-contrast CT scan. There is a large isodense suprasellar mass with heavy calcification on the left side. (b) Sagittal T_1-weighted and (c) axial T_2-weighted MRI scans. The tumour is hyperintense on both sequences, typical of the 'engine-oil' cysts. The dense calcification is seen as low signal within the tumour on both T_1- and T_2-weighted scans.

tein contained. Protein-rich cysts containing so-called 'engine oil' return a high signal on T_1-weighted sequence and are also relatively high on the T_2weighted sequence. Enhancement following gadolinium injection has the same distribution as with CT.

16.5.2 RATHKE POUCH CYSTS

These have a similar origin to craniopharyngioma. Although cysts of the pars intermedia have been reported in up to 26% of routine autopsy series, clinically symptomatic ones

282

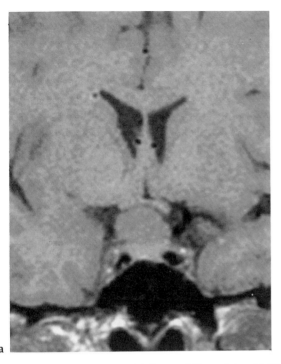
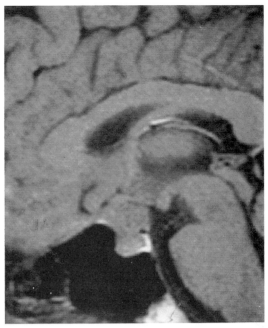

b

a

Fig. 16.8 Meningioma. (a) Coronal T$_1$-weighted MRI scan. There is a suprasellar mass nearly isointense with, but separable from, the pituitary tissue elevating the optic chiasm. The carotid arteries are not displaced. (b) Sagittal T$_1$-weighted MRI scan. The mass projects forwards onto the planum sphenoidale and there is pheumosinus dilatans.

are very much less common. They arise within the pituitary fossa and may become large. On CT, they have a density similar to that of CSF but, depending on their contents, may be isodense with brain. In this they are similar to cystic craniopharyngiomas, and enhancement occurs in only half the cases [19]. Calcification occurs in about 6%. On MRI, the cysts are indistinguishable from cystic craniopharyngiomas. They return high signal on both T$_1$- and T$_2$-weighted sequences in about half the cases, and low signal on T$_1$- and high signal on T$_2$-weighted sequences in the remainder.

16.5.3 MENINGIOMA

Approximately 10% of meningiomas occur in the parasellar region [20]. They may arise

in the sphenoid wing or petrous apex and extend medially or forwards to encroach on the cavernous sinus and sellar region, or primarily from the dura in the region of the planum sphenoidale where they can cause hyperostosis and pneumosinus dilatans [21] (Fig. 16.8).

They sometimes reach a large size, but virtually never cause obstruction to the foramen of Monro. Sometimes they are broad-based and may cover the diaphragma sellae. In this situation, a normal pituitary fossa usually differentiates them from tumours arising within the sella.

On CT, the majority are hyperdense homogeneous masses which enhance after intravenous contrast. On non-contrasted MRI, the tumour usually returns a similar signal to that of grey matter on T$_1$-weighted MRI

283

sequences. On T_2-weighted sequences, the signal may be isointense with brain or it may be slightly hyperintense. Masses in this region can usually be clearly identified on both scans. Diagnosis is not usually difficult where the mass is broad-based and the sella is normal, but where doubt persists dural enhancement adjacent to the tumour suggests a meningioma. Although this sign is not specific and can be seen with many types of pathology [22,23], the 'flare' or 'tail' sign adjacent to a tumour in this region is highly suggestive [24,25]. MRI is more sensitive than CT to small tumours, which can be obscured by artefact caused by dense surrounding bone. Calcification may also obscure the tumour on CT, but the matrix itself produces a signal on MRI and even the smallest tumours should not be missed.

16.5.4 CHIASMATIC/HYPOTHALAMIC GLIOMA

Tumours arising in the region of the optic chiasm and hypothalamus are common in children. Those that commence in the hypothalamus grow rapidly and may reach a large size before imaging is undertaken. These children frequently present during infancy with failure to thrive (Fig. 16.9).

Tumours that arise primarily in the optic chiasm frequently occur as an expression of neurofibromatosis and are usually smaller and sometimes extend to involve the adjacent optic nerves and tracts (Figs 16.10 and 16.11). Their behaviour differs from the typical hypothalamic glioma. They are usually slow growing and cause early visual symptoms. Imaging reveals the site of origin. Because of their different behaviour, differentiation between these two tumours is usually simple, particularly when there is enlargement of optic nerves or extension along the optic tracts. These tumours can usually be appreciated on CT, although minimal density ab-

normalities and lack of definition of the suprasellar regions may confuse, but are better localized on MRI.

On CT, hypothalamic gliomas are usually large, low-density masses which may obstruct the foramen of Monro. Intravenous contrast usually causes dense homogeneous enhancement. On MRI, they return low signal on T_1- and high signal on T_2-weighted sequences. Multiplanar imaging provides the necessary anatomical detail and intravenous contrast is rarely required.

Tumours arising in the optic chiasm are frequently isodense with brain on CT. They may be missed if the scan is not of sufficient quality to allow a clear appreciation of the suprasellar cistern. Extension forwards or backwards along the optic pathway is often difficult to appreciate. Some enhancement occurs in about two-thirds of cases [26]. With the use of appropriate sequences, MRI provides a more complete study than CT and demonstrates the full extent of the tumour both into the orbit and posteriorly, even occasionally as far as optic radiation. Multiplanar imaging is required: T_1-weighted sequences in axial, sagittal and coronal planes demonstrate the extent of the tumour within the chiasm and optic nerves, while T_2-weighted sequences may demonstrate high signal foci along the optic tracts. Since many of these patients have neurofibromatosis type 1, gliotic regions within the brain substance, particularly in basal ganglia, may also be identified. Therefore, not all the lesions seen on the T_2-weighted sequence are an expression of the tumour itself.

16.5.5 HYPOTHALAMIC HAMARTOMA

This is usually a small sessile or pedunculated mass of non-neoplastic tissue of neural origin, which frequently causes precocious puberty. It arises from the tuber cinereum in the floor of the third ventricle [27]. It usually projects down into the interpeduncular cis-

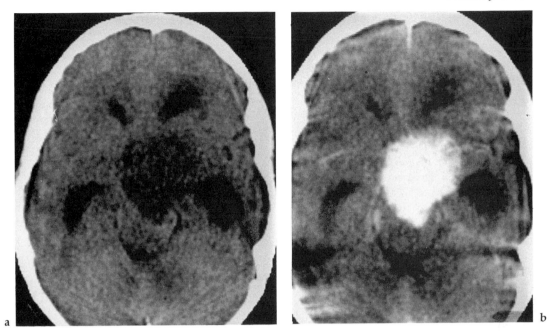

Fig. 16.9 Hypothalamic glioma. (a) Pre-contrast and (b) post-contrast CT scans. There is a large low density enhancing mass, which indents the brainstem and obstructs the foramen of Monro.

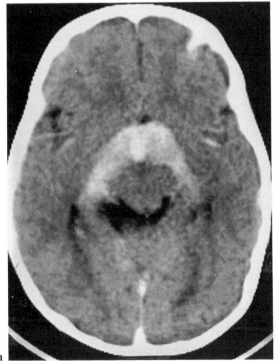

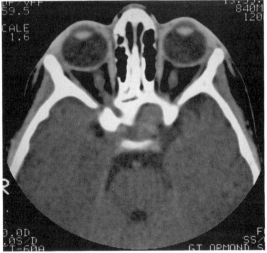

Fig. 16.10 Optic pathway glioma. (a) Post-contrast CT scan showing a large enhancing mass extending posterolaterally along both swollen optic tracts to the geniculate bodies and beyond into the anterior parts of the optic radiation. (b) The tumour extends into both optic nerves and is expanding the left optic canal.

285

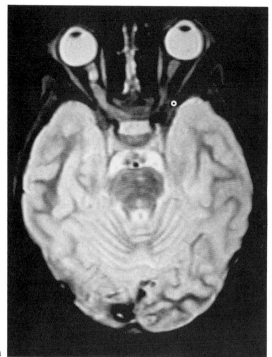

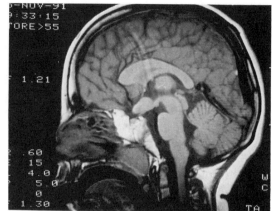

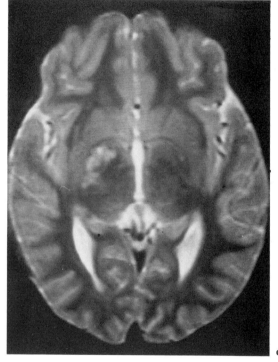

Fig. 16.11 Optic pathway tumour. (a) Axial proton density weighted, (b) sagittal T_1-weighted, and (c) axial T_2-weighted MRI scans showing similar appearances to Fig. 16.10. The multiplanar imaging of MRI facilitates the demonstration of the tumour.

tern and rarely becomes larger than about 2 cm. Although calcification, fat and cysts have been reported [28], these are very rare and the mass is typically isodense. Since the hypothalamic hamartoma does not enhance on either CT or MRI, it requires high quality imaging, particularly on CT, where its density can lead to the mass being missed if it is not surrounded by CSF and the normal suprasellar cistern cannot clearly be identified (Fig. 16.12).

Coronal CT scanning seldom improves diagnosis. The examination of choice again is MRI in the sagittal and coronal planes. The majority of tumours return a signal identical to grey matter on T_1-weighted sequences [29], but occasionally biopsy-proven hamartomas have been reported to be hyperintense on T_2-weighted sequences [30].

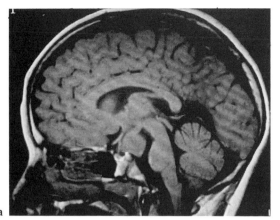

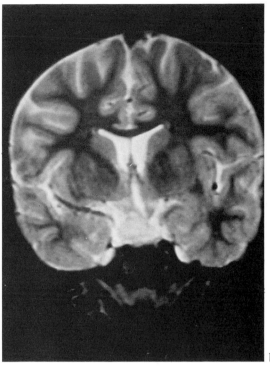

Fig. 16.12 Hypothalamic hamartoma. (a) Sagittal T$_1$-weighted and (b) coronal T$_2$-weighted MRI scans. There is a round mass projecting from the region of the tuber cinereum into the suprasellar cistern. It is isointense with grey matter on both sequences.

16.5.6 GERMINOMA

The most common site for germinomas is the pineal region, but approximately 20% of them are situated in the suprasellar cistern [31]. Some of these result from metastases into the subarachnoid space, but in other cases where there is no evidence of a pineal tumour it is thought that they arise from totipotent cells or cell rests. However, they have a similar appearance to the post-third ventricular lesions on CT and MRI. They may metastasize into the subarachnoid space, where they either form nodular lesions or sheets of tumour cells. In the suprasellar region they usually appear on the pre-contrast CT scan, as a moderate sized isodense mass with dramatic enhancement after intravenous contrast. On MRI, they return a slightly hypointense signal on T$_1$- and hyperintense signal on T$_2$-weighted sequences; they also enhance after gadolinium. Although these masses are usually as well seen on CT as on MRI, an isolated mass does not have any specific diagnostic features. The multiplanar capabilities of MRI do allow a more extensive evaluation of the subarachnoid space within the cranial cavity and in the upper cervical spine during the same study. The finding of another lesion suggests the diagnosis.

16.5.7 ARACHNOID CYST

The suprasellar cistern is a common site for an arachnoid cyst. It usually remains silent until it reaches a large size and obstructs the foramen of Monro (Fig. 16.13).

The majority appear to be closed, but contrast cisternography demonstrates delayed filling of the cyst. Imaging with CT and MRI demonstrates the size of the mass at diag-

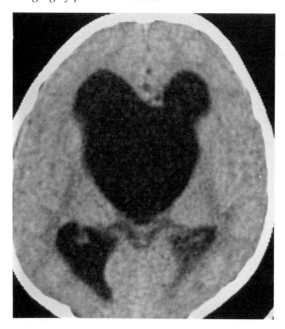

Fig. 16.13 Arachnoid cyst. Axial CT scan demonstrating a large CSF density mass obstructing the foramen of Monro and producing the 'Mickey Mouse' appearance. The third ventricle is flattened and cannot be seen.

nosis, and its contents, which consist of CSF, indicate its nature. Therefore, on CT the cyst appears as a rounded mass in the suprasellar cistern, and because it is of long standing it often truncates the dorsum sellae. It has sometimes been mistaken for an enlarged third ventricle, but its width is usually considerably greater than the width of even the largest third ventricle which, in this situation, is elevated, compressed and small.

The ventricle is not visible on CT, but can usually be seen on MRI. The cyst returns low intensity on T_1- and high intensity on T_2-weighted sequences typical of CSF. It naturally does not enhance. The diagnosis, therefore, can be made on CT or MRI. The size and appearance of the lesion with either modality usually secures the diagnosis.

16.6 VASCULAR AND ISCHAEMIC CONDITIONS

There are a number of conditions affecting the parasellar region which have a vascular basis to their aetiology. These are considered together.

16.6.1 ANEURYSM

Aneurysms arising from the terminal portion of the internal carotid arteries may enlarge and act as a mass. Giant aneurysms are those over 25 mm in diameter. The highest incidence is around the age of 50 and they account for about 5% of all aneurysms [32]. Those that arise within the cavernous sinus expand this structure and may erode the bone medially, extending into the pituitary fossa. They seldom bleed [33,34], but rupture into the cavernous sinus leads to a caroticocavernous fistula. Those that arise from the supraclinoid segment lie in the subarachnoid space and behave like suprasellar masses. Less commonly, they erode the pituitary fossa, although the pressure effects of pulsation may truncate the dorsum sellae.

On CT, masses that lie in the suprasellar region are usually rounded and are isodense or slightly hyperdense on the plain scan. There may be circumferential calcification in the wall, and after intravenous contrast the patent part of the mass will show dramatic enhancement. Many of these aneurysms, however, are partially thrombosed and this part of the mass obviously does not enhance. Occasionally, the majority of the aneurysm is thrombosed and only a small enhancing lumen remains. Those which arise within the cavernous sinus may be more difficult to diagnose. Expansion into the pituitary fossa can occur with many masses in this region, and since the cavernous sinus itself enhances after intravenous contrast it is impossible on CT to separate the aneurysm from the surrounding sinus. Furthermore, beam hardening artefact adjacent to the bone often degrades image quality. There should be little difficulty suggesting the diagnosis with large erosive masses, but in those which have yet to attain a significant size, diagnosis relies on angiography.

On MRI, the appearance will depend on the extent of thrombosis. In those aneurysms which have a patent lumen, there is a rounded mass of signal void, which is partly caused by movement of blood through the slice and partly by dephasing due to turbulence within the aneurysm. This is particularly well seen on T_2-weighted spin echo sequences, but can also be appreciated on T_1-weighted sequences. Intravenous gadolinium does not play a role in this condition, the rapidity of flow and the rapid dephasing usually preventing any enhancing effect due to gadolinium. Since many of these aneurysms are partially thrombosed, the clot can be identified on MRI as regions of high signal on both T_1- and T_2-weighted sequences. The former is due to recent clot, and the latter due to regions of older thrombosis. There are also areas of hypointensity on the T_2-weighted sequences due to haemosiderin deposition in macrophages. This, in addition to any signal void due to flowing blood, simplifies the diagnosis.

The majority of large suprasellar aneurysms can be diagnosed as easily with CT as with MRI. Those that lie within the cavernous sinus, however, are more satisfactorily demonstrated by MRI, since the multiplanar facility and the properties of flowing and clotted blood, both in the aneurysm and in adjacent vessels, clearly render this a superior imaging tool to CT.

16.6.2 PITUITARY APOPLEXY

The clinical triad of severe headache, hypotension and visual loss due to haemorrhagic necrosis of pituitary tissue is rare. Apart from pregnancy, a number of precipitating factors have been incriminated, including raised intracranial pressure, radiation therapy, trauma and diabetes [35]. The incidence varies in the published literature, but is probably less than 10% of pituitary adenomas, although clinically unsuspected haemorrhage occurs in about 25% of cases on histological examination [36,37]. Acute necrosis practically never occurs unless the pituitary gland is abnormal and almost all patients have an enlarged sella [38].

Herniation of CSF below the diaphragma sellae may occur as a sequel to this condition, and if the fossa is not grossly expanded the appearance could be mistaken for the common 'empty sella'. However, the asymmetrical shape and large size of the pituitary fossa usually indicates an underlying macroadenoma. The CT and MRI appearances will depend upon the stage of the process. In the acute stage, sudden visual loss indicates the anatomical region of the pathology. Haemorrhage is the hallmark of diagnosis, and in the first two or three days the diagnosis is more easily arrived at by CT, since there is likely to be hyperdensity within the pituitary tissue [39]. During this period, the early changes of haemorrhage seen on MRI, namely hypointensity on T_2-weighted sequences, is more difficult to appreciate. CT changes will persist between five and seven days after the onset when change from oxyhaemoglobin to methaemoglobin will lead to hyperintensity on T_1-weighted sequences (Fig. 16.14). This has been reported to persist for up to 15 months [36], long after CT evidence of haemorrhage has disappeared, leaving only changes that cannot be differentiated from necrosis [40]. Similar high intensity contents can be encountered in some craniopharyngioma cysts containing high concentrations of cholesterol [41], and CT may be required to search for calcification. CT and MRI, therefore, have a complementary role in this condition.

289

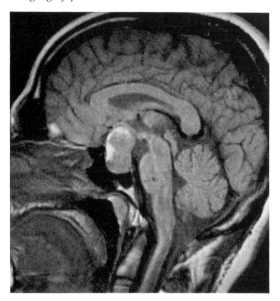

Fig. 16.14 Pituitary apoplexy: six months of failing vision with one month of rapid deterioration. Sagittal T_1-weighted MRI scan. There is enlargement of the pituitary fossa with a suprasellar tumour extension. Most of the tumour is isointense, but areas of hyperintensity due to methaemoglobin are seen anteriorly.

16.7 INFLAMMATORY PROCESSES

16.7.1 PITUITARY ABSCESS

This condition is rare. It does not occur in normal pituitary tissue but has been documented in macroadenomas and craniopharyngiomas, although it virtually never follows transsphenoidal surgery. The clinical features are difficult to differentiate from those of macroadenoma. Systemic sepsis is uncommon and the insidious development of this condition means that the diagnosis is rarely made before exploration. CT and MRI features are similar. There may be an area of central necrosis with peripheral enhancement on post-contrast scans. However, areas of necrosis within a macroadenoma are also not uncommon, so that differentiation from the more common pathology is difficult.

16.7.2 TUBERCULOUS GRANULOMAS

Tuberculous granulomas are part of generalized tuberculous meningitis. The suprasellar cistern is the most frequently affected region, and large masses of granulation tissue often surround the basal vessels, optic chiasm and intracranial optic nerves (Fig. 16.15).

This condition may be indolent and can persist for many years, even with adequate therapy. On plain CT, there is obliteration of the suprasellar cistern, which is either isodense or hyperdense. Small flecks of calcification are not infrequent. Intravenous contrast demonstrates nodular enhancement, within which are sometimes central non-enhancing areas of necrosis. There is usually more extensive basal enhancement, and other granulomata may be identified elsewhere. There is usually hydrocephalus. Involvement of the basal vessels can lead to

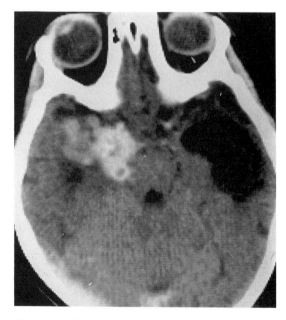

Fig. 16.15 Tuberculous granulation tissue. Post-contrast CT scan demonstrates a mass of enhancing tissue above the right cavernous sinus extending into the right middle fossa.

vascular occlusion and cerebral ischaemia, particularly in childhood, when low density infarcts may be apparent in the basal ganglia and capsules.

All these changes are also seen on MRI scans, with basal enhancement apparent on post-gadolinium scans. The inflammatory process that spreads to involve the leptomeninges leads to superficial venous infarction, which produces areas of high signal on non-contrast T_2-weighted scans, particularly on the inferior and medial surfaces of the temporal lobes.

16.7.3 PITUITARY-HYPOTHALAMIC AXIS

Patients with lesions affecting the pituitary-hypothalamic axis frequently present with diabetes insipidus. Head injury and surgery are responsible for about 50% of cases, and a further 25% are accounted for by other specific causes, such as tumours (primary and secondary), Langerhans cell histiocytosis, pituitary apoplexy, sarcoidosis and other conditions [42–44]. In many patients scans are normal, but in those with diabetes insipidus swelling and enhancement occur and there is loss of the normal posterior pituitary high signal on MRI [45].

16.8 MISCELLANEOUS

16.8.1 EMPTY SELLA

The superior surface of the pituitary is normally confined by the diaphragma sellae. This dural layer is, however, frequently deficient and CSF is present below the interclinoid line. The incidence of this finding depends much on the method of assessment, but has been reported to be as low as 5.5% [46] and as high as 58% [47], the latter study being undertaken on autopsy material. A true incidence of about 20% is probably a more accurate figure [48].

The pituitary stalk is identified projecting down into the sella immediately in front of the dorsum sellae. It can be clearly seen on axial and coronal CT scans [4] but is more elegantly demonstrated on MRI. Normal pituitary tissue is identified below. Differentiation from a cystic pituitary tumour depends on this finding. The optic chiasm and nerves follow a direct path between the hypothalamus and the optic canals. Herniation of the chiasm into an enlarged chiasm probably does not occur in the normal patient, but it indicates downward displacement of the anterior third ventricle as a result of previous hydrocephalus.

16.8.2 GROWTH HORMONE DEFICIENCY SYNDROMES

Children suffering from growth hormone deficiency may have a normal pituitary fossa, but more commonly there is radiological evidence of the biochemical dysfunction on plain films, CT or MRI. Two main forms occur – partial and complete. In patients with partial growth hormone deficiency, the sella has a normal shape or is slightly small and on scanning there is moderate reduction in the volume of pituitary tissue [49]. There is a normal pituitary stalk and the bright neurohypophysis is usually normally situated. The sella is frequently partly empty. All these features are clearly demonstrated on MRI and on reformatted, thin section, post-contrast CT scans [50]. In the group of patients with total growth and multiple hormone deficiency, the sella may be smaller. The residual pituitary tissue is often very small [49], but some tissue can be seen in up to 60% of patients [50]. The pituitary stalk is also small, and may not be visible.

Radiological features of these two conditions have been clarified by MRI. The gland and stalk can usually be demonstrated on CT reformats, but the adenohypophyses and neurohypophyses cannot be separated. MRI, however, provides more detailed assessment of the pituitary structure. In patients with isolated and multiple growth hormone deficiencies, there is usually a small amount of anterior pituitary tissue demonstrated as isointense signal on T_1-weighted sequences [51]. The posterior pituitary, which is normally seen as a high intensity region in the normal scan on T_1-weighted sequences, is ectopic and situated at the base of the hypothalamus in a high proportion of patients with multiple hormone deficiencies and pituitary dwarfism [52].

REFERENCES

1. Bonneville, J.-F., Cattin, F., Portha, C., Cuerin, E., Clere, P. and Bartholomot, B. (1986) Computed tomographic demonstration of the posterior pituitary. *Am. J. Roentg.*, **146**, 263–6.

2. Mark, K.P., Haughton, V.M., Hendrix, L.E., Daniels, D.L., Williams, A.L., Czervionke, L.F. and Asleson, R.J. (1991) High intensity signals within the posterior pituitary fossa: a study with fat suppression MR techniques. *AJNR*, **12**, 529–32.

3. Kucharczyk, W., Leninski, R.E., Kucharczyk, J. and Henkelman, R.M. (1990) The effect of phospholipid vesicles on the NRM relaxation of water: an explanation for the MR appearances of the neurohypophysis. *AJNR*, **11**, 693–700.

4. Haughton, V.M., Rosenbaum, A.E., Williams, A.L. and Drayer, B. (1980) Recognising the empty sella by CT: the infundibulum sign. *AJNR*, **1**, 527–9.

5. Parsons Sheffer, J. (1924) Some points in the regional anatomy of the optic pathway, with especial reference to tumours of the hypophysis cerebri and resulting ocular changes. *Anat. Rec.*, **28**, 243–79.

6. Bull, J. (1956) The normal variations in the position of the optic recess of the third ventricle. *Acta Radiol.*, **46**, 72–80.

7. Costello, R.T. (1936) Subclinical adenoma of the pituitary gland. *Am. J. Path.*, **12**, 205–15.

8. Swanson, H.A. and de Boulay, G. (1976) Borderline variants of the normal pituitary fossa. *Br. J. Radiol.*, **48**, 366–9.

9. Kirsky, P.A., Newton, T.H. and Horton, B.H. (1981) Sellar contour anatomic polytomographic correlation. *Am. J. Roentg.*, **137**, 213–16.

10. Muhr, C., Bergstrom, K., Grimelius, L. and Larsson, S.G. (1981) A parallel study of the roentgen anatomy of the sellar tursica and the history of pathology of the pituitary gland in 205 autopsy specimens. *Neuroradiology*, **21**, 55–65.

11. Hemminghytt, S., Kalcoff, R.K., Daniels, D.L., Williams, A.L., Grogan, J.P. and Horton, V.M. (1983) Computed tomographic study of hormone secreting microadenomas. *Radiology*, **146**, 65–9.

12. Chambers, E.F., Turskay, P.A., Lamasters, D. and Newton, T.H. (1982) Regions of low density in the contrast enhanced pituitary gland normal and pathologic processes. *Radiology*, **144**, 109–33.

13. Kucharczyk, W., Davies, D.O., Kelly, W.M., Sze, G., Norman, D. and Newton, T.H. (1986) Pituitary adenomas: high resolution MR imaging at 1.5T. *Radiology*, **161**, 761–5.

14. Marcovitz, S., Wee, R., Chan, J. and Hardy, J. (1987) Diagnostic accuracy of pre-operative CT scanning in the evaluation of pituitary ACTH secreting adenomas. *AJNR*, **8**, 641–4.

15. Newton, D.R., Dillon, W.P., Norman, D., Newton, T.H. and Wilson, C.B. (1989) Gadolinium-DTPA enhanced MR imaging of pituitary adenomas. *AJNR*, **10**, 949–54.

16. Bonneville, J.-F., Cattin, F., Moussa Bacha, K. and Portha, C. (1983) Dynamic computed tomography of the pituitary gland: the 'Tuft sign'. *Radiology*, **149**, 145–8.

17. Kazner, E., Wende, S., Grummet, T., Stochdorph, O., Felix, R. and Claussen, C. (ed.) *Computed Tomography and Magnetic Resonance Tomography of Intracranial Tumours*, Springer-Verlag, London, p. 327.

18. Harwood-Nash, D.C. and Fitz, C.R. (1976) *Neuroradiology of Infants and Children*, C.V. Mosby, St Louis, pp. 668–78.

19. Volker, J.L., Campbell, R.L. and Muller, J. (1991) Clinical radiographic and pathological features of symptomatic Rathke cleft cysts. *J. Neurosurg.*, **74**, 535–44.

20. Russell, D.S. and Rubenstein, L.J. (1989) *Pathology of Tumours of the Nervous System*, 5th edn, Williams and Wilkins, Baltimore.

21. Wiggli, Q. and Oberson, R. (1975) Pneumosinus dilatons and hyperostosis: early signs of meningiomas on the anterior diasmatic angle. *Neuroradiology*, **8**, 217–21.

22. Phillips, M., Ryals, T.J., Yuh, W.T.C. and Kambho, S. (1989) Evaluation of meningeal enhancement with GdDTPA. Presented at the 75th Scientific Meeting of the Radiological Society of America, Chicago.

23. Wilms, G., Lammens, M., Marchal, G., Demaerel, Ph., Verplancke, J., van Calenbergh, F., Goffin, J., Plets, C. and Baret, A.L. (1991) Prominent dural enhancement adjacent to non-meningiomatous malignant lesions on contrast enhanced MR images. *AJNR*, **12**, 761–4.

24. Aoki, S., Sasaki, Y., Machida, T. and Tanioka, H. (1990) Contrast enhanced MR images in patients with meningioma: importance of enhancement of the dura adjacent to the tumour. *AJNR*, **11**, 935–9.

25. Tien, R.D., Yang, P.J. and Chu, P.K. (1991) 'Dural fail sign': a specific MR sign for meningioma? *JCAT*, **15**, 64–6.

26. Gonzales, C.F., Grossman, C.B. and Masdew, J.C. (ed.) (1985) *Head and Spine Imaging*, Wiley, New York, p. 505.

27. Hochman, H.I., Judge, D.M. and Reichlin, S. (1981) Precocious puberty and hypothalamic hamartoma. *Pediatrics*, **67**, 236–44.

28. Burton, E.M., Ball, W.S., Crone, K. and Dolan, L.M. (1989) Hamartoma of the tuber cinereum: a comparison of MR and CT findings in 4 cases. *AJNR*, **10**, 497–501.

29. Boyko, O.B., Curnes, J.T., Oakes, W.J. and Burger, P.C. (1991) Hamartomas of the tuber cinereum: CT, MR and pathologic findings. *AJNR*, **12**, 309–14.

30. Nishio, S., Pujiwara, S., Aiko, Y., Takeshita, I. and Fukui, M. (1989) Hypothalamic hamartoma. Report of two cases. *J. Neurosurg.*, **70**, 640–5.

31. Jellinger, K. (1973) Primary intrasellar germ cell tumours. *Acta Neuropathol.*, **25**, 291–306.

32. Morley, T.P. and Barr, H.W.K. (1968) Giant intracranial aneurysms: diagnosis course and management. *Clin. Neurosurg.*, **16**, 73–94.

33. Sarwar, M., Batnitsky, S. and Schechter, M. (1976) Tumorous aneurysm. *Neuroradiology*, **12**, 79–97.

34. O'Neill, M., Hope, T. and Thomson, G. (1980) Giant intracranial aneurysms: diagnosis with special reference to computed tomography. *Clin. Radiol.*, **31**, 27–39.

35. Reid, R.L., Quigley, M.E. and Yen, S.S.C. (1985) Pituitary apoplexy. A review. *Archs Neurol.*, **42**, 712–19.

36. Glick, R.P. and Tiesa, J.A. (1990) Subacute pituitary apoplexy: clinical and magnetic resonance imaging characteristics. *Neurosurgery*, **27**, 214–19.

37. Ostrov, S.G., Quencer, R.M., Hoffman, J.C., Davis, P.C., Hass, A.N. and David, N.J. (1989) Haemorrhage within pituitary adenomas; how often associated with pituitary apoplexy syndrome. *AJNR*, **10**, 503–10.

38. Fitzpatrick, D., Tolis, G., McGarry, E.E. and Taylor, S. (1980) Pituitary apoplexy – the importance of skull roentgenograms and computed tomography. *J. Am. Med. Ass.*, **244**, 59–61.

39. Post, M.J.D., David, N.J., Glaser, J.S. and Safran, A. (1980) Pituitary apoplexy: diagnosis by computed tomography. *Radiology*, **134**, 665–70.

40. Davis, P.C., Hoffman, J.C., Tindall, G.T. and Braun, I.F. (1985) CT–surgical correlation in pituitary adenomas: evaluation in 113 patients. *AJNR*, **6**, 711–16.

41. Pusey, E., Kortman, K.E., Flannigan, R.D., Tsuruda, J. and Bradley, W.G. (1987) MR of craniopharyngiomas: tumour delineation and characterisation. *AJNR*, **8**, 439–44.

42. Moses, A.M. (1985) Clinical and laboratory observations in the adult with diabetes insipidus and related syndrome. *Front. Horm. Res.*, **13**, 156–75.

43. Tien, R.D., Newton, T.H., McDermott, M.W., Dillon, W.P. and Kucharczyk, J.K. (1990) Thickened pituitary stalk on MR features in patients with diabetes insipidus and Langerhans cell histiocytosis. *AJNR*, **11**, 703–8.

44. Veldhuis, J. and Hammond, J. (1980) Endocrine function after spontaneous infarction of the human pituitary: report, review and appraisal. *Endocr. Rev.*, **1**, 100–7.

45. Tien, R., Kucharczyk, K.J. and Kucharczyk, W. (1991) MR imaging of the brain in patients with diabetes insipidus. *AJNR*, **12**, 533–42.

46. Busch, W. (1961) Die morphologie der sella turcica und ihre Beziehungen zur Hypophyse. *Archs Path. Anat.*, **320**, 437–58.

47. Kaufman, B. and Chamberlain, Jr, W.B. (1972) The ubiquitous 'empty' sella turcica. *Acta Radiol.*, **13**, 413–25.

48. Hall, K. and McAllister, V.L. (1980) Metrizamide cisternography in pituitary and juxta pituitary lesions. *Radiology*, **134**, 101–8.

49. Kuroiwa, T., Okabe, Y., Hasuo, K., Yasumori, K., Mizushima, A. and Masuda, K. (1991) MR imaging of pituitary dwarfism. *AJNR*, **12**, 161–4.

50. Stanhope, R., Hindmarsh, P., Kendall, B. and Brook, C.G.D. (1986) High resolution CT scanning of the pituitary gland in growth disorders. *Acta Paediat. Scand.*, **75**, 779–86.

51. Abrahams, J.J., Trefelner, E. and Boulware, S.D. (1991) Idiopathic growth hormone deficiency: MR findings in 35 patients. *AJNR*, **12**, 155–60.

52. Kelly, W.M., Kucharczyk, W., Kucharczyk, J., Kjos, B., Peck, W.W., Norman D. and Newton, T.H. (1988) Posterior pituitary ectopia; an MR feature of pituitary dwarfism. *AJNR*, **9**, 455–60.

17

Investigation of hyponatraemia

P.M. BOULOUX

17.1 INTRODUCTION

Hyponatraemia is a common biochemical abnormality in clinical practice and its origin can in most instances be ascertained with some simple investigations. It is defined as a plasma sodium less that $135\,mmol\,l^{-1}$, and may be present in between 15% and 22% of both acutely [1] and chronically hospitalized patients. Minor degrees of hyponatraemia ($<5\,mmol\,l^{-1}$) are common in hospital populations, when compared with healthy control subjects [2].

Hyponatraemia is dangerous when it reflects hypo-osmolality of body solutes. However, there are two situations in which hyponatraemia is not associated with true plasma hypo-osmolality. The first is 'pseudo-hyponatraemia', caused by marked elevation in lipids or proteins in plasma. In such cases the concentration of sodium per litre of plasma water is actually normal, but the concentration of sodium per litre plasma appears artefactually decreased because of the increased fraction of lipid or protein in the plasma relative to the plasma water. In such cases, direct measurement of plasma osmolality is spuriously low. This is because osmolality measurement is based on the colligative properties of solute particles in solution and will not be significantly affected by increased lipids or protein. Measurement of sodium by ion specific electrode will also yield normal results in such circumstances.

The second situation occurs when high concentrations of effective solutes other than sodium are present in extracellular fluid (ECF), thereby causing relative decreases in plasma sodium, despite an unchanged effective osmolality of the ECF. This occurs in severe hyperglycaemia [3]. Misdiagnosis of hypo-osmolality can, in such cases, be avoided by correcting the measured plasma Na^+ by approximately $1.5\,mmol\,l^{-1}$ for every $5\,mmol\,l^{-1}$ of increased plasma glucose above the normal range [4]. This correction cannot be effected in situations where there are large amounts of unmeasured solutes such as mannitol, radiographic contrast media, ethanol, etc. In such case, direct measurement of plasma osmolality is best carried out; however, even in this situation, the measurement may not yield the true effective osmolality since in the case of ethanol the unmeasured solute permeates freely across cells.

If the calculated effective plasma osmolality ($Posm\ (mosm\,kg^{-1}\ H_2O = 2 \times Na^+)$ $(mmol\,l^{-1})$ + glucose $(mmol\,l^{-1})$) is less than $275\,mosm\,kg^{-1}$, significant hypo-osmolality is present. The absence of a significant discrepancy between the measured total plasma osmolality and the calculated effective plasma osmolality confirms the presence of significant hyponatraemia. If there is a discrepancy between these two values, further testing is required to exclude pseudohyponatraemia.

17.2 PATHOGENESIS OF HYPONATRAEMIA (Table 17.1)

The presence of significant hyponatraemia and hypo-osmolality always signifies an excess of water relative to sodium and other extracellular solutes. Since water moves freely between extracellular and intracellular volumes, hyponatraemia generally indicates an excess of water relative to total body solutes.

Table 17.1 Causes of hyponatraemia

Salt depletion
1. Renal solute loss
   Diuretic therapy
   Solute diuresis (glucose, mannitol)
   Mineralocorticoid deficiency
   Salt wasting nephropathy (e.g. polycystic
      kidneys, interstitial nephritis)

2. Non-renal salt loss
   Haemorrhage
   Skin loss by sweating, burns
   Gastrointestinal loss (vomiting, diarrhoea,
      pancreatitis, intestinal obstruction)

Dilutional mechanism
Impaired renal water excretion

1. Increased proximal reabsorption
   Congestive cardiac failure
   Cirrhosis
   Nephrotic syndrome
   Hypothyroidism

2. Decreased distal dilution
   SIADH
   Glucocorticoid deficiency

3. Excess water intake
   Primary polydipsia

This can occur by two mechanisms: sodium depletion in excess of concurrent water depletion, or simply by the dilutional effects of increased total water.

17.2.1 SODIUM DEPLETION

This can occur following loss of ECF, following diuretic therapy, salt-wasting nephropathy (e.g. polycystic disease, interstitial nephritis) and mineralocorticoid deficiency. Nonrenal solute losses include such causes as haemorrhage, cutaneous losses (sweating, burns), diarrhoea, vomiting, intestinal obstruction and pancreatitis. With marked ECF depletion, signs of hypovolaemia are present, with reduced tissue turgor, tachycardia and postural hypotension.

17.2.2 WATER EXCESS

Most cases of hyponatraemia encountered in hospital practice result from increases in total body water. This can theoretically result from impaired renal free water excretion or excessive water intake. However, the former accounts for the vast majority of the hyponatraemic disorders because normal kidneys have sufficient diluting capacity to allow excretion of 20–30 l of free water per day [5]. Thus, dilutional hyponatraemia usually indicates some abnormality of renal free water excretion. Such abnormalities occur via mechanisms operating at either the proximal or distal tubule.

Any disorder that causes a decrease in glomerular filtration rate in the absence of significant ECF losses is usually an oedema forming state, associated with secondary hyperaldosteronism. Such conditions (e.g. severe hypothyroidism) will lead to increased absorption of both sodium and water in the proximal tubule and in this case the ability to excrete free water will be limited because of decreased delivery of tubular fluid to the distal nephron. Disorders causing solute depletion by non-renal means also produce the same effect, which then contributes to subsequent water retention.

17.3 DIFFERENTIAL DIAGNOSIS OF HYPONATRAEMIA

The evaluation depends on the results of a careful history (especially with regard to medication), clinical assessment of extracellular volume status (to ascertain whether hypovolaemia is present), a neurological evaluation, plasma electrolytes, urea, glucose, creatinine, calculated effective osmolality and/or directly measured plasma osmolality, and simultaneous urinary electrolytes and osmolality.

17.3.1 HYPOVOLAEMIC HYPONATRAEMIA (DECREASED ECF)

In this context, extracellular sodium depletion is present. If urinary sodium is low, then non-renal causes of sodium depletion should be evaluated. If urinary sodium is high, renal causes of sodium depletion should be considered, diuretic therapy being the most common. Adrenal insufficiency should also be considered; hyperkalaemia, low bicarbonate and raised urea and creatinine may then be present.

17.3.2 INCREASED ECF VOLUME WITH OEDEMA AND ASCITES

The hyponatraemia in this case suggests depletion of intravascular volume. Because of secondary hyperaldosteronism, the urinary sodium concentration is low, unless the patient has been put on diuretics, or is experiencing a solute diuresis (e.g. polyuria due to glycosuria). There is non-osmotic stimulation of AVP production, with water retention as a consequence [6]. This appears to be the pathogenic mechanism operating in cases of cirrhosis of the liver.

17.3.3 EUVOLAEMIC HYPONATRAEMIA

Here, the determination of urinary sodium is particularly important. A low urinary sodium suggests a depletional hypo-osmolality secondary to ECF losses, with subsequent volume replacement with water or other hypotonic fluids.

A high urinary sodium in euvolaemic hyponatraemia usually indicates a distally mediated dilutional hypo-osmolality, such as the syndrome of inappropriate antidiuresis (SIADH). Glucocorticoid deficiency can closely mimic the SIADH syndrome. This is because it can cause both elevated antidiuretic

Table 17.2 Criteria for diagnosis of SIADH

Major criteria
1. Low effective plasma osmolality (Posm $<275\,\mathrm{mOsm\,kg^{-1}}$) or corrected plasma sodium $<135\,\mathrm{mmol\,l^{-1}}$
2. Inappropriate urinary concentration (Uosm $>100\,\mathrm{mOsm\,kg^{-1}}$ at some level of plasma hypo-osmolality
3. Normal plasma and extracellular volume (i.e. no clinically detectable hypovolaemia or hypervolaemia)
4. Elevated urinary sodium concentration on a normal salt and water intake
5. Hypothyroidism and hypoadrenalism excluded, and no recent diuretic therapy

Supportive evidence
1. Abnormal water load test (inability to excrete at least 90% of a $20\,\mathrm{ml\,kg^{-1}}$ water load in 4 hours and failure to dilute urine osmolality to less than $100\,\mathrm{mOsm\,kg^{-1}}$
2. Plasma vasopressin level inappropriately elevated
3. Inability to correct plasma osmolality with therapeutic attempts at volume expansion, but improvement following fluid restriction

---

hormone (ADH) levels (due to ECF depletion) as well as having a direct effect on the distal nephron, to prevent maximal urinary dilution even in the absence of ADH. The diagnosis is made be a short Synacthen test.

17.3.4 SYNDROME OF INAPPROPRIATE DIURESIS (Table 17.2)

This is the commonest cause of euvolaemic hyponatraemia, accounting for 14%–40% of cases of hyponatraemia [3,7]. The diagnosis depends upon the demonstration of:

1. True ECF hypo-osmolality, pseudohyponatraemia and hyperglycaemia having been excluded.
2. Urinary osmolality must be inappropriate for plasma hypo-osmolality. This does not require the urine osmolality to be greater than plasma osmolality – rather the urine is not maximally dilute (with normal renal function, this means a urine osmolality less than $100 \, \text{mosm kg}^{-1}$).
3. Clinical euvolaemia must be present.
4. Renal salt wasting must be present. However, the usefulness of this is limited by:
   (a) urinary sodium is also high in renal causes of salt depletion such as diuretic use or in Addison's disease;
   (b) patients with SIADH also develop low urinary salt excretion if they become hypovolaemic, with sometimes follows severe salt and water restriction.
5. Thyroid and adrenal dysfunction should be ruled out.

Aetiology of SIADH

A number of disorders can be associated with SIADH (Table 17.3)

Tumour related SIADH is the most common, particularly small cell carcinoma of the bronchus. The tumour may be small, and in unexplained cases of SIADH, a meticulous search for this tumour should be made, with sputum cytology, computerized tomography (CT) scanning and bronchoscopy, even if the chest X-ray is normal.

Central nervous system tumours account for the next most common group of SIADH. There are long and polysynaptic pathways from the brainstem cardiovascular centres (inhibitory) and osmoreceptors (stimulatory) to the magnocellular neurons that synthesize ADH, and several intracranial pathologies

Table 17.3 Aetiology of SIADH

Neoplasms: thoracic tumours
Small cell carcinoma bronchus
Mesothelioma
Thymoma
Hodgkin's Lymphoma

CNS disorders
Tumours
Brain abscess
Subdural haematoma
Encephalitis
SLE
Guillain–Barré syndrome
Spinal cord lesions
Head trauma
Pituitary stalk section

Drugs: stimulation of ADH release
Nicotine
Phenothiazines
Tricyclics
Vincristine
Narcotics

Uncertain mechanisms
Chlorpropamide
Colchicine
Cyclophosphamide
Carbamazepine

Pulmonary disease
Tuberculosis
Pneumonia
Lung abscess
Positive pressure ventilation

can disrupt these pathways, provoking inappropriate ADH secretion. Thirdly, drug induced SIADH is increasingly recognized as a common cause of this diagnosis. Chlorpropamide appears to possess both direct posterior pituitary stimulant effects, as well as some direct renal effects [8]. Finally, it is noteworthy that one of the most potent causes of bioactive ADH secretion, nausea, even when chronic, is rarely if ever associated with hyponatraemia. This is most likely related to the disinclination of patients to drink fluids under such circumstances. However, aggressive therapy with intravenous fluids in nauseous patients can lead to significant hyponatraemia, particularly in the setting of chemotherapy administration.

REFERENCES

1. Flear, C.T.G., Gill, G.V. and Burn, J. (1981) Hyponatraemia: mechanisms and management. *Lancet*, **ii**, 26–31.
2. Owen, J.A. and Campbell, D.G. (1968) A comparison of plasma electrolyte and urea values in healthy persons and in hospital patients. *Clin. Chim. Acta*, **22**, 611–18.
3. Anderson, R.J., Chung, H.-M., Kluge, R. and Schreier, R.W. (1985) Hyponatraemia: a prospective analysis of its epidemiology and the pathogenic role of vasopressin. *Ann. Intern. Med.*, **102**, 164–8.
4. Katz, M.A. (1973) Hyperglycaemic induced hyponatraemia – calculation of expected serum sodium depression. *New Engl. J. Med.*, **289**, 843–4.
5. Robertson, G.L. (1986) Diseases of the posterior pituitary. In *Endocrinology and Metabolism* (ed. P. Felig, J.D. Baxter, A.E. Broadus and L.A. Frohman), McGraw-Hill, New York, pp. 338–85.
6. Schreier, R.W. (1988) Pathogenesis of sodium and water retention in high output and low output cardiac failure, nephrotic syndrome, cirrhosis and pregnancy. *New Engl. J. Med.*, **319**, 1065–72.
7. Kleinfeld, M., Casimir, M. and Borro, S. (1979) Hyponatraemia as observed in a chronic disease facility. *J. Am. Geriat. Soc.*, **27**, 156–61.
8. Miller, M. and Moses, A.M. (1976) Drug induced states of impaired water excretion. *Kidney Int.*, **10**, 96–103.

Index

page numbers in **bold** refer to figures, those in *italic* refer to tables